Cancer Drug Discovery and Development

Series Editor
Beverly A. Teicher, Bethesda, MD, USA

Cancer Drug Discovery and Development is the definitive book series in cancer research and oncology, providing comprehensive coverage of specific topics in the field. The aim of the series is to cover the process of drug discovery, preclinical models in cancer research, specific drug target groups and experimental and approved therapeutic agents across volumes.

Volumes are current and timely, anticipating areas where experimental agents are reaching FDA approval. Each volume is edited by an expert in the related field and chapters are authored by renowned scientists and physicians in their fields of interest. All volumes undergo single blind peer review and review by the series editor prior to acceptance and publication in the series. Cancer Drug Discovery & Development is indexed in SCOPUS.

More information about this series at https://link.springer.com/bookseries/7625

Armin Ghobadi • John F. DiPersio
Editors

Gene and Cellular
Immunotherapy for Cancer

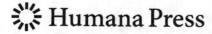 Humana Press

Editors
Armin Ghobadi
Department of Medicine,
Division of Oncology
Washington University School of Medicine
St. Louis, MO, USA

John F. DiPersio
Department of Medicine Pathology &
Immunology, Division of Oncology
Washington University School of Medicine
Saint Louis, MO, USA

ISSN 2196-9906   ISSN 2196-9914   (electronic)
Cancer Drug Discovery and Development
ISBN 978-3-030-87851-1   ISBN 978-3-030-87849-8   (eBook)
https://doi.org/10.1007/978-3-030-87849-8

This Humana imprint is published by the registered company Springer Nature Switzerland AG
The registered company address is: Gewerbestrasse 11, 6330 Cham, Switzerland

Preface

Genetically modified cellular immunotherapies and T-cell bispecifics are changing the landscape of cancer treatment. Approval of five CAR-T products and a T-cell engager by the US Food and Drug Administration (FDA) for hematologic malignancies represents the start of a wave of cellular therapies that will dramatically change how we treat cancer in the near future. These advances have resulted in a high level of enthusiasm among scientific community, clinicians, and industry for developing effective immunotherapies for hematological malignancies and solid tumors. This book will cover two broad categories of gene and cellular therapies: (1) Cellular-based immunotherapies: CAR-T, TCR-T, TIL, viral CTLs, NK cells; (2) T/NK cell engagers including BiTEs, DARTs, TanAbs, and others. The first two chapters present a review of the biologic basis of innate and adaptive immunity and a history of cellular therapy. We then review each treatment category comprehensively covering the whole spectrum of the bench to bedside preclinical and clinical studies. There is a substantial emphasis on CAR-T therapies followed by chapters focused on regulatory aspects of gene and cellular immunotherapy, manufacturing including point-of-care manufacturing of genetically modified cellular therapies and a roadmap to outpatient cellular therapy. This book provides a comprehensive source for readers involved in or interested in the nuts and bolts of gene and cellular therapies. We have prepared this book as a comprehensive review in a single volume for trainees and basic and clinical researchers in academic centers and the industry. In light of the rapid evolution of this field, we are planning to update this book every 4 years.

St. Louis, MO, USA   Armin Ghobadi
St. Louis, MO, USA   John F. DiPersio

Acknowledgments

We want to thank contributors who are all well-respected experts in the field of gene and cellular therapy. We appreciate Joel Eissenberg for the copy editing of multiple chapters, Larissa Albright, acquisitions editor, Springer; Deepak Ravi, product development editor; and Matt Wyczalkowski for illustrating the majority of figures for this book; they were instrumental in bringing this project to the finish line. Finally, we thank our wives and families for their support during the design, implementation, and completion of this project.

Armin Ghobadi, MD
John F. DiPersio, MD, PhD

Contents

Part I
Overview

The History of Cellular Therapies

Zachary D. Crees and Armin Ghobadi

Abstract The approval of multiple CAR-T cell and T cell engaging products for lymphoma, leukemia and multiple myeloma in recent years, in addition to hundreds of active clinical trials in cancer using these platforms, marks the start of a new era in gene and cellular therapy for cancer. However, these remarkable achievements in medicine are built upon thousands of years of advancement in the understanding of cancer and immunity with rapid acceleration in the last few decades. In this chapter, we will broadly review historical aspects of gene and cellular therapy development, focusing on major milestones.

Keywords Gene and cellular therapy history · Hippocrates · Mohammed ibn Zakariya al-Razi · Rudolph Virchow · William Coley · Ilya Metchnikoff · Paul Ehrlich · Allogeneic hematopoietic cell transplantation · Donor lymphocyte infusions (DLI) · Tumor infiltrating lymphocytes (TILs) · Chimeric antigen receptor T-cells (CAR-T) · T-cell receptor engineered T-cells (TCR-T) · Viral cytotoxic T-lymphocytes (viral CTLs) · Natural killer (NK) cells · Dual-targeting immune cell engaging therapies · Pillars of cancer care

Introduction

Historical descriptions of cancer have been found in ancient Egyptian texts dating as early as ~1600 B.C., with the term "carcinoma" first attributed to the Greek physician Hippocrates around the fourth-fifth century B.C [1, 2]. Additionally, one of the earliest observations of acquired immunity was reported as early as

Z. D. Crees · A. Ghobadi (✉)
Department of Medicine, Division of Oncology, Washington University School of Medicine, Saint Louis, MO, USA
e-mail: arminghobadi@wustl.edu

© Springer Nature Switzerland AG 2022
A. Ghobadi, J. F. DiPersio (eds.), *Gene and Cellular Immunotherapy for Cancer*, Cancer Drug Discovery and Development,
https://doi.org/10.1007/978-3-030-87849-8_1

3

~900 A.D. by the Persian physician and scientist Mohammed ibn Zakariya al-Razi, when he postulated that prior infection with smallpox seemed to confer resistance to future infection [3]. However, it was not until the late nineteenth century that the burgeoning field of pathology, bolstered by technical advances in microscopy, enabled the histopathologic features of cancer to be more fully explored. In 1863, Rudolph Virchow described the presence of leukocyte infiltration of neoplastic tissues, marking one of the earliest reports of cellular immunoreactivity to malignant cells [4]. In 1891, William Coley published a report on the use of injections of streptococcal organisms to produce tumor shrinkage in sarcoma, hypothesizing that the immune response to a bacterial infection could promote anti-tumor responses [5]. While Coley's research was met with criticism for methodologic inconsistencies and a lack of independent reproducibility, his work marked one of the first reports of immunotherapy to successfully treat cancer at a time when many of the basic functions of the immune system had yet to be described [6]. Meanwhile, during the late 1800's and into the early 1900's, Ilya Metchnikoff published seminal research in which he described the process of phagocytosis by macrophages and leukocytes, providing important groundwork for our current understanding of cellular immunity. During the same period, Paul Ehrlich and others advanced research on the formation of antibodies and humoral immunity. Notably, Ehrlich applied his research to the field of oncology, proposing that the immune system was capable of "immune surveillance" of malignant tissues. In 1908, both Metchnikoff and Ehrlich were jointly awarded the Nobel Prize in Physiology or Medicine in recognition of their pioneering work on the fundamental mechanisms of cellular and humoral immunity [7].

Over the ensuing century, additional scientific discoveries continued to lay the foundations for cancer immunotherapy by elucidating fundamental humoral and cell-mediated effector functions of the innate and adaptive immune system, along with the complex mechanisms whereby the immune system recognizes and eliminates cancer cells. Beginning in the 1990's, technological advances enabled modern medicine to translate these scientific discoveries into effective immunotherapeutic approaches to treat cancer. Since that time, immunotherapy has quickly risen to become the latest pillar in the treatment paradigm of cancer therapeutics, along with surgery, radiation, chemotherapy, and targeted/precision therapies (Fig. 1).

Embedded within the pillar of immunotherapy lies a unique group of immunotherapies more accurately characterized as gene and cellular immunotherapies. As of 2021, the development of gene and cellular therapies stands as one of the most promising recent developments in cancer therapeutics for a wide array of both hematologic and solid malignancies. However, the realization of safe and effective gene- and cellular-based treatments for cancer has been a long journey marked by numerous milestones which warrant recognition (Fig. 2).

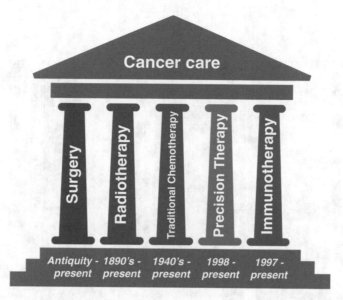

Fig. 1 Pillars of cancer care

Allogeneic Hematopoietic Cell Transplantation

The development of **allogeneic hematopoietic cell transplantation (HCT)** and recognition of the associated "graft-versus-tumor" (GvT) effect serves as one of the earliest and most successful forms of cellular therapy to date. Following World War II, the discovery of radiation-induced bone marrow damage led to rapid scientific advances in the understanding of endogenous hematopoiesis. In 1957, Thomas et al. published early reports on the safety of bone marrow infusions in conjunction with lethal doses of radiation and high-dose chemotherapy for the treatment of various malignancies [8]. Subsequent research in the field of HCT for the treatment of multiple hematologic malignancies has paved the way for development of adoptive cellular immunotherapies by expanding the current understanding of alloreactivity, conditioning regimens, GvT interactions, histocompatibility, and the key effector functions of various immune cell subsets.

Donor Lymphocyte Infusions

Capitalizing on the growing appreciation of the GvT effect of allogeneic lymphocytes to produce long-term remissions following allogeneic HCT in the treatment of acute myeloid leukemia (AML), Kolb et al. published in 1990 on the efficacy of allogeneic **donor lymphocyte infusions (DLI)** as a form of adoptive cellular therapy (ACT) for the treatment of patients with chronic myeloid leukemia (CML)

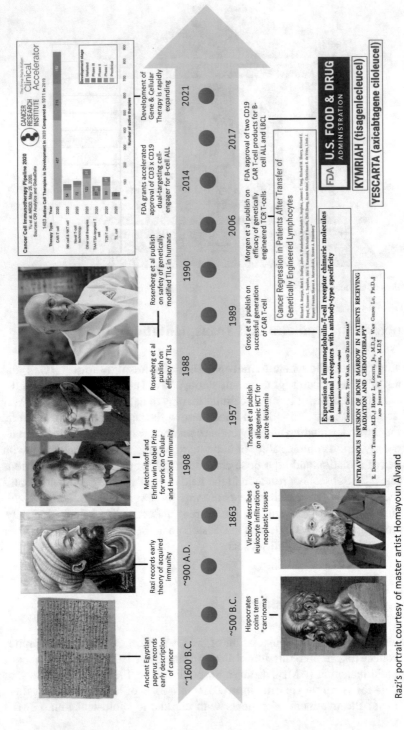

Razi's portrait courtesy of master artist Homayoun Alvand

Fig. 2 Milestones in cellular therapy development

relapsing after allo-HCT [9]. Additional research has revealed the clinical efficacy of DLI in different malignancies to be somewhat variable, highlighting the complexity of both host and donor immune surveillance as well as the ability of different malignancies to evade immune surveillance. Nevertheless, the use of DLI has led to valuable advances in understanding of important concepts relevant to gene- and cellular therapies, including the cellular composition of the product, selection of optimal cell doses, and the role of immunosuppressive therapies in modulating the therapeutic effects and toxicities of cellular therapy.

Chimeric Antigen Receptor T-Cells

The first report of a genetically engineered T-cell which expressed a chimeric antigen receptor (CAR) containing the variable antigen-recognition domains of an antibody connected to the constant transmembrane and intracellular signaling domains of a T-cell receptor (TCR) was made by Yoshihisa Kuwana, Yoshikazu Kurosawa and colleagues in 1987 [10]. In 1989, Gideon Gross and Zelig Eshhar at the Weissman Institute published subsequent work further detailing the generation and functionality of genetically engineered CAR T-cells [11]. Notably, these CAR T-cells were capable of recognizing antigen in the absence of major histocompatibility complex (MHC) presentation and activating T-cell effector functions. Further technical improvements in transduction efficiency, manufacturing processes and optimal preparative conditioning regimens advanced the clinical development of CAR-T cells. Meanwhile, further refinement of the CAR constructs via modification to the single-chain variable fragment (scFv) domains, the transmembrane domains, and most notably the intracellular endodomains by adding costimulatory domains (e.g. CD28 or 41BB) has resulted in improved clinical efficacy. In 2017, data from pivotal clinical trials evaluating two separate CD19 CAR T-cell therapies for the indications of relapsed/refractory acute lymphoblastic leukemia (ALL) and large B-cell lymphoma (LBCL) led to their United States Food and Drug Administration (FDA) approval [12, 13]. Since that time, additional CAR-T products have been FDA approved for mantle cell lymphoma (MCL), multiple myeloma (MM) and numerous CAR-based therapies are under active clinical development [14].

Tumor Infiltrating Lymphocytes

In the 1980's, Steven Rosenberg and collaborators further characterized the presence of a repertoire of **tumor infiltrating lymphocytes (TILs)** in melanoma tumors which exhibited anti-tumor reactivity. They subsequently published pre-clinical data on the efficacy of ACT using TILs extracted from tumors, expanded ex-vivo and re-infused into animals. In 1988, they reported data on the first-in human trial of ACT in metastatic melanoma, where TIL re-infusion resulted in >50% response rates [15]. Rosenberg and colleagues then proceeded in 1990 to use a retroviral gene-transduced TIL to monitor location and persistence of TILs in vivo, marking the first-in-human use of a gene-edited cellular therapy in the treatment of cancer [16]. This pioneering work established TILs as an effective cellular therapy platform for melanoma, while also demonstrating the safety of genetically modified cellular therapies. However, despite the groundbreaking nature of TIL therapy many tumor types do not contain TILs, thus limiting the broad clinical utility of TILs and necessitating the development of additional cellular therapy platforms.

T-Cell Receptor Engineered T-Cells

Beginning in the 1980's and continuing on into the present, various groups have contributed to the development of **genetically engineered TCRs** with enhanced antigen specificity and binding affinity capable of recognizing selected cancer antigens of interest, especially intracellular antigens, within the context of MHC. One method published in 2006 by Morgan et al., described the transduction of such genetically modified TCRs with specificity against the tumor-associated antigens (TAAs) gp100, MART-1, NY-ESO-1, and p53 into T-cells isolated from peripheral blood [17]. Since that time, this approach has allowed for the development of numerous engineered TCR T-cells against multiple TAAs which are in various stages in clinical development. These trials have not only highlighted the potential clinical benefit of genetically engineered cellular therapies, but also illustrated important lessons regarding the potential for serious, life-threatening immune-mediated toxicities and the need for careful selection of antigen targets to minimize risk of "on-target" but "off-tumor" toxicity to normal tissues expressing similar antigens.

Viral Cytotoxic T-Lymphocytes

Viral Cytotoxic T-Lymphocytes (CTLs) have long been recognized as a naturally occurring subset of virus specific T-lymphocytes resulting from systemic viral infections which demonstrate the ability to target and kill virally infected cells. However, following the wide-spread clinical use of allo-HCT and concomitant immunosuppression, viral infections were increasingly recognized as significant sources of morbidity and mortality among HCT patients. In addition, it was also observed that patients receiving an allo-HCT from donors with pre-existing cytomegalovirus (CMV)-specific CTLs experienced lower rates of CMV reactivation following allo-HCT. In the 1990's with the increasing use of DLI, it was also noted that DLI was capable of eliminating Epstein–Barr virus (EBV)-associated post-transplant lymphoproliferative disorders (PTLDs) following allo-HCT. Subsequent research demonstrated that isolation and adoptive transfer of EBV-specific CTLs was effective in reducing EBV viremia and appeared to reduce the risk of EBV-associated PTLD. In 2007, Haque et al. reported clinical outcomes evaluating EBV-specific CTLs to treat PTLD, with 52% response rates and a duration of response of more than 6 months [18]. Since that time, multiple additional clinical trials have been completed or are currently underway evaluating viral-specific CTLs for EBV+ PTLD and other viral infections.

Natural Killer Cells

In 1975, Kiessling et al. first reported on the presence of "naturally occurring killer lymphocytes", or **Natural Killer (NK) cells,** isolated from the spleens of mice which were capable of robust leukemia cell lysis [19]. Throughout the 1990's and 2000's, seminal work conducted by Kärre, Ljunggren, Moretta and many others helped to characterize the diverse repertoire of NK cell receptors which mediate the unique function of NK cells, such as Killer Ig-like receptors (KIRs), Natural Cytotoxicity Receptors (NCRs) and non-HLA class I-specific activating receptors [20–22]. We now understand NK cells represent a unique subset of specialized effector lymphocytes which have the ability to directly kill malignant cells and virally infected cells through multiple mechanisms; while also being capable of interacting with various different innate and adaptive immune cells to promote a multi-faceted anti-tumor immune response. Early clinical development of NK cells as a platform for ACT demonstrated the effectiveness of donor-derived alloreactive NK cells in conjunction with allo-HCT for the treatment of leukemia [23]. Subsequent efforts employing various strategies including adoptive transfer of cytokine stimulated NK cells, combining NK cell infusions with monoclonal antibodies (mAbs) and transduction of CARs into NK cells (CAR-NKs) have all shown promise in early clinical development.

Dual-Targeting Immune Cell Engaging Therapies

Similar to the aforementioned cellular therapies, the clinical development of **dual-targeting immune cell engagers** spans decades. Beginning in the 1980s, descriptions began to emerge of hetero-conjugated monoclonal antibodies with two different antigen-recognition domains capable of inducing a cytotoxic immune response to target antigens in the absence MHC presentation. However, early manufacturing of such dual-targeting cell engaging molecules was technically challenging and cost-prohibitive for large-scale clinical use. Nevertheless, technical advances and improved production costs facilitated further development of various dual-targeting cell engagers through the 1990's and 2000's. In 2014, the FDA granted accelerated approval for blinatumomab, a CD3 x CD19 bi-specific T-cell engager (BiTE), for the indication of relapsed/refractory B-cell ALL. Confirmatory data in

2017 from a Phase III, international, randomized study led to the first full FDA approval of a dual-targeting cell engager therapy for the treatment of cancer [24]. Additional studies investigating the modified dual-targeting platforms known as immune-mobilizing monoclonal TCR Against Cancer (ImmTAC), dual-affinity retargeting (DART) proteins and NK-cell engaging molecules have shown clinical activity in specific tumor types.

Disclosures AG reports participation in advisory board meetings of Kite, Amgen, BMS, Atara, and Wugen. AG has received research funding from Kite and Amgen.

References

1. Allen JP. The art of medicine in ancient Egypt. New York: New Haven: Metropolitan Museum of Art ; Yale University Press; 2005.
2. Early History of Cancer | American Cancer Society [Internet]. [cited 2021 Mar 2]; https://www.cancer.org/cancer/cancer-basics/history-of-cancer/what-is-cancer.html
3. Band IC, Reichel M. Al Rhazes and the beginning of the end of smallpox. JAMA Dermatol. 2017;153(5):420.
4. Virchow R. Die krankhaften Geschwulste. Dreissing Vorlesungen gehalten wahrend des Wintersemesters 1862-1867 an der Universitat zu Berlin, vol. 1-3. Berlin: A. Hirschwald; 1863-1865.
5. Coley WB II. Contribution to the knowledge of sarcoma. Ann Surg. 1891;14(3):199–220.
6. McCarthy EF. The toxins of William B. Coley and the treatment of bone and soft-tissue sarcomas. Iowa Orthop J. 2006;26:154–8.
7. The Nobel Prize in Physiology or Medicine 1908 [Internet]. NobelPrize.org. [cited 2021 Mar 2]; https://www.nobelprize.org/prizes/medicine/1908/summary/
8. Thomas ED, Lochte HL, Lu WC, Ferrebee JW. Intravenous infusion of bone marrow in patients receiving radiation and chemotherapy. N Engl J Med. 1957;257(11):491–6.
9. Kolb H, Mittermuller J, Clemm C, et al. Donor leukocyte transfusions for treatment of recurrent chronic myelogenous leukemia in marrow transplant patients. Blood. 1990;76(12):2462–5.
10. Kuwana Y, Asakura Y, Utsunomiya N, et al. Expression of chimeric receptor composed of immunoglobulin-derived V regions and T-cell receptor-derived C regions. Biochem Biophys Res Commun. 1987;149(3):960–8.
11. Gross G, Waks T, Eshhar Z. Expression of immunoglobulin-T-cell receptor chimeric molecules as functional receptors with antibody-type specificity. Proc Natl Acad Sci. 1989;86(24):10024–8.
12. Neelapu SS, Locke FL, Bartlett NL, et al. Axicabtagene Ciloleucel CAR T-cell therapy in refractory large B-cell lymphoma. N Engl J Med. 2017;377(26):2531–44.
13. Schuster SJ, Bishop MR, Tam CS, et al. Tisagenlecleucel in adult relapsed or refractory diffuse large B-cell lymphoma. N Engl J Med. 2019;380(1):45–56.
14. Wang M, Munoz J, Goy A, et al. KTE-X19 CAR T-cell therapy in relapsed or refractory mantle-cell lymphoma. N Engl J Med. 2020;382(14):1331–42.
15. Rosenberg SA, Packard BS, Aebersold PM, et al. Use of tumor-infiltrating lymphocytes and Interleukin-2 in the immunotherapy of patients with metastatic melanoma. N Engl J Med. 1988;319(25):1676–80.
16. Rosenberg SA, Aebersold P, Cornetta K, et al. Gene transfer into humans—immunotherapy of patients with advanced melanoma, using tumor-infiltrating lymphocytes modified by retroviral gene transduction. N Engl J Med. 1990;323(9):570–8.

17. Morgan RA, Dudley ME, Wunderlich JR, et al. Cancer regression in patients after transfer of genetically engineered lymphocytes. Science. 2006;314(5796):126–9.
18. Haque T, Wilkie GM, Jones MM, et al. Allogeneic cytotoxic T-cell therapy for EBV-positive posttransplantation lymphoproliferative disease: results of a phase 2 multicenter clinical trial. Blood. 2007;110(4):1123–31.
19. Kiessling R, Klein E, Wigzell H. "Natural" killer cells in the mouse. I. Cytotoxic cells with specificity for mouse Moloney leukemia cells. Specificity and distribution according to genotype. Eur J Immunol. 1975;5(2):112–7.
20. Ljunggren H-G, Kärre K. In search of the 'missing self': MHC molecules and NK cell recognition. Immunol Today. 1990;11:237–44.
21. Moretta A, Bottino C, Vitale M, et al. Receptors for HLA class-I molecules in human natural killer cells. Annu Rev Immunol. 1996;14(1):619–48.
22. Moretta A, Bottino C, Vitale M, et al. Activating receptors and Coreceptors involved in human natural killer cell-mediated cytolysis. Annu Rev Immunol. 2001;19(1):197–223.
23. Ruggeri L. Effectiveness of donor natural killer cell alloreactivity in mismatched hematopoietic transplants. Science. 2002;295(5562):2097–100.
24. Kantarjian H, Stein A, Gökbuget N, et al. Blinatumomab versus chemotherapy for advanced acute lymphoblastic Leukemia. N Engl J Med. 2017;376(9):836–47.

Basics of Immunity

Brian T. Edelson

Abstract This chapter will serve as a brief review of immunology for oncologists. No single chapter can fully describe the complexity of the immune system and so the goal here will be to simply serve as a refresher. Innate and adaptive immunity will be concisely reviewed, with a brief description of the cells of each system. Focus will then be paid to the how T cells are activated and function. Finally, basic principles of T cell-mediated immunity to tumors will be presented. These foundational concepts will be useful for understanding later chapters which largely deal with the purposeful engineering of immune cells for adoptive cellular therapies. An attempt has been made to highlight recent review articles for further reading, with an emphasis on those that involve tumor immunology.

Keywords Innate immunity · Adaptive immunity · B cells · T cells · Natural killer (NK) · Natural killer T (NKT) cells · CD4+ cells · CD8+ cells · T helper (Th1, Th2, Th17) · T follicular helper (Tfh) · T regulatory cells (Treg) · Mucosal-associated invariant T (MAIT) cells · γδ T cells · Myeloid-derived suppressor cells (MDSCs) · Innate lymphoid cells (ILCs) · Cytotoxic T lymphocytes (CTLs) · B cell receptor (BCR) · T cell receptor (TCR) · Dendritic cells (DCs) · Antigen presenting cells (APCs) · Major histocompatibility (MHC) class I and class II molecules · Pathogen-associated molecular patterns (PAMPs) · Pathogen recognition receptors (PRRs) · Toll-like receptors (TLRs) · Tumor microenvironment (TME)

Innate Vs. Adaptive Immunity

The responses of the immune system to injury or infection that occur within the first minutes to hours are collectively called the innate immune response. These systems are evolutionarily old, and mainly serve the functions of pathogen recognition and

B. T. Edelson (✉)
Department of Pathology and Immunology, Washington University School of Medicine,
St. Louis, MO, USA
e-mail: bedelson@wustl.edu

© Springer Nature Switzerland AG 2022
A. Ghobadi, J. F. DiPersio (eds.), *Gene and Cellular Immunotherapy for Cancer*, Cancer Drug Discovery and Development,
https://doi.org/10.1007/978-3-030-87849-8_2

rapid pathogen attack. Components of innate immunity exist in all human cell types, although a specialized set of immune cells, both tissue-resident and blood-circulating, also contributes in important ways. Components of innate immunity alert other cells to the presence of a pathogen, such that they can be mobilized to the site of invasion, or their cell-intrinsic defenses can be strengthened in preparation for an upcoming encounter with the pathogen. Aspects of the innate immune system are also active in processes that don't involve pathogen invasion per se, including normal growth and organ development, responses to sterile wounding, physiologic interactions with the microbiome, and autoimmune responses. In the setting of tumor development, growth, and metastasis, cellular and soluble components of the innate immune system play important roles in both tumor promotion and restriction.

Adaptive immunity refers to the processes whereby lymphocytes of both the B cell and T cell lineages engage with antigens and carry out effector functions, again typically aimed at pathogen clearance. Unlike innate immune cells, which are typically more promiscuous in their recognition of common pathogen components or damaged cells, B and T cells are exquisitely antigen-specific and are called to duty only in the very special circumstance when their cognate antigen is involved. B and T cell development takes place in the bone marrow and thymus, respectively, in orchestrated processes whereby each cell is endowed with a single antigen-specific receptor [a B cell receptor (BCR) or T cell receptor (TCR)] in an anticipatory manner, such that the collection of B and T cells provides an immense repertoire of specificities for recognition of the universe of pathogens. By anticipatory, here, I mean that the instruction for which unique antigen-receptor a particular B or T cell comes to express developmentally is not instructed by any encounter with cognate antigen itself. B and T cell development occurs in a manner whereby self-reactive cells are eliminated. This "central" tolerance system is not always complete, however, and so mechanisms of "peripheral" tolerance are also in place to assure that, in most cases, self-reactive lymphocytes are held in check.

One other important concept in understanding adaptive immunity is that the process is clonal. A single B or T cell retains its unique BCR or TCR throughout its lifespan, and this antigen-receptor specificity is retained by progeny of the cell that arise through cell division. This is termed clonal expansion. For T cells, the TCR expressed by a single T cell clone is completely immutable, even upon T cell proliferation. B cells, however, can make limited changes to the sequence of their BCR upon activation through a process called somatic hypermutation, in which amino acid changed arise in specific regions of the BCR. These changes are subtle, and ideally result in B cell progeny with BCRs that display heightened affinity for cognate antigen, a process called affinity maturation.

The Stereotypical Immune Response to a Pathogen

Here, I will describe a stereotypical immune response to an invading pathogen, as it illustrates many of the concepts important to understanding how immune responses occur more broadly. In general, the innate and adaptive immune systems work together, which each feeding information to the other through soluble components and cellular interactions. Upon initial encounter with a pathogen, innate immune cells and soluble pathogen recognition systems like the complement proteins serve as initial sentinels to warn and prepare other host cells, but also make attempts to initially contain the pathogen and limit its spread. Effector systems of the innate response include molecules directly toxic to the pathogen, phagocytosis of the invading organisms, and mobilization of cell-autonomous defenses like the type I interferon (IFN) system. These systems also alert B and T cells that a pathogen has been encountered and create a set of conditions for optimal priming of naïve B and T cell responses. Priming typically occurs in the lymph nodes draining a breached tissue, or in the spleen, in the case of blood-borne pathogens. Intact pathogens, or components of the pathogen, reach lymph nodes via afferent lymphatic vessels, sometimes carried by migratory innate immune cells. In an amazingly efficient process, rare B and T cells with specificities for antigens of the invading pathogen engage these antigens, are activated through cell signaling cascades, proliferate, and take on effector phenotypes as directed by signals they receive from innate immune cells.

Priming of antigen-specific, naïve T cells requires specialized antigen presentation by dendritic cells (DCs, a specialized innate immune cell type). Antigen presentation is a process whereby antigen presenting cells (APCs) partially catabolize protein antigens and display short peptide fragments of these antigens on their surface in complexes with major histocompatibility (MHC) molecules (Fig. 1). Pathogen recognition by innate immune cells can sense the type of pathogen encountered via recognition of pathogen-associated molecular patterns (PAMPs). PAMPs are recognized at the cell surface, within endosomal compartments, and within the cytosol by an array of pathogen recognition receptors (PRRs), including multiple Toll-like receptors (TLRs) and a diverse set of cytosolic sensors. Distinct cytokine signals arising from antigen-presenting DCs based on the PAMPs detected drive specialized T cell responses, such that distinct effector T cell "subsets" develop.

In the cortex of lymph nodes, antigen-activated B and T cells also communicate with each other through soluble proteins called cytokines and through cell-cell interactions within the lymph node to orchestrate effects on the proliferating B cells, including adaptation to antibody secretion, optimization of antibody affinity (somatic hypermutation/affinity maturation) and isotype (a process called isotype switching), and the development of antigen-specific long-lived memory B cells and plasma cells. The complexities of B cell responses to antigens will not be covered further here.

Following T cell activation in lymph nodes, a process which usually takes 5–7 days, effector T cells are recruited to sites of infection by chemokine signals created by innate immune cells. Here, effector T cells orchestrate an inflammatory reaction which ideally can eliminate the pathogen with minimal tissue damage. This reaction includes both recruitment of more innate immune cells, signals to the non-immune cells that make up the tissue, direct cytotoxicity of infected cells, and eventually signals that restore homeostasis and promote healing. While this T cell-mediated reaction is occurring, memory T cells are also forming to provide a

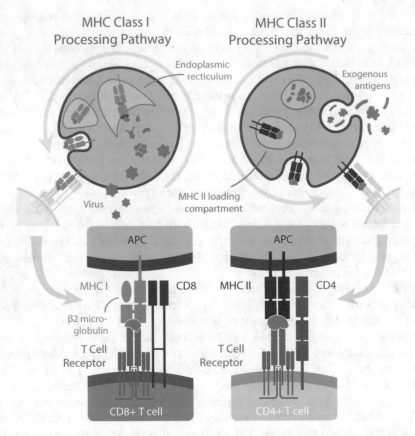

Fig. 1 Antigen presentation pathways. The MHC class I processing pathway (left) involves limited catabolism of cytosolic proteins into peptides which are then transported into the endoplasmic reticulum for loading onto MHC class I molecules. These MHC class I-peptide complexes traffic to the cell surface for presentation to TCRs on CD8+ T cells. The MHC class II processing pathway (right) involves limited catabolism of exogenous protein antigens within vesicular compartments. Peptides are loaded onto MHC class II molecules in the MHC II loading compartment. MHC class II-peptide complexes traffic to the cell surface for presentation to TCRs on CD4+ T cells

reservoir of antigen-specific T cells which have the properties of longevity and more rapid and robust activation for future encounters with the same pathogen. Following elimination of antigen, the large population of antigen-specific effector T cells that has formed through clonal expansion is markedly reduced, leaving behind a more modest but still important population of memory T cells. Notably, in chronic infections where antigen cannot be fully eliminated, T cell activation persists through repeated encounters with peptide-presenting APCs. T cells in this situation take on an "exhausted" phenotype, becoming recalcitrant to repeated stimulation and less robust in their cytokine secretion and cytotoxic activity.

Cells of the Innate Immune System

Here, I will briefly describe the major cell types of the innate immune system. Note that some effector arms of the innate immune system, including complement, will not be covered.

Granulocytes. These can be divided into neutrophils, basophils, and eosinophils. They are myeloid cells that produced in the bone marrow and traffic via the blood to sites of inflammation. Each of these has specialized granules which can be deployed upon cell signaling and which contain compounds toxic to microbes. There are examples of these cells playing roles in the immune response to cancer as regulators of the tumor microenvironment (TME), sometimes in a manner that promotes tumor growth or immune evasion, and at other times playing tumoricidal roles [1, 2]. Different tumor types may have different interactions with these cells. Neutrophils, in particular, have been associated with establishment of the pre-metastatic niche [3]. Furthermore, neutrophil-like myeloid-derived suppressor cells (MDSCs), sometimes called granulocytic or polymorphonuclear MDSCs, have been described that also can suppress anti-tumor adaptive immune responses [4].

Cells of the mononuclear phagocyte system. This collection of mononuclear cells encompasses monocytes, macrophages, and DCs. Monocytes are blood-circulating myeloid cells that form in the bone marrow and possess the properties of cell migration, phagocytosis, pathogen recognition, cytokine production, and antigen presentation [5]. Upon pathogen encounter and/or activation by inflammatory cytokines, these cells can differentiate into various forms of cells that morphologically resemble the other cells of this lineage, creating significant nomenclature issues in the field (e.g. so-called inflammatory macrophages or monocyte-derived DCs) [6]. Monocyte responses to tumors, like granulocytes, can probably be both pro- and anti-tumoral, and monocyte-like MDSCs also have been identified and characterized [4].

Macrophages refer to a set of tissue-resident large phagocytes present in all organs in the steady state. Organs are seeded during embryogenesis with macrophage progenitors from either the yolk-sac or fetal liver, and in most organs mature macrophages are self-renewing [7]. In different organs, macrophages take on distinct features in response to environmental cues, such that historically these cells have been given diverse names (e.g. microglia, alveolar macrophages, red pulp macrophages of the spleen, Kupffer cells of the liver) and have been appreciated for their morphologic differences. Tissue-resident macrophages are important in tissue homeostasis and can respond to pathogens by enhanced phagocytosis, microbicidal activity, and cytokine production. These cells can also present antigenic peptides via surface MHC molecules to T cells. To different degrees in different organs, tissue-resident macrophages are replaced with age by blood-monocyte derived cells in the steady state. Monocytes respond to environmental cues and adopt the phenotype of embryonically derived macrophages, such that in adults, tissue-resident macrophages represent a mixture of cells derived from embryonic precursors and monocytes [8]. Tumors contain a complex array of macrophages, including some derived from their organ's originally resident macrophage population, and others derived from blood monocytes that have entered the tumor [9]. It is common for

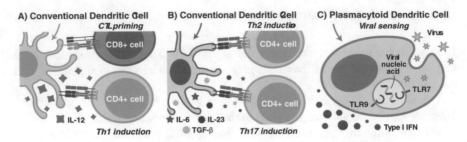

Fig. 2 Dendritic cell subsets and functions. Three subsets of DCs, (A) cDC1s, (B) cDC2s, and (C) pDCs, are shown performing their classic functions. cDC1s prime CTL responses and provide the cytokine signals needed for the instruction of Th1 cell responses. cDC2s provide the cytokine signals needed for the instruction of Th2 cell and Th17 cell responses. pDCs recognize viral nucleic acids and are rapid producers of type I IFNs

macrophages in tumors to be designated "tumor-associated macrophages", typically referring to cells with tumor-supporting characteristics, although this is an oversimplification that does not appreciate their heterogeneity [10].

DCs are bone-marrow derived cells present in all tissues and exist in three basic subsets, conventional DC1s (cDC1s), cDC2s, and plasmacytoid DCs (pDCs) [11] (Fig. 2). These subsets also exist in lymphoid organs. The two cDC subsets are premier APCs and, based on their collection of ligands for T cell-expressed costimulatory receptors and their cytokine production, are especially capable of priming naïve T cells. cDC1s are important in the priming of CD8+ T cells [12], with cDC2s having been thought to have a stronger role in priming CD4+ T cells [13, 14]. cDC1s possess a specialized antigen presentation pathway called cross presentation, in which exogenous protein antigens captured through pinocytosis or phagocytosis can be catabolized to peptides presented on MHC class I molecules, the group of MHC molecules that presents peptide to CD8+ T cells [15]. In all other cell types, including non-hematopoietic cells, MHC class I-presented peptides derive from cytosolic protein antigens. cDCs of both subsets also perform typical antigen processing of exogenous protein antigens to present peptides on MHC class II molecules to CD4+ T cells. cDC presentation of tumor antigens is exceptionally important in the context of T cell immunity to tumors, with recognition that in some cases cDC1s are uniquely required for CD8+ T cell priming and T cell-mediated clearance of model immunogenic tumors [12]. Newer data also suggests cDC1s play an important role in priming CD4+ T cell responses to tumor antigens, with CD4+ T cells subsequently "licensing" cDC1s to optimally prime anti-tumor CD8+ T cell responses [16]. pDCs are specialized cells with a unique collection of pathogen recognition receptors and which produce large amounts of type I IFNs upon receptor signaling. This response is thought to be a means of rapidly responding to viruses. A role for pDCs in tumor immunity is unclear. Several attempts have been made to harness the power of DCs as cell-based therapeutics for the induction of a T cell response to tumor antigens [17]. In most cases, the cells used were dendritic in nature, but not *bona fide* cDCs. Rather, they were cells derived from blood monocytes following in vitro treatment with hematopoietic growth factors. Such monocyte-derived DCs may retain some of the antigen-presenting properties and T cell priming abilities of *bona fide* cDCs, and therefore could be useful therapeutics. There continues to be interest in harnessing the power of cDCs to initiate or augment anti-tumor T cell responses.

Mast cells. These myeloid cells are rich in connective and mucosal tissues and are heavily loaded with secretory granules. They are best recognized for their role in allergic responses following triggering by Fc epsilon receptor-bound IgE in response to allergens. They can also respond to other diverse ligands including complement components and PAMPs. Their granules contain heparin, histamine, and proteases but they also release lipid mediators and cytokines that altogether can initiate a rapid and robust inflammatory response. Mast cells have been identified as a component of certain human tumors, and in different cases have been suggested to be pro- or anti-tumoral [18].

Innate and innate-like lymphocytes. Several types of innate and innate-like lymphocyte lineages have been identified with diverse functions. In general, many of these cell types are tissue-resident and some express a characteristic semi-invariant BCR or TCR for recognition of non-peptide ligands. These cells have homeostatic functions in tissues, but also are fast-acting and are important in the early phases of immune encounters with pathogens. This broad topic is beyond the scope of this chapter, but a few cell types deserve mention. Innate B cells, including B-1 cells and marginal zone B cells, secrete natural IgM important in the earliest phases of a primary immune response and may have immunoregulatory properties [19]. Innate-like lymphocytes (also called unconventional T cells) include natural killer T (NKT) cells, mucosal-associated invariant T (MAIT) cells, and γδ T cells [20]. These cell types secrete cytokines and/or display cytotoxic function in response to activation of their semi-invariant TCRs by specific ligands which are often derived from the microbiota [21]. Whether they play roles in immune responses to tumors remains unclear [22]. Finally, classical natural killer (NK) cells and innate lymphoid cells (ILCs) are non-TCR-expressing lymphocytes which share properties of cytotoxicity and cytokine production with T cells. NK cells utilize an array of activating and inhibitory ligands to sense cells experiencing various forms of cell stress and can be potent cytotoxic cells. NK cells are thought to be a component of tumor immunosurveillance [23]. ILCs exist as three tissue-resident subsets (ILC1, ILC2, and ILC3) that secrete distinct cytokines and have roles in tissue homeostasis [24]. Their roles in cancer are less clear. Importantly, and related to the chapters that follow, attempts are being made to harness the therapeutic potential of innate lymphocytes, especially NK cells, for the treatment of cancer [25].

Cells of the Adaptive Immune System

B cells. These lymphocytes develop in the bone marrow through a process of antigen receptor gene rearrangement of the immunoglobulin heavy and light chain genes, a process called V(D)J rearrangement [26, 27]. Developing B cells proceed through a series of defined stages in which their rearranged immunoglobulin genes are tested for function, but also for self-reactivity. Naïve, mature B cells emerge from this process that are selective for non-self antigens with each B cell expressing a unique BCR that contains 2 identical antigen-binding regions. In naïve B cells these BCR molecules utilize specific constant regions determined by gene rearrangements of the heavy chain locus, such that these cells express BCRs of the IgD and IgM isotype. Transmembrane BCR proteins associate with short transmembrane proteins that contain cytosolic tails which can be phosphorylated upon BCR engagement by antigen. Naïve B cells circulate through the blood and lymphoid tissues scanning for their cognate antigen. Upon antigen binding, cell signaling pathways are triggered, largely involving phosphorylation events, leading to complex changes in transcription, metabolism, and cytoskeletal structure [28]. This process is called B cell activation. Antigen-activated B cells proliferate clonally and take on various phenotypes including forms that secrete immunoglobulin. Secreted immunoglobulin maintains the antigen specificity and basic structure of the transmembrane BCR, but instead does not express a transmembrane portion, allowing the protein to traffic intracellularly for glycosylation and ultimately secretion. B cells that receive T cell help in the form of cytokines and cell-cell interactions in the lymph node undergo complex phenotypic changes to result in clonal production of memory B cells and long-lived plasma cells, a process termed the germinal center reaction [29, 30]. This topic is beyond the scope of this chapter.

T cells. These lymphocytes develop from dedicated progenitors that leave the bone marrow and travel to the thymus for completion of development. Here, T cell precursors undergo v(D)J recombination to ultimately express a mature TCR and the associated transmembrane signaling molecules (generally referred to as the CD3 complex). During this process selection occurs such that T cells with high reactivity for self-peptides presented by MHC molecules on thymic APCs are eliminated (negative selection). Further, only T cells with low affinity recognition for self-peptide with MHC molecules receive survival signals (positive selection). T cells with TCRs that are ignorant (i.e. have no recognition) of self-peptide/MHC are eliminated by apoptosis.

During this education process in the thymus, TCRs with low affinity for self-peptide and MHC class I molecules take on the phenotype of "cytotoxic T lymphocytes' (CTLs) and express the surface protein CD8. Likewise, other TCRs with low affinity for self-peptide and MHC class II molecules direct cells to become CD4-expressing "helper" T cells. As reviewed earlier, each naïve T cell that develops expresses a single TCR specificity that has a unique reactivity with a foreign (but not yet "seen") peptide in the context of one self MHC molecule (this is referred to as MHC restriction).

T Cell Activation and Effector Functions

CD8+ T cells are recognized for their ability to rapidly kill target cells through a process that involves perforin and granzyme secretion in response to TCR recognition of cognate antigenic peptide presented by an MHC class I molecule. TCR signaling and costimulation, most notably through CD28 binding to B7 molecules during priming by DCs, results in a phenotypic change in CD8+ T cells to become effector cells with increased perforin- and granzyme- containing granules and heightened cytokine secretion. CD8+ T cell proliferation is rapid, such that antigen-specific clones expand by several logs over the first week of an immune response to a pathogen. Many of these effector CD8+ T cells will eventually die by apoptosis after pathogen clearance, although some responding CD8+ T cells will phenotypically change during an immune response to become a heterogenous set of long-lived memory cell types. CD8+ T cells responding to chronic stimulation, in the form of non-resolving chronic infections or tumor antigens, however, undergo further phenotypic changes to become "exhausted" [31]. This phenotype is characterized by metabolic alterations, lower cytotoxicity, and lower cytokine secretion (particularly IL-2, TNFα, and IFNγ). Exhausted T cells express a collection of negative costimulatory molecules, the most recognized of which is PD-1. Enhanced negative costimulation and chronic cytokine stimulation by IL-10 and TGFβ contribute to T cell exhaustion.

CD4+ T cells orchestrate immune responses through their elaboration of cytokines and their direct interaction with antigen presenting B cells. They play important roles in the establishment of CD8+ T cell memory, as well. Upon activation through TCR signaling and costimulation, CD4+ T cells expand clonally (Fig. 3). During priming by DCs, instructive cytokines determine the gene expression profile of activated CD4+ T cells, such that they take on stereotypical "T helper subset" phenotypes through the actions of specific transcription factors. Activated CD4+ T cells have been divided into five basic subsets (Th1, Th2, Th17, Tfh, and Treg). Th1, Th2, and Th17 cells are marked by the production of their hallmark cytokines IFNγ, IL-4, and IL-17A, respectively [32, 33]. Each of these subsets is tailored to the response to a specific pathogen type (intracellular pathogens for Th1 cells,

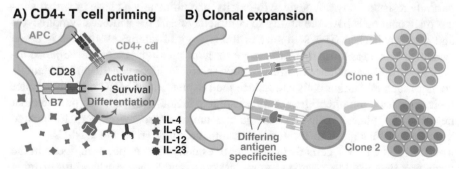

A) CD4+ T cell priming   **B) Clonal expansion**

Fig. 3 Activation and expansion of CD4+ T cells. (A) CD4+ T cell priming requires three signals. The TCR recognizes cognate MHC class II peptide complexes on the surface of the APC. Costimulatory molecules like CD28 signal in response to binding of their ligands. Cytokine receptors signal in response to secreted cytokines. Together these signals lead to activation, survival, and differentiation of the CD4+ T cell. (B) Different CD4+ T cells, each with specificity for a distinct peptide ligand, will proliferate in response to these activating signals to generate expanded clones

helminths for Th2 cells, and extracellular bacteria and fungi for Th17 cells). T fol-licular helper (Tfh) cells play a specific role in the germinal center response by providing signals to activated B cells to instruct their somatic hypermutation and isotype switching. T regulatory cells (Tregs) play an immunoregulatory role in sup-pressing autoreactive cells through a variety of mechanisms including elaboration of immunosuppressive cytokines. Beyond these five basic subsets, other T helper cell subsets have been recognized based on their production of specific inflamma-tory cytokines, but these, in general, are not as well characterized. Each of the T helper cell subsets can play important roles in tumors in different contexts and can recognize tumor antigens [34].

Basics Principles of T Cell-Mediated Immunity to Cancer and Immune Evasion

Immunosurveillance is the process whereby the immune system can recognize can-cer cells and eliminate them before they progress to tumor formation or effects on health. This is understood to be the domain of classical T cells and requires func-tioning antigen presenting cells and the action of innate immune cells to allow effec-tive T cell priming and effector function. There are also roles for innate-like lymphocytes and ILCs in the recognition of tumor cells through changes in tumor cell expression of MHC molecules and stress ligands which serve to activate NK cells, NKT cells, and γδ T cells [35–37]. A three-phase process encompassing an elimination phase, an equilibrium phase, and an escape phase has been described to explain the interaction of lymphocytes with tumor cells ultimately tumor growth. The initial phase involves successful elimination of malignant cells upon first rec-ognition, a second phase in which malignant cells develop alterations to become partially resistant to lymphocyte cytotoxicity, and ultimately a phase in which vari-ant malignant cells have the ability to completely resist the action of lymphocytes and grow unchecked. This sculpting of the biology of tumor cells by the immune system to select for those that can escape immune pressure is termed immunoedit-ing [38–40]. The avoidance of immune recognition includes genetic and epigenetic changes such that tumor cells can reduce their expression of MHC molecules, alter their expression tumor antigens, express soluble factors or membrane proteins that negatively regulate T cells, or change the tumor microenvironment to include immune cells that result in T cell suppression, including Tregs and MDSCs.

CD4+ and CD8+ T cells recognize peptides derived from tumor antigens in the same way they would recognize foreign peptides, and DCs are critical for priming of these T cell responses. Tumor antigens can be divided into three basic types that are important to recognize when designing or utilizing adoptive cell therapy. Tumor-associated antigens are overexpressed normal proteins that either play a role in oncogenesis or represent a protein expressed at high levels by both tumor cells and normal cells of the same origin ("differentiation" antigens). T cells are normally tolerant to these antigens, but they can be useful targets of certain forms of immunotherapy. Tumor-restricted antigens, also referred to as "cancer-testes" antigens, are proteins which are normally only expressed on germ cells but become aberrantly expressed on tumor cells. These can be immunogenic and can be recognized by T cells. Tumor-specific antigens are either viral proteins expressed in tumor cells by oncogenic viruses or mutated self-proteins. This latter group, termed neoantigens, encompass either peptides derived from oncogenic proteins or "passenger" mutations to non-oncogenic proteins such that the amino acid changes result in a peptide that can be presented by MHC molecules and recognized as foreign by T cells. Neoantigenic peptides presented by MHC class I molecules to CD8+ T cells have garnered the most attention, but similar peptides exist that are presented by MHC class II molecules to CD4+ T cells. Optimal anti-tumor T cell responses require the priming of both types of T cells, and tumors with a higher mutational burden possess more neoantigens. Neoantigen-based cancer vaccines offer the promise of identifying neoantigens in a personalized fashion and delivering a vaccine that could prime or boost T cells specific to these peptides [41].

Finally, a few words on the three most prominent forms of cancer immunotherapy, immune checkpoint blockade, T/NK cell engagers, and adoptive T cell therapy [42]. Immune checkpoint blockade refers to monoclonal antibody-based therapeutics which block negative costimulatory molecule signaling on T cells. The most prominent negative costimulatory molecules expressed on T cells to date are CTLA4 and PD-1, and agents targeting these have been remarkably successful at inducing profound anti-tumor responses in a subset of patients in a variety of cancer types. These work, in general, through enhanced activation of T cells and increased proliferation, effector function, and memory cell development. They may also have negative effects on Tregs such that the tumor microenvironment becomes more amenable to the action of effector T cells. Other negative costimulatory molecules on T cells are also of considerable interest as targets for novel checkpoint inhibitors.

T/NK cell engagers are engineered multi-functional antibody-like proteins with at least one antigen-binding site specific for a T cell or NK cell activating receptor and at least one antigen-binding site specific for a surface-expressed tumor-associated antigen. T/NK engagers coordinate an interaction between a lymphocyte and a tumor cell to promote direct tumor cell killing.

Adoptive T cell therapy refers broadly to the injection of patient-derived or allogenic T cells aimed at promoting an anti-tumor response. "Donor lymphocyte infusions" can be a component of allogeneic hematopoietic stem cell transplantation and mediate graft vs. tumor effects. Other forms of adoptive T cell therapy include the in vitro expansion and reinfusion of patient-derived tumor-infiltrating lymphocytes (TILs) that target tumor antigens, TCR gene-modified T cells (TCR-T), viral specific cytotoxic lymphocytes (viral CTLs), NK cells, and chimeric antigen receptor T cells (CAR-T cells). In particular, the last few years has seen an explosion in interest in CAR-T cells and related forms of engineered cells that are the subject of many of the subsequent chapters in this volume. These cells are being designed with specificity for new target antigens that may allow them to target solid tumors and are being modified to enhance their trafficking, function, and longevity. Challenges for both immune checkpoint blockade-based therapies, T/NK cell engagers, and adoptive cell therapies include patient selection, serious immune-mediated adverse events, high cost, and treatment resistance. These challenges are being tackled by numerous basic, translational, and clinical studies, and the future is bright for cancer immunotherapy.

References

1. Duhan V, Smyth MJ. Innate myeloid cells in the tumor microenvironment. Curr Opin Immunol. 2021;69:18–28.
2. Mattei F, Andreone S, Marone G, et al. Eosinophils in the tumor microenvironment. Adv Exp Med Biol. 2020;1273:1–28.
3. Jablonska J, Lang S, Sionov RV, Granot Z. The regulation of pre-metastatic niche formation by neutrophils. Oncotarget. 2017;8:112132–44.
4. Veglia F, Sanseviero E, Gabrilovich DI. Myeloid-derived suppressor cells in the era of increasing myeloid cell diversity. Nat Rev Immunol. 2021;1:1–14. (Epub ahead of print)
5. Guilliams M, Mildner A, Yona S. Developmental and functional heterogeneity of monocytes. Immunity. 2018;49:595–613.
6. Guilliams M, Ginhoux F, Jakubzick C, et al. Dendritic cells, monocytes and macrophages: a unified nomenclature based on ontogeny. Nat Rev Immunol. 2014;14:571–8.
7. T'Jonck W, Guilliams M, Bonnardel J. Niche signals and transcription factors involved in tissue-resident macrophage development. Cell Immunol. 2018;330:43–53.
8. Liu Z, Gu Y, Chakarov S, Bleriot C, et al. Fate mapping via Ms4a3-expression history traces monocyte-derived cells. Cell. 2019;178:1509–25.
9. Zhu Y, Herndon JM, Sojka DK, et al. Tissue-resident macrophages in pancreatic ductal adenocarcinoma originate from embryonic hematopoiesis and promote tumor progression. Immunity. 2017;47:323–38.
10. DeNardo DG, Ruffell B. Macrophages as regulators of tumour immunity and immunotherapy. Nat Rev Immunol. 2019;19:369–82.
11. Anderson DA 3rd, Dutertre CA, Ginhoux F, Murphy KM. Genetic models of human and mouse dendritic cell development and function. Nat Rev Immunol. 2021;21:101–15.
12. Hildner K, Edelson BT, Purtha WE, et al. Batf3 deficiency reveals a critical role for CD8alpha+ dendritic cells in cytotoxic T cell immunity. Science. 2008;322:1097–100.
13. Dudziak D, Kamphorst AO, Heidkamp GF, et al. Differential antigen processing by dendritic cell subsets in vivo. Science. 2007;315:107–11.
14. Binnewies M, Mujal AM, Pollack JL, et al. Unleashing Type-2 dendritic cells to drive protective antitumor CD4+ T cell immunity. Cell. 2019;177:556–71.
15. Gros M, Amigorena S. Regulation of antigen export to the cytosol during cross-presentation. Front Immunol. 2019;10:41.
16. Ferris ST, Durai V, Wu R, et al. cDC1 prime and are licensed by CD4+ T cells to induce antitumour immunity. Nature. 2020;584:624–9.
17. Fu C, Zhou L, Mi QS, Jiang A. DC-based vaccines for cancer immunotherapy. Vaccines (Basel). 2020;8:706.
18. Aponte-López A, Muñoz-Cruz S. Mast cells in the tumor microenvironment. Adv Exp Med Biol. 2020;1273:159–73.
19. Grasseau A, Boudigou M, Le Pottier L, et al. Innate B cells: the archetype of protective immune cells. Clin Rev Allergy Immunol. 2020;58:92–106.
20. Pellicci DG, Koay HF, Berzins SP. Thymic development of unconventional T cells: how NKT cells, MAIT cells and γδ T cells emerge. Nat Rev Immunol. 2020;20:756–70.
21. Constantinides MG. Interactions between the microbiota and innate and innate-like lymphocytes. J Leukoc Biol. 2018;103:409–19.

22. Chou C, Li MO. Re(de)fining innate lymphocyte lineages in the face of cancer. Cancer Immunol Res. 2018;6:372–7.
23. Molgora M, Cortez VS, Colonna M. Killing the I\invaders: NK cell impact in tumors and antitumor therapy. Cancers (Basel). 2021;13:595.
24. Branzk N, Gronke K, Diefenbach A. Innate lymphoid cells, mediators of tissue homeostasis, adaptation and disease tolerance. Immunol Rev. 2018;286:86–101.
25. Cortés-Selva D, Dasgupta B, Singh S, Grewal IS. Innate and innate-like cells: the future of chimeric antigen receptor (CAR) cell therapy. Trends Pharmacol Sci. 2021;42:45–59.
26. Wang Y, Liu J, Burrows PD, Wang JY. B cell development and maturation. Adv Exp Med Biol. 2020;1254:1–22.
27. Chi X, Li Y, Qiu X. V(D)J recombination, somatic hypermutation and class switch recombination of immunoglobulins: mechanism and regulation. Immunology. 2020;160:233–47.
28. Tanaka S, Baba Y. B cell receptor signaling. Adv Exp Med Biol. 2020;1254:23–36.
29. Elsner RA, Shlomchik MJ. Germinal center and extrafollicular B cell responses in vaccination, immunity, and autoimmunity. Immunity. 2020;53:1136–50.
30. Ise W, Kurosaki T. Plasma cell differentiation during the germinal center reaction. Immunol Rev. 2019;288:64–74.
31. McLane LM, Abdel-Hakeem MS, Wherry EJ. CD8 T cell exhaustion during chronic viral infection and cancer. Annu Rev Immunol. 2019;37:457–95.
32. Zhu X, Zhu J. CD4 T helper cell subsets and related human immunological disorders. Int J Mol Sci. 2020;21:8011.
33. Dong C. Cytokine regulation and function in T cells. Annu Rev Immunol. 2021;11:51. (Epub ahead of print)
34. Alspach E, Lussier DM, Miceli AP, et al. MHC-II neoantigens shape tumour immunity and response to immunotherapy. Nature. 2019;574:696–701.
35. Guillerey C. NK cells in the tumor microenvironment. Adv Exp Med Biol. 2020;1273:69–90.
36. Fujii SI, Shimizu K. Immune networks and therapeutic targeting of iNKT cells in cancer. Trends Immunol. 2019;40:984–97.
37. Willcox CR, Mohammed F, Willcox BE. The distinct MHC-unrestricted immunobiology of innate-like and adaptive-like human γδ T cell subsets - nature's CAR-T cells. Immunol Rev. 2020;298:25–46.
38. Dunn GP, Old LJ, Schreiber RD. The three Es of cancer immunoediting. Annu Rev Immunol. 2004;22:329–60.
39. Schreiber RD, Old LJ, Smyth MJ. Cancer immunoediting: integrating immunity's roles in cancer suppression and promotion. Science. 2011;331:1565–70.
40. Mittal D, Gubin MM, Schreiber RD, Smyth MJ. New insights into cancer immunoediting and its three component phases—elimination, equilibrium and escape. Curr Opin Immunol. 2014;27:16–25.
41. Blass E, Ott PA. Advances in the development of personalized neoantigen-based therapeutic cancer vaccines. Nat Rev Clin Oncol. 2021;20:1–15. (Epub ahead of print)
42. Waldman AD, Fritz JM, Lenardo MJ. A guide to cancer immunotherapy: from T cell basic science to clinical practice. Nat Rev Immunol. 2020;20:651–68.

Part II
CAR-T

Biology of CAR-T Cells

Trisha R. Berger, Alexander Boardman, Renier Brentjens, and Marcela V. Maus

Abstract Chimeric antigen receptors (CARs) are engineered receptors that redirect immune cells to target cancer cells. CAR-T cells have had impressive results in patients with hematologic malignancies, leading to the FDA approval of five CAR-T cells for relapsed or refractory B cell malignancies. The components of these CARs (the extracellular antigen-binding domain, hinge and transmembrane region, co-stimulatory domains, and activation domain) were methodically designed to optimize cell activation and improve cell persistence. Using different domains or making minor modifications to the domain sequence greatly changes the CAR-T cell's efficacy. Despite their success thus far, many patients develop CAR-T cell-associated toxicities and relapse from CAR-T cell therapy. Next-gen CAR-T cells aim to reduce toxicity and prevent relapse through refining antigen targeting, regulating assembly or activation of the CAR components, preventing anti-CAR immunity, and/or armoring the cell to respond to its surroundings. While the FDA approved CAR-T cells target two B cell antigens, CD19 and B cell maturation antigen (BCMA), additional targets for B cell malignancies, other hematologic cancers, and solid tumors are rapidly emerging. Antigens shared across tumor types that have been or are currently being tested in clinical trials are discussed.

Keywords Cellular therapy · Chimeric antigen receptor · Immunotherapy · CAR components · Next-gen CAR-T cell · Antigen-binding domain · Costimulatory domains · Armored CAR · Target antigens · Logic-gated CAR

T. R. Berger · M. V. Maus (✉)
Cellular Immunotherapy Program, Massachusetts General Hospital Cancer Center and Harvard Medical School, Boston, MA, USA
e-mail: mvmaus@mgh.harvard.edu

A. Boardman · R. Brentjens
Cellular Therapeutics Center, Department of Medicine, Memorial Sloan-Kettering Cancer Center, New York, NY, USA

© Springer Nature Switzerland AG 2022
A. Ghobadi, J. F. DiPersio (eds.), *Gene and Cellular Immunotherapy for Cancer*, Cancer Drug Discovery and Development,
https://doi.org/10.1007/978-3-030-87849-8_3

Overall Anatomy and Design of CAR-T Cells

Chimeric antigen receptor (CAR)-T cells are lymphocytes that are genetically engineered to express an antigen receptor and signaling domains that reprogram the T cell to activate in response to binding a specific target. Engineered T cell therapies, an emerging branch of immuno-oncology, have achieved impressive response rates and durable remissions in patients with hematologic malignancies. Following their FDA approval, CAR-T cell research rapidly expanded, with new and innovative designs improving their function. Each component of the CAR has a specific function in antigen binding, signaling, and persistence—factors that influence CAR-T cell anti-tumor efficacy.

First, Second, and Third Generation CARs

CARs are composed of four major domains: antigen binding, hinge, transmembrane and intracellular signaling. Each domain plays a role in recognizing the CAR target and relaying this signal to activate the T cell. Determining the optimal components to drive CAR-T cell function is a major area of CAR-T cell research. First generation CARs contained an extracellular antigen binding domain composed of the single-chain variable fragment (scFv) of an antibody sequence attached to a transmembrane domain and CD3ζ intracellular signaling domain from the endogenous T cell receptor (Fig. 1a, b) [1–3]. These CARs were designed so that when the scFv region binds its target antigen, CD3ζ transduces an activating signal for the T cell to expand, kill the target cell, and persist for long-term tumor control. However, clinical trials using first generation CARs showed little efficacy in patients due to limited expansion and persistence of the CAR-T cells [4].

To improve their function, second generation CARs were developed with additional intracellular signaling domains aimed at boosting the activation signal. Second-generation CARs typically contain either a CD28 or 4-1BB co-stimulatory domain placed between the transmembrane domain and CD3ζ Fig. 1b [5, 6]. Either combination implemented in CD19-targeted CAR-T cells demonstrated anti-tumor efficacy in patients, with profound and durable responses achieved for relapsed or refractory B cell leukemia [7–9]. These results led to the FDA approval of two

---

Fig. 1 (continued) Third generation CAR-T cells feature multiple co-stimulatory domains. (**c**) The improved efficacy of second generation CARs led to the FDA approval of four CD19-targeted and one BCMA targeted engineered T cell therapies in 2017, including CD28-containing Axicabtagene ciloleucel and 4-1BB-containing Tisagenleleucel. Brexucabtagene autoleucel, approved for use in mantle cell lymphoma in 2020, uses the same CAR construct as axi-cel, but differs in the method of T cell isolation. Lisocabtagene maraleucel uses a 4-1BB costimulatory domain with a CD28 transmembrane domain and contains a 1:1 mixture of transduced CD4 and CD8 T cells. Idecabtagene vicleucel, approved this year for use in multiple myeloma, is another second generation CAR with an anti-BCMA scFv and a 4-1BB costimulatory domain

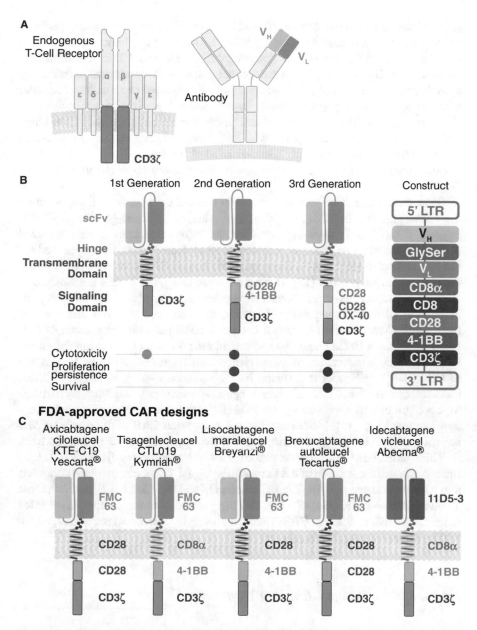

Fig. 1 Schematic of CAR design by generation. (**a**) Canonical chimeric antigen receptor (CAR) constructs contain an extracellular binding domain derived from an antibody single-chain variable fragment (scFv) sequence, including variable light (V_L) and variable heavy (V_H) regions of the antigen binding fragment (Fab) of an antibody. Intracellular signaling domains are derived from sequences in the endogenous T cell receptor (TCR) and vary by generation (**b**). First generation CAR-T cells contain only CD3ζ sequence, however, resulting T cell expansion and persistence is inadequate for clinical use. Second generation constructs harbor an additional co-stimulatory sequence—typically either CD28 or 4-1BB—and have shown improved efficacy and persistence in humans.

second-generation CAR-T cells in 2017 (Fig. 1c). Axicabtagene ciloleucel (axi-cel, brand name Yescarta, manufactured by Kite Pharma Inc.) is composed of a CD19-specific scFv, CD28 hinge and transmembrane domain, CD28 costimulatory domain, and CD3ζ activation domain. Axi-cel is approved for relapsed or refractory large B-cell lymphoma [10], and more recently for relapsed or refractory follicular lymphoma. Tisagenleleucel (tisa-cel, brand name Kymriah, manufactured by Novartis) harbors the same scFv and activation domain but contains a CD8 hinge and transmembrane domain with a 4-1BB costimulatory domain. Tisa-cel is approved for pediatric and young adult relapsed or refractory B-cell acute lympho-blastic leukemia (ALL) and adult relapsed or refractory large B-cell lymphoma [11, 12].

Since then, three more second generation CAR-T cells have been approved by the FDA (Fig. 1c). In 2020 and 2021, two additional second-generation CD19-targeted CAR-T cells were approved by the FDA. Brexucabtagene autoleucel (brexu-cel, brand name Tecartus, manufactured by Kite Pharma Inc), approved for use in mantle cell lymphoma, is identical to the axi-cel CAR construct, but varies in the manufacturing process [13]. During manufacturing, the T cells are isolated to ensure that no leukemia or lymphoma cells are included in the product. Lisocabtagene maraleucel (liso-cel, brand name Breyanzi, manufactured by Juno Therapeutics Inc./Bristol-Myers Squibb) harbors a similar 4-1BB costimulatory domain as tisa-cel, but also has a CD28 hinge and transmembrane domain [14]. During the manu-facturing process, genetically modified lymphocytes are allocated into a 1:1 mixture of CD4:CD8 T cells prior to infusion into the patient. Finally, in March of 2021, idecabtagene vicleucel (ide-cel, brand name Abecma, manufactured by Bristol-Myers Squibb) was approved by the FDA for treatment of relapsed or refractory multiple myeloma [15]. Ide-cel is a second generation CAR with an anti-BCMA scFv, a 4-1BB costimulatory domain, and a CD8 α hinge and transmembrane domain.

Third generation CARs contain two co-stimulatory domains adjacent to CD3ζ to further enhance the strength of the intracellular signal. Other costimulatory domains that have been tested in CAR-T cells include OX40 [16], CD27 [17], and inducible T cell co-stimulator (ICOS) [18] (Fig. 2). The type of costimulatory domain included in the CAR renders different CAR-T cells with varying functional properties, which will be discussed later in this section.

Extracellular Antigen-Binding Domains

The extracellular segment of the CAR is classically composed of an scFv that binds to the target antigen (Fig. 2). The scFv contains variable light (V_L) and variable heavy (V_H) regions of an antibody specific to the target antigen connected by a flex-ible linker. The affinity of the scFv for its target antigen influences the strength of the activation signal relayed to the T cell, with higher affinity leading to greater activation. When the binding affinity is low, CAR-T cells can discern between cells with overexpression or normal expression of the target antigen [19–21]. This is

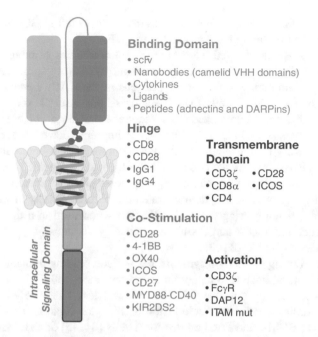

Fig. 2 CAR domain components. Chimeric antigen receptor (CAR) proteins consist of an extracellular antigen-binding domain, a hinge, a transmembrane domain, a co-stimulatory domain, and an activation domain. The extracellular portion of the CAR is most often composed of a single-chain variable fragment (scFv) molecule, though camelid nanobodies and humanized natural ligands or cytokines have been used. The intracellular regions, which function in activation upon antigen binding, typically harbor a T cell activation domain derived from the CD3ζ chain of the T cell receptor. Co-stimulatory domains often include CD28 or 4-1BB and can influence CAR-T cell memory, phenotype, and metabolism. Other co-stimulatory domains have been tested including OX40, CD27, and inducible T cell co-stimulator (ICOS). The activation domain, composed of CD3ζ, DAP12, or other sequences, contains immunoreceptor tyrosine-based activation motif (ITAM) regions that can be mutated to attenuate downstream activity

advantageous if the target is found on both normal and tumor cells. On the other hand, an scFv with high binding activity can lead to overactivation of the T cell, resulting in activation-induced cell death (AICD) [22, 23] or toxicity [24, 25]. The organization of the V_L and V_H within the CAR construct can also affect the binding activity of the scFv, with the V_L-linker-V_H orientation (versus V_H-linker-V_L) typically having greater binding activity [26].

The linker is traditionally composed of repeated glycine and serine residues, allowing for flexibility and solubility respectively. The length of the linker affects the binding activity of the scFv, since it determines the distance between the V_L and V_H. Depending on the composition, some scFvs have the tendency to dimerize or multimerize without interacting with their target antigen, leading to activation-independent or "tonic" signaling of the CAR. This can result in CAR-T cell exhaustion or activation-induced cell death (AICD) [27, 28]. The length of the linker can also affect this clustering, as longer linkers tend to decrease dimerization [26, 29].

Linkers with different compositions, such as the Whitlow linker [30], have also been used to enhance the stability and affinity of the scFv.

The scFv is usually derived from monoclonal antibodies of mouse origin, and thus can be recognized as foreign by the immune system. In some cases, patients have developed immunity to the mouse portions of the CAR, thereby limiting the persistence of the CAR-T cells [31]. To address this issue, several CARs were developed with a fully humanized scFv sequence that does not trigger rejection [32–38]. However, some instances of anti-CAR immunity have been reported even with a human scFv [39]. Camelid antibodies, composed of a single domain heavy chain (V_{HH}, also known as nanobodies), have low immunogenic potential due to high sequence homology with human V_H fragments and may circumvent immune rejection [40]. CARs using V_{HH} demonstrate high binding affinity to various tumor antigens and efficiently trigger T cell activation when used in a third generation CAR construct with CD28 and OX40 costimulatory domains [41, 42] or a second generation CAR with CD28 [43].

Rather than using antibody fragments, the antigen binding domain can be engineered from natural ligands to receptors found on cancer cells. Natural ligands are attractive because they are also fully human and less likely to elicit rejection. Previously studied candidates include tumor receptor ligands, such as APRIL, which binds to BCMA and TACI on myeloma cells [44, 45] or T1E, which binds to ErbB receptors on various tumors [46]. These CARs are referred to as "promiscuous" because they can bind multiple antigens with a single receptor. Immobilized cytokines (called zetakines) may also serve as the binding domain in the CAR construct and have been shown to bind natural receptors expressed on tumor cells [47].

Hinge and Transmembrane Domain

The extracellular antigen-binding domain is connected to the transmembrane domain through a hinge, also known as a spacer (Fig. 2). Most CAR designs use immunoglobulin (Ig)-like hinges, either derived from IgG or from native T-cell molecules. IgG-derived hinges can be targeted by myeloid cells or other lymphoid cells with Fc gamma receptors (FcγR) against the CH2 IgG domain. This interaction can lead to AICD of the CAR-T cell and decreased engraftment in animal models [48–50]. However, mutating or removing the CH2 prevents interaction with FcγR and restores CAR-T cell function in vivo [48, 51, 52]. On the other hand, T cell derived hinges are commonly composed of domains from CD28 or CD8 [53, 54].

Hinge length and flexibility play important roles in CAR activation, since a specific distance between the interacting cells is required for an immune synapse to form. The length of the hinge influences flexibility. For example, longer hinges provide more flexibility to target epitopes of the target antigen that are closer to the cell membrane [55, 56] or with complex glycosylation [57]. Alternatively, short hinges are best for tumor antigen epitopes near the amino terminal of the target protein, which are easily accessible [22, 55].

The transmembrane portion anchors the CAR to the cell membrane through a hydrophobic α helix, usually derived from CD3ζ, CD28, CD4, or CD8α. Though it is the least studied of all the CAR components, the transmembrane domain has a significant role in the stability and function of the CAR-T cell [58, 59]. CD28 provides more stability, whereas a CD3ζ transmembrane domain can associate the CAR with other molecules of the native TCR/CD3 complex [58, 60].

Costimulatory Domains

CARs are designed with one or multiple costimulatory domains intracellular to the transmembrane domain (Fig. 2). Costimulatory domains were added to second-generation CARs, since signaling from the CD3z domain alone was insufficient to activate resting T cells [61]. As discussed previously, the primary costimulatory domains used in CARs are 4-1BB and CD28. Both are used in FDA-approved CAR-T cells and we now recognize that the activity and function of these products vary depending on which costimulatory domain is used [62, 63]. For example, CAR-T cells with a 4-1BB costimulatory domain tend to expand more slowly and persist longer compared to those with a CD28 costimulatory domain, which expand rapidly but are more prone to T cell exhaustion [10, 64]. In patients, CD28 CAR-T cells are usually undetectable within 3 months [7, 65], while 4-1BB CAR-T cells are detectable for several years [66]. This discrepancy is thought to be due to the constitutive association of the tyrosine kinase LCK with the CD28 costimulatory domain, resulting in a high magnitude of protein phosphorylation upon activation. In contrast, 4-1BB CAR-T cells show a lesser degree of phosphorylation, which may result in decreased sensitivity to triggering in the setting of low antigen density [67]. The costimulatory domains also influence the CAR-T cell memory phenotype and metabolism. CAR-T cells bearing a 4-1BB domain have a more central memory phenotype and exhibit fatty acid metabolism while those with a CD28 domain have an effector-like memory phenotype and primarily undergo glycolytic metabolism [67–71].

Most studies directly comparing costimulatory domains have been conducted in mice, though two small studies investigated products with different domains in the same patient. In the first of these clinical studies, patients with B cell malignancies were simultaneously injected with first and second generation CD19-targeted CAR-T cells. Serum FACS analyses revealed improved expansion and enhanced persistence among second-generation CAR-T cells, suggesting more favorable pharmacokinetics [72]. The same group similarly compared second and third-generation CARs (with both CD28 and 4-1BB) in patients and showed further improved expansion and persistence with the addition of the 4-1BB domain [73].

Alternative costimulatory domains have been tested in CAR-T cells in preclinical models but have not yet been tested in clinical trials. These include OX40 [16, 74, 75], CD27 [17], ICOS [18], MYD88 and CD40 [76], and killer cell immunoglobulin-like receptor SDS2 (KIR2DS2) combined with an immunotyrosine-based activation motif-containing adapter (DAP12) [77]. CD27 has been shown to enhance CAR-T cell survival compared to CD28 [17]. ICOS drives a Th1/Th17 phenotype in CD4+ T cells and increases in vivo T cell persistence compared to CD28 or 4-1BB [18]. When ICOS is used in combination with 4-1BB in a third generation CAR, T cells exhibit greater antitumor effects and increased persistence in vivo compared to second generation CAR-T cells [59].

Activation Domains

The activation domain, the most distal intracellular portion of the CAR, is most commonly composed of the CD3ζ sequence (Fig. 2). It contains three immunoreceptor tyrosine-based activation motifs (ITAMs) that are phosphorylated when the CAR is activated by the target antigen. ZAP70 is subsequently recruited to initiate a signaling cascade similar to that of the endogenous T cell receptor [78]. Mutating the ITAM motifs in CD3ζ can optimize activation, prevent exhaustion, and create a central memory phenotype without sacrificing effector functions in a preclinical model [79]. These ITAM-mutant 1XX CAR-T cells are the subject of several ongoing clinical investigations in patients (NCT04464200; NCT04577325). In a different strategy, a second generation CAR using DAP12 in combination with 4-1BB demonstrated comparable tumor killing but decreased cytokine-mediated systemic toxicity, relative to 4-1BB-CD3ζ CARs, in a xenograft mouse model [80].

Next-Gen Modifications

Next-generation CAR-T cells are engineered with creative designs to combat factors that limit efficacy in patients. Three common mechanisms of treatment failure include antigen escape, CAR-T cell-associated toxicities, and limited persistence in vivo, which can be in part due to suppression in the tumor microenvironment (TME.) Next-gen CAR-T cell modifications can enhance tumor cell killing, mitigate toxicities, and overcome suppression.

Multi-Targeted CARs

As more patients have been treated with CAR-T cells, a common mechanism of relapse is antigen escape—where the tumor downregulates or mutates the target antigen, resulting in outgrowth of antigen-negative tumor cells [81, 82]. In fact, up to 25% of ALL patients treated with CD19-targeted CAR-T cells relapse with CD19-negative disease [64, 83]. To overcome this limitation, CARs targeting more than one tumor antigen have been developed to increase tumor cell elimination and decrease the potential for antigen negative tumor outgrowth. In addition to promiscuous CARs discussed previously, multi-targeted CAR-T cells use two or more antigen binding domains to target multiple antigens simultaneously. This can be achieved through the transduction of multiple CAR constructs into the same T cell, either via the same [84] or separate construct(s) [85], or coadministration of separately transduced CAR-T cells [86–88] (Fig. 3a). Alternatively, two scFvs specific to different target antigens can be expressed in tandem and attached to a single intracellular signaling domain [89–91] (Fig. 3a). Each of these combinations has required optimization of the CAR design, including the use of different configurations of the linker and antigen binding variable regions [92, 93].

CAR-T cells can also target multiple tumor antigens by secretion of a bispecific T cell engagers (Fig. 3b). T cell engagers are composed of two scFvs in tandem: one specific to a tumor antigen and the other to the CD3 domain of the TCR. Upon binding the tumor antigen, T cell engagers can recruit endogenous T cells in the tumor microenvironment to kill tumor cells. T cell engagers have known efficacy when delivered as monotherapy, though significant cytokine-mediated toxicity can occur [94]. Local secretion by CAR-T cells enables antigen targeting without systemic dissemination of the antibody or downstream immune-related adverse effects (irAEs) due to target antigen expression in normal tissue [95].

Self- or Triggered-Assembly of CARs

Several methods of indirect antigen binding have been devised to allow for a single CAR-To target different antigens. These "universal" CARs allow the same CAR design to be used across different tumor types. This can be achieved through the use of a bridging molecule that binds to a tumor-associated antigen and provides a complimentary binding domain for the CAR. For example, an scFv can be linked to a leucine zipper that binds to a cognate leucine zipper CAR (also known as a SUPRA CAR) [96]. When the leucine zippers interact, the CAR self-assembles, and the T cell is activated. A variation of this strategy is to use a tagged tumor antigen antibody with an anti-tag CAR, such as a biotinylated antibody and a CAR with an avidin binding domain [97, 98] or a fluorescein (FITC)-tagged antibody and a FITC-binding CAR [99]. Similarly, CARs can be engineered with a CD16 binding domain that recognizes the Fc constant region of tumor-specific antibodies when bound to their target antigen [100]. These methods are highly dependent on T cell persistence and the half-life of the adaptor.

Adaptor systems can also improve the safety of CAR-T cells by enabling dynamic control of cell activation. Among the safety issues posed by CD19-directed CAR-T cells is overactivation of the T cells leading to cytokine release syndrome (CRS) or immune cell-associated neurotoxicity syndrome (ICANS). The ability to rapidly turn off CAR-T cells when toxicity becomes apparent can circumvent these potentially fatal irAEs in patients. Low molecular weight adapters can be designed

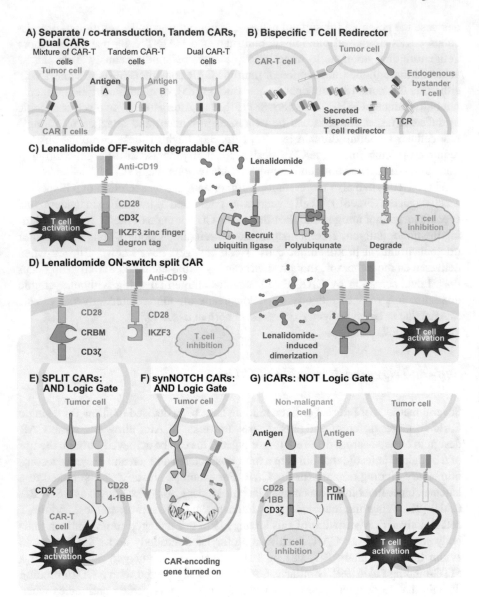

Fig. 3 Next generation CAR-T cell modifications. Chimeric antigen receptor (CAR)-T cells can be designed to evade tumor antigen escape and mitigate off tumor effects. (**a**) Antigen escape can be evaded by infusing a mixture of CAR-T cell products targeting different antigens or multi-targeted CAR-T cells designed to target multiple tumor antigens either via the same or different CAR constructs or (**b**) CAR-T cells engineered to secrete bi-specific T cell engagers which recruit endogenous T cells to engage in tumor killing. (**c**) To improve safety, one approach is to turn "OFF" the CAR by attaching a zinc finger degron motif to the C-terminus, which binds lenalidomide. When lenalidomide is added, a ubiquitin ligase is recruited, which targets the CAR for degradation and inactivates the CAR-T cell. (**d**) Triggered assembly CARs improve safety by enabling dynamic control of CAR-T cell activation via exogenously administered agents. In one

to bridge FITC to a molecule that will bind a receptor on the tumor cell, such as folate and the folate receptor. When coadministered with FITC-binding CAR-T cells, this adaptor molecule induced tumor killing in a mouse model [101]. Importantly, cessation of adaptor infusion or administration of a competing ligand halted cytokine-mediated toxicity [101]. A similar system uses a tumor-specific antibody fragment (Fab) containing a neo-epitope peptide that will bind to a CAR with an scFv specific to the neoantigen (termed a switch CAR) [102]. When this strategy was implemented using a Fab against CD19 in a xenograft model of B cell leukemia, it enabled dose-adjusted tuning of activity with comparable efficacy and lower systemic cytokine levels relative to standard CD19-targeted CAR-T cells [102].

CAR-T cell activation can also be controlled through the addition of small molecules that trigger CAR assembly. One version of an "ON-switch" CAR uses a split CAR with an antigen-binding domain that assembles with the intracellular signaling domain only in the presence of a heterodimerizing small molecule. This CAR, nicknamed a remote-control CAR [103], provides a tunable system to control the CAR-T cell activation. Another "ON-switch" CAR, termed a SWIFF-CAR, uses a CAR construct linked by a protease site to a protease that is connected to a degron. In the absence of a protease inhibitor, the protease will cleave the site, disconnecting the CAR and allowing its expression on the cell membrane. Conversely, in the presence of a protease inhibitor, this activity is blocked and the CAR construct is targeted for proteolytic degradation by the degron [104]. Another degron-based system directly targets the CAR for degradation by including a C-terminal zinc finger degron motif that recruits a ubiquitin ligase in the presence of lenalidomide, thus targeting it for degradation (Fig. 3c) [105]. Lenalidomide, which is FDA-approved for treating multiple myeloma and non-Hodgkin lymphoma, can be used in a similar system to activate CAR expression on the T cell surface. A split CAR can be engineered with one subunit containing the extracellular antigen-binding and CD28 intracellular domains connected to the zinc finger degron and the other subunit made up of CD28 and CD3ζ domains flanking a CRBN lenalidomide binding motif (normally found as part of the E3 ubiquitin ligase complex.) In this system, addition of lenalidomide induces dimerization of the CAR and activation in the presence of target antigen (Fig. 3d) [105].

Fig. 3 (continued) example, lenalidomide-binding (CRBN) and zinc finger degron (IKZF3) domains can be engineered into SPLIT CARs to enable dimerization and thus activation only in the presence of lenalidomide. (**e**) Logic-gated CAR-T cells can mitigate on-target off-tumor effects by introducing another layer of specificity. Multi-targeted SPLIT CARs activate only when two tumor antigens are bound by separate scFvs. (**f**) Conditional expression of a CAR against one antigen is activated by binding of a separate synthetic Notch (synNotch) receptor against a different tumor antigen. (**g**) CAR-T cells can inactivate upon binding to an antigen on non-malignant cells. Thus, activation depends on binding to one tumor antigen but not the other in a "NOT" logic gate approach. (iCAR, inhibitory chimeric antigen receptor; ITIM, immunoreceptor tyrosine- based inhibitory motif; PD-1, programmed cell death 1)

Logic-Gated and Drug-Controlled CARs

When targeting multiple antigens, CAR-T cells can be designed to activate via binding of either one antigen, both antigens, or one antigen but not the other. According to Boolean logic, the former can be referred to as "OR" gate CARs. While "OR" gate CARs address the challenge of variable antigen expression and tumor heterogeneity, the risk of on-target off-tumor effects remains a concern due to their ability to bind two antigens that may be expressed on normal tissue. To mitigate this toxicity, multi-target CAR-T cells have been engineered to activate only when both antigens are recognized, referred to as "AND" gate CARs [106]. Dual activation can be achieved by using a split-CAR construct in which the scFv targeting one antigen is linked to the CD3ζ domain and the scFv targeting the other antigen is linked to CD28 and 4-1BB. Only when both scFvs are bound to their target antigens will the CARs cluster together and transduce an activation signal (Fig. 3e) [106–108].

Another strategy for regulation of CAR-T cells is the synNotch system, which utilizes a synthetic notch receptor (synNotch) with a tumor-specific extracellular antigen binding domain linked to an intracellular transcription factor (Fig. 3f). Upon binding to its target antigen, the receptor is cleaved, and the transcription factor is triggered to move into the nucleus to induce transcription of a separate construct, encoding a CAR against a different tumor antigen [109]. Implementation of this complex "AND" gate exhibited safe anti-tumor efficacy in a solid tumor model [110] but had significant on-target off-tumor effects in a hematologic tumor model, felt to be due to co-localization of dual and single antigen expressing cells [111]. Recently, synNotch receptors have been used to create a three-antigen "AND" gate that is composed of three sequentially linked CARs. This system is capable of selectively eliminating tumor cells expressing all three tumor antigens, while ignoring tumors expressing only two of the target antigens in a bilateral tumor mouse model [112].

Inhibitory CARs use a "NOT" gate approach, through which CAR-T cell activation depends on the presence of one antigen and the absence of another (Fig. 3g). In this system, a canonical CAR construct targeting a tumor-associated antigen is paired with a separate CAR tethered to an inhibitory intracellular domain, usually from CTLA-4 or PD-1. CAR-T cell binding to the latter target antigen transduces downstream dephosphorylation (and therefore inactivation) of the intracellular domain of the first CAR [113]. This results in CAR-T cell inactivation upon binding to antigen on non-malignant cells.

CAR-T cell activation can also be dynamically regulated using drug-controlled systems to rapidly turn off downstream activity. It was recently discovered that dasatinib, which is FDA-approved for the treatment of chronic myeloid leukemia and ALL, inhibits LCK binding to CD3ζ and therefore inhibits CAR intracellular signaling [114]. Although the use of dasatinib for treatment of CRS in patients has not been reported, in mouse models of lymphoma, dasatinib reduced mortality from CRS by reversibly limiting CAR-T cell activation [114]. CAR-T cells can also be engineered to express non-signaling receptors, such as the extracellular and transmembrane domains of EGFR or CD20, which can be targeted with monoclonal antibodies cetuximab and rituximab respectively [115–118]. Administration of the corresponding drug results in antibody-mediated CAR-T cell destruction. The clinical utility of this approach is limited by its slow kinetics, which is unable to rapidly reverse CRS symptoms.

More rapid off switches have been designed, including the suicide switch inducible caspase 9 system (iCasp9), which uses the pro-apoptotic caspase 9 protein fused to a modified form of the FK506 binding protein FKBP1A. Administration of a biologically inert small molecule (AP1903) triggers dimerization of Caspase 9, resulting in CAR-T cell apoptosis. Use of this switch in genetically modified donor lymphocytes enabled reversal of acute graft versus host disease (GVHD) in leukemia patients after allogeneic hematopoietic stem cell transplants [119] and was shown to eliminate T cells within 30 minutes.

Armored CARs

CAR-T cell efficacy can also be significantly limited by the hostile tumor microenvironment (TME), comprised of anti-inflammatory cytokines and immune cells that directly suppress T cell function. Armored CAR-T cells (alternatively referred to as fourth generation CAR-T cells, Fig. 4) are designed to dampen the suppression signal, transform it into an activation signal, or recruit bystander immune effectors to promote tumor cell targeting. For example, armored CAR-T cells expressing dominant negative (dn) cytokine receptors, such as dnTGFβRII [120], can effectively deplete locally secreted cytokines, such as TGFβ. Alternatively, CARs engineered with a switch receptor, such as the TGFRβR linked to a second-generation CAR intracellular signaling domain, converts an inhibitory stimulus to an activating signal [121]. Switch receptors can also transduce homeostatic signals by expressing a CAR with the IL-4 receptor ectodomain linked to an IL-7, IL-2, or IL-15 receptor intracellular signaling domain [122–124].

T cell function can be suppressed by direct binding to inhibitory ligands, such as PD-L1, expressed on tumor cells and tumor-associated myeloid cells [125]. Binding of PD-L1 to its receptor (PD-1) on T cells promotes T cell exhaustion diminishes CAR-T cell persistence [125]. Several armored CARs have been designed to combat this pathway, including expressing a dnPD-1 receptor [126], using a PD-1 switch receptor with a CD28 intracellular signaling domain [127], engineering the CAR to secrete an anti-PD-1 antibody [128] or a blocking scFv [129, 130], and silencing PD-1 expression using short hairpin RNAs [126] or CRISPR-Cas9 [131, 132] (Fig. 4a). CAR-T cells that secrete anti-PD-1 antibodies or scFvs exhibit autocrine and paracrine effects, thereby bolstering the endogenous and CAR-T cell-mediated anti-tumor response.

More recently, CAR-T cells have been engineered to express co-stimulatory ligands, such as the proinflammatory marker CD40 ligand (CD40L) and 4-1BB ligand (4-1BBL) to foster a more supportive TME (Fig. 4b). CD40L is expressed on

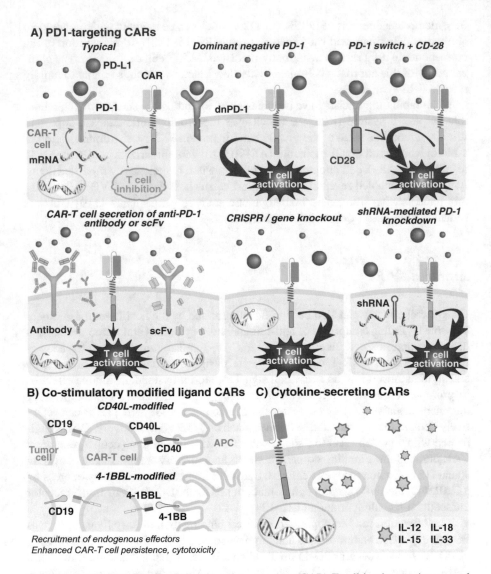

Fig. 4 Armored CAR-T cells. Chimeric antigen receptor (CAR)-T cell in vivo persistence and anti-tumor efficacy can be inhibited by anti-inflammatory cells and cytokines in the tumor microenvironment (TME). Armored CAR-T cells are designed to combat these barriers by attenuating suppressive signals or by promoting endogenous immune effectors and inflammatory cytokines. For example, (**a**) CAR-T cells can circumvent inhibitory immune checkpoint signaling via targeting of the programmed cell death 1 (PD-1) pathway. This can be accomplished via knockdown of PD-1, engineered dominant-negative PD-1 or PD-1 switch receptors, or direct secretion of anti-PD-1 antibodies. (**b**) CAR-T cells can be engineered to express peptides that recruit endogenous effector T cells and foster a supportive microenvironment such as CD40 ligand (CD40L) or 4-1BB ligand (4-1BBL). (**c**) Finally, CAR-T cells may promote an inflammatory milieu by direct expression and secretion of cytokines. (APC, antigen-presenting cell; CSR, chimeric switch receptor; DNR, dominant negative receptor; scFv, single-chain variable fragment; shRNA, short hairpin RNA

activated T cells and binds to CD40 receptor on antigen presenting cells (APCs). Interaction of CD40L with its cognate receptor results in APC activation and downstream secretion of proinflammatory cytokines. CAR-T cells expressing either membrane bound or soluble CD40L activate APCs in the TME and promote endogenous (non-CAR)-T cells to recognize and eliminate tumor cells [133, 134]. CAR-T cells co-expressing membrane-bound 4-1BBL exhibited enhanced persistence and decreased expression of exhaustion markers in a murine lymphoma model [135]. These were later used in a phase I clinical trial in patients with relapsed or refractory B cell NHL, and demonstrated a complete response rate of 59% with durable remission achieved in 29% of patients [65, 136].

CAR-T cells can be programmed to secrete their own cytokines, which promotes proliferation, survival, and antitumor activity of T cells while also altering the immune milieu of the TME [137]. (Fig. 4c). Cytokines such as IL-12, IL-15, and IL-18, can promote T cell persistence and expansion. IL-12 secreting CAR-T cells exhibit enhanced expansion and persistence, have greater cytotoxicity, and are more resistant to apoptosis and suppression by PD-1 [138]. A clinical trial of these armored CAR-T cells is currently underway in patients with ovarian cancer (NCT02498912) [139]. IL-15 similarly promotes expansion, antitumor activity, and persistence of CAR-T cells when secreted [140–142], or tethered to the cell membrane [143], but has demonstrated little effect on the surrounding TME. IL-18 also enhances functionality of CAR-T cells in humanized mouse models, while altering the TME by increasing the abundance of proinflammatory macrophages, depleting anti-inflammatory macrophages and T regulatory cells, and recruiting endogenous T cells [13, 144, 145]. Cytokine-secreting CAR-T cells can, however, promote CRS in animal models despite the fact that secretion predominantly occurs locally. So far, pre-clinical models have confirmed this strategy to be safe with minimal systemic toxicity at lower doses.

CAR Targets

The ideal CAR-T cell target antigen is expressed exclusively on cancer cells, with minimal or absent expression on normal cells to mitigate unwanted on-target off-tumor toxicities. Four of the five FDA-approved CAR-T cells target CD19, a membrane-bound protein expressed on both normal and malignant B cells. Patients treated with these therapies develop B cell aplasia and hypogammaglobulinaemia, though this adverse effect is tolerable with periodic intravenous immunoglobulin replacement. CARs have been designed to target many different tumor antigens, including additional targets in hematologic malignancies and novel targets in solid tumors. At the time of this publication, there are over 500 active clinical trials investigating CAR-T cell therapies for cancer registered with the United States National Library of Medicine.

Hematologic Malignancies

CAR-T cell design to date has primarily focused on hematologic malignancies. In addition to the five FDA approved CAR-T cells, there have been a number of trials focused on improving the function and expanding the use of CAR-T cells targeting CD19. Additional clinical trials for CD19-targeted CAR-T cells are underway in patients with multiple myeloma [146, 147] and mantle cell and follicular lymphoma [148]. Additional B cell malignancy targets are being explored to overcome CD19 antigen escape that occurs after CAR-T cells are administered. CAR-T cells targeting both CD19 and CD20 or CD22 are being investigated as individually transduced CAR-T cells that are co-administered or in tandem CAR designs [86, 92, 149–151]. Another tandem CAR showing promising results in preclinical models targets CD79b in addition to CD19 [152].

CAR-T cells targeting B-cell maturation antigen (BCMA) hold great promise in the treatment of multiple myeloma. BCMA expression is restricted to terminally differentiated B cells and plasma cells but is also found on multiple myeloma cells [153]. Two CAR-T cells targeting BCMA, bb2121 (ide-cel) [154, 155] and JNJ-4528 [156, 157], were granted breakthrough therapy designations by the FDA and ide-cel was approved for treatment of relapsed or refractory multiple myeloma in 2021 [15]. Despite this success, evidence of antigen escape has been observed with BCMA-negative relapses [158, 159], and immune rejection of the mouse scFV of BCMA-targeted CAR-T cells has also been a therapeutic obstacle [160]. To overcome these limitations, CAR-T cells targeting dual antigens or using alternative antigen binding domains have been developed for multiple myeloma. In addition to BCMA, transmembrane activator and CAML interactor (TACI) can be targeted by CARs using a natural ligand that binds both BCMA and TACI, which has demonstrated anti-tumor activity in preclinical models [44, 45]. BCMA-targeting CAR-T cells with camelid V_{HH} or fully human antigen binding domains have also been developed [156, 160–162]. Additional targets being explored for multiple myeloma include CD38, CD138, CS1 (*SLAMF7*), immunoglobulin kappa light chain, CD44v6, CD56, Lewis Y, CD229, and others [162, 163]. Many of these are also being explored for the treatment of other B cell malignancies [164]; however, most have overlapping expression on normal tissues, which may limit their therapeutic potential. Another target, G protein-coupled receptor, class C group 5 member D (GPRC5D), is expressed both on hair follicles and myeloma cells but has been safely targeted by CAR-T cells, eradicating multiple myeloma in a BCMA antigen escape model without significant off-tumor effects [165].

Individual targets are also being explored in T cell malignancies and acute myeloid leukemia (AML). CAR-T cells targeting CD37, an antigen expressed by B and T cell malignancies, have shown efficacy in xenograft mouse models [166], and a phase I trial of CAR37 cells is ongoing (NCT04136275). Other targets for T cell malignancies include CD5 [167] and CD7 [168]. CAR-T cell development for AML has been difficult due to the lack of surface target antigens unique to tumor cells [169]. The most common targets used in clinical trials for AML are CD33, also expressed on hematopoietic stem and progenitor cells (HSPCs) and in the lung, skin, and prostate [169], and CD123, with lower HSPC expression. CD33-targeting antibody-drug conjugates caused significant toxicities when administered in patients [170], whereas a CD33-targeted CAR-T cell reduced marrow blasts in one patient for 9 weeks with only minor toxicities [171]. More recently, a unique approach of knocking out CD33 in HSPCs and performing a bone marrow transplant along with the CD33-CAR was successful in a preclinical model [172]. A similar approach has been taken with CD5 and CD7, to prevent fratricide of T cells when targeting a T cell antigen [173, 174]. The first few patients treated with CD123 CAR-T cells experienced severe toxicities, but there are still ongoing clinical trials (NCT03672851, NCT04265963, NCT04014881).

Solid Tumors

Identifying CAR-T cell targets for solid tumors is challenging, in part due to tumor antigen heterogeneity and simultaneous expression on normal tissues. Many targets are being explored for numerous types of solid tumors [175]. We will discuss a subset of antigens shared across different tumor types that have been or are currently being tested in clinical trials.

One very promising target, EGFRvIII, is uniquely expressed on tumor cells as a mutated form of the epidermal growth factor receptor (EGFR) lacking the ligand binding domain. It is a neoantigen expressed on several tumor types including glioblastoma, medulloblastoma, non-small cell lung carcinoma, and breast, colon, ovarian, head and neck, and metastatic prostate cancer [176]. EGFRvIII-targeted CAR-T cells have unfortunately not shown promising response rates in phase I trials in glioblastoma patients [177, 178]. Post-treatment tumor biopsies in these patients demonstrated infiltration of suppressive regulatory CD4+ T cells and a decrease in EGFRvIII protein expression, suggesting TME-mediated immunosuppression and antigen escape as mechanisms of treatment failure [177]. Given that EGFR is overexpressed in glioblastoma and other cancers, CAR-T cell targeting EGFRvIII were designed to secrete a T cell engager specific to EGFR and showed promising results with no off-tumor toxicity after injection locally in a xenograft mouse model [95].

Another member of the EGFR family, HER2, has also been explored as a CAR-T cell target. While HER2 is overexpressed in multiple tumor types, including glioblastoma, breast cancer, and GI malignancies, it is also widely expressed on normal tissues [179]. A clinical trial of CAR-T cells targeting HER2 in glioblastoma patients demonstrated safety, without dose-limiting toxicity, in a trial of 17 patients [180], but limited anti-tumor effect was observed. Another studied target in glioblastoma is IL-13Rα2, which is overexpressed in tumors but also found in normal tissues [181]. CAR-T cells targeting IL-13Rα2 were engineered with an IL-13 zetakine as the antigen binding domain and showed impressive tumor killing in a patient after direct tumor injection and intrathecal infusion [182]. CARs targeting HER2 and IL-13Ra2 in tandem or in a tricistronic CAR-T cell also targeting ephrin-A2

(EphA2) have been developed to overcome tumor heterogeneity and antigen escape, showing promising results in preclinical models [84, 89]. HER2 and IL-13Ra2 are also being targeted by CAR-T cells in other types of tumors, including sarcoma, colorectal cancer, and melanoma.

Other promising targets for CAR-T cells in solid tumors are mesothelin, B7-H3, and MUC1. Mesothelin, a cell-surface antigen highly expressed in lung, pancreatic, ovarian, and other cancers, has been used as a target in multiple CAR-T cell pre-clinical studies and showed promising efficacy [183]. Several clinical trials of mesothelin-targeting CAR-T cells are ongoing [184, 185]. B7-H3 is an immune checkpoint molecule with low surface expression that has been studied as a CAR-T cell target. To minimize on-target off-tumor toxicity, B7-H3 CARs were designed with an scFv recognizing only high concentration of target antigen, a strategy that showed safe anti-tumor activity in pre-clinical models of pediatric brain tumors and sarcomas [186, 187]. MUC1, a glycoprotein expressed in many normal tissue types, is also expressed as a unique isoform in certain cancers and represents a potential neoantigen target. CAR-T cells targeting Tn-MUC1 have demonstrated anti-tumor efficacy in xenograft mouse models [188] and there are several clinical trials underway for CAR-T cells targeting MUC1 in esophageal, breast, and non-small cell lung cancer (NCT03706326, NCT03525782, NCT04020575).

Though CAR-T cells are designed to target antigens on the surface of cancer cells and initiate a T cell response in a non-MHC restricted manner, there are many intracellular antigens that are unique to tumor cells but are out of reach for CAR-T cells. One way to overcome this is to design a CAR with an antigen binding domain based on an antibody that binds to a specific peptide epitope of a tumor antigen presented on an MHC. For example, NY-ESO-1 is a cancer testis antigen that is expressed in the cytoplasm of a wide range of tumors but is not expressed in normal somatic cells [189]. CAR-T cells specific to an NY-ESO-1 peptide in the context of HLA-A*0201 have shown efficacy in mouse models of melanoma [190] and multiple myeloma [191]. This approach has the potential to vastly expand the range of target antigens for CAR-T cells by making them accessible to more neoantigens and opening new avenues for cancer immunotherapy.

References

1. Hwu P, Shafer GE, Treisman J, et al. Lysis of ovarian cancer cells by human lymphocytes redirected with a chimeric gene composed of an antibody variable region and the fc receptor gamma chain. J Exp Med. 1993;178:361–6.
2. Hwu P, Yang JC, Cowherd R, et al. In vivo antitumor activity of T cells redirected with chimeric antibody/T-cell receptor genes. Cancer Res. 1995;55:3369–73.
3. Stancovski I, Schindler DG, Waks T, Yarden Y, Sela M, Eshhar Z. Targeting of T lymphocytes to Neu/HER2-expressing cells using chimeric single chain Fv receptors. J Immunol. 1993;151:6577–82.
4. Kershaw MH, Westwood JA, Parker LL, et al. A phase I study on adoptive immunotherapy using gene-modified T cells for ovarian cancer. Clin Cancer Res. 2006;12:6106–15.

5. Krause A, Guo HF, Latouche JB, Tan C, Cheung NK, Sadelain M. Antigen-dependent CD28 signaling selectively enhances survival and proliferation in genetically modified activated human primary T lymphocytes. J Exp Med. 1998;188:619–26.
6. Vandenberghe P, Freeman GJ, Nadler LM, et al. Antibody and B7/BB1-mediated ligation of the CD28 receptor induces tyrosine phosphorylation in human T cells. J Exp Med. 1992;175:951–60.
7. Brentjens RJ, Riviere I, Park JH, et al. Safety and persistence of adoptively transferred autologous CD19-targeted T cells in patients with relapsed or chemotherapy refractory B-cell leukemias. Blood. 2011;118:4817–28.
8. Kalos M, Levine BL, Porter DL, et al. T cells with chimeric antigen receptors have potent antitumor effects and can establish memory in patients with advanced leukemia. Sci Transl Med. 2011;3:95ra73.
9. Porter DL, Levine BL, Kalos M, Bagg A, June CH. Chimeric antigen receptor-modified T cells in chronic lymphoid leukemia. N Engl J Med. 2011;365:725–33.
10. Neelapu SS, Locke FL, Bartlett NL, et al. Axicabtagene Ciloleucel CAR T-cell therapy in refractory large B-cell lymphoma. N Engl J Med. 2017;377:2531–44.
11. Maude SL, Frey N, Shaw PA, et al. Chimeric antigen receptor T cells for sustained remissions in leukemia. N Engl J Med. 2014;371:1507–17.
12. Schuster SJ, Svoboda J, Chong EA, et al. Chimeric antigen receptor T cells in refractory B-cell lymphomas. N Engl J Med. 2017;377:2545–54.
13. Avanzi MP, Yeku O, Li X, et al. Engineered tumor-targeted T cells mediate enhanced antitumor efficacy both directly and through activation of the endogenous immune system. Cell Rep. 2018;23:2130–41.
14. Abramson JS, Palomba ML, Gordon LI, et al. Lisocabtagene maraleucel for patients with relapsed or refractory large B-cell lymphomas (TRANSCEND NHL 001): a multicentre seamless design study. Lancet. 2020;396:839–52.
15. Munshi NC, Anderson LD Jr, Shah N, et al. Idecabtagene Vicleucel in relapsed and refractory multiple myeloma. N Engl J Med. 2021;384:705–16.
16. Pule MA, Straathof KC, Dotti G, Heslop HE, Rooney CM, Brenner MK. A chimeric T cell antigen receptor that augments cytokine release and supports clonal expansion of primary human T cells. Mol Ther. 2005;12:933–41.
17. Song DG, Ye Q, Poussin M, Harms GM, Figini M, Powell DJ Jr. CD27 costimulation augments the survival and antitumor activity of redirected human T cells in vivo. Blood. 2012;119:696–706.
18. Guedan S, Chen X, Madar A, et al. ICOS-based chimeric antigen receptors program bipolar TH17/TH1 cells. Blood. 2014;124:1070–80.
19. Chmielewski M, Hombach A, Heuser C, Adams GP, Abken H. T cell activation by antibody-like immunoreceptors: increase in affinity of the single-chain fragment domain above threshold does not increase T cell activation against antigen-positive target cells but decreases selectivity. J Immunol. 2004;173:7647–53.
20. Liu X, Jiang S, Fang C, et al. Affinity-tuned ErbB2 or EGFR chimeric antigen receptor T cells exhibit an increased therapeutic index against Tumors in mice. Cancer Res. 2015;75:3596–607.
21. Caruso HG, Hurton LV, Najjar A, et al. Tuning sensitivity of CAR to EGFR density limits recognition of Normal tissue while maintaining potent antitumor activity. Cancer Res. 2015;75:3505–18.
22. Hudecek M, Lupo-Stanghellini MT, Kosasih PL, et al. Receptor affinity and extracellular domain modifications affect tumor recognition by ROR1-specific chimeric antigen receptor T cells. Clin Cancer Res. 2013;19:3153–64.
23. Watanabe K, Terakura S, Uchiyama S, et al. Excessively high-affinity single-chain fragment variable region in a chimeric antigen receptor can counteract T-cell proliferation. Blood. 2014;124:4799.

24. Ghorashian S, Kramer AM, Onuoha S, et al. Enhanced CAR T cell expansion and prolonged persistence in pediatric patients with ALL treated with a low-affinity CD19 CAR. Nat Med. 2019;25:1408–14.
25. Lynn RC, Feng Y, Schutsky K, et al. High-affinity FRbeta-specific CAR T cells eradicate AML and normal myeloid lineage without HSC toxicity. Leukemia. 2016;30:1355–64.
26. Desplancq D, King DJ, Lawson AD, Mountain A. Multimerization behaviour of single chain Fv variants for the tumour-binding antibody B72.3. Protein Eng. 1994;7:1027–33.
27. Long AH, Haso WM, Shern JF, et al. 4-1BB costimulation ameliorates T cell exhaustion induced by tonic signaling of chimeric antigen receptors. Nat Med. 2015;21:581–90.
28. Ajina A, Maher J. Strategies to address chimeric antigen receptor tonic Signaling. Mol Cancer Ther. 2018;17:1795–815.
29. Singh N, Frey NV, Engels B, et al. Single chain variable fragment linker length regulates CAR biology and T cell efficacy. Blood. 2019;134:247.
30. Whitlow M, Bell BA, Feng SL, et al. An improved linker for single-chain Fv with reduced aggregation and enhanced proteolytic stability. Protein Eng. 1993;6:989–95.
31. Turtle CJ, Hanafi LA, Berger C, et al. CD19 CAR-T cells of defined CD4+:CD8+ composition in adult B cell ALL patients. J Clin Invest. 2016;126:2123–38.
32. Brudno JN, Lam N, Vanasse D, et al. Safety and feasibility of anti-CD19 CAR T cells with fully human binding domains in patients with B-cell lymphoma. Nat Med. 2020;26:270–80.
33. Mirzaei HR, Jamali A, Jafarzadeh L, et al. Construction and functional characterization of a fully human anti-CD19 chimeric antigen receptor (huCAR)-expressing primary human T cells. J Cell Physiol. 2019;234:9207–15.
34. Sommermeyer D, Hill T, Shamah SM, et al. Fully human CD19-specific chimeric antigen receptors for T-cell therapy. Leukemia. 2017;31:2191–9.
35. Lanitis E, Poussin M, Hagemann IS, et al. Redirected antitumor activity of primary human lymphocytes transduced with a fully human anti-mesothelin chimeric receptor. Mol Ther. 2012;20:633–43.
36. Song DG, Ye Q, Poussin M, Liu L, Figini M, Powell DJ Jr. A fully human chimeric antigen receptor with potent activity against cancer cells but reduced risk for off-tumor toxicity. Oncotarget. 2015;6:21533–46.
37. Alabanza L, Pegues M, Geldres C, et al. Function of novel anti-CD19 chimeric antigen receptors with human variable regions is affected by hinge and transmembrane domains. Mol Ther. 2017;25:2452–65.
38. Smith EL, Staehr M, Masakayan R, et al. Development and evaluation of an optimal human single-chain variable fragment-derived BCMA-targeted CAR T cell vector. Mol Ther. 2018;26:1447–56.
39. Hege KM, Bergsland EK, Fisher GA, et al. Safety, tumor trafficking and immunogenicity of chimeric antigen receptor (CAR)-T cells specific for TAG-72 in colorectal cancer. J Immunother Cancer. 2017;5:22.
40. Harmsen MM, De Haard HJ. Properties, production, and applications of camelid single-domain antibody fragments. Appl Microbiol Biotechnol. 2007;77:13–22.
41. Jamnani FR, Rahbarizadeh F, Shokrgozar MA, et al. T cells expressing VHH-directed oligoclonal chimeric HER2 antigen receptors: towards tumor-directed oligoclonal T cell therapy. Biochim Biophys Acta. 1840;2014:378–86.
42. Sharifzadeh Z, Rahbarizadeh F, Shokrgozar MA, et al. Genetically engineered T cells bearing chimeric nanoconstructed receptors harboring TAG-72-specific camelid single domain antibodies as targeting agents. Cancer Lett. 2013;334:237–44.
43. Rajabzadeh A, Rahbarizadeh F, Ahmadvand D, Kabir Salmani M, Hamidieh AA. A VHH-based anti-MUC1 chimeric antigen receptor for specific retargeting of human primary T cells to MUC1-positive cancer cells. Cell J. 2021;22:502–13.
44. Lee L, Draper B, Chaplin N, et al. An APRIL-based chimeric antigen receptor for dual targeting of BCMA and TACI in multiple myeloma. Blood. 2018;131:746–58.
45. Schmidts A, Ormhoj M, Choi BD, et al. Rational design of a trimeric APRIL-based CAR-binding domain enables efficient targeting of multiple myeloma. Blood Adv. 2019;3:3248–60.

46. Davies DM, Foster J, Van Der Stegen SJ, et al. Flexible targeting of ErbB dimers that drive tumorigenesis by using genetically engineered T cells. Mol Med. 2012;18:565–76.
47. Brown CE, Aguilar B, Starr R, et al. Optimization of IL13Ralpha2-targeted chimeric antigen receptor T cells for improved anti-tumor efficacy against glioblastoma. Mol Ther. 2018;26:31–44.
48. Hudecek M, Sommermeyer D, Kosasih PL, et al. The nonsignaling extracellular spacer domain of chimeric antigen receptors is decisive for in vivo antitumor activity. Cancer Immunol Res. 2015;3:125–35.
49. Hombach A, Hombach AA, Abken H. Adoptive immunotherapy with genetically engineered T cells: modification of the IgG1 fc 'spacer' domain in the extracellular moiety of chimeric antigen receptors avoids 'off-target' activation and unintended initiation of an innate immune response. Gene Ther. 2010;17:1206–13.
50. Almasbak H, Walseng E, Kristian A, et al. Inclusion of an IgG1-fc spacer abrogates efficacy of CD19 CAR T cells in a xenograft mouse model. Gene Ther. 2015;22:391–403.
51. Jonnalagadda M, Mardiros A, Urak R, et al. Chimeric antigen receptors with mutated IgG4 fc spacer avoid fc receptor binding and improve T cell persistence and antitumor efficacy. Mol Ther. 2015;23:757–68.
52. Watanabe N, Bajgain P, Sukumaran S, et al. Fine-tuning the CAR spacer improves T-cell potency. Onco Targets Ther. 2016;5:e1253656.
53. Kochenderfer JN, Feldman SA, Zhao Y, et al. Construction and preclinical evaluation of an anti-CD19 chimeric antigen receptor. J Immunother. 2009;32:689–702.
54. Milone MC, Fish JD, Carpenito C, et al. Chimeric receptors containing CD137 signal transduction domains mediate enhanced survival of T cells and increased antileukemic efficacy in vivo. Mol Ther. 2009;17:1453–64.
55. Guest RD, Hawkins RE, Kirillova N, et al. The role of extracellular spacer regions in the optimal design of chimeric immune receptors: evaluation of four different scFvs and antigens. J Immunother. 2005;28:203–11.
56. James SE, Greenberg PD, Jensen MC, et al. Antigen sensitivity of CD22-specific chimeric TCR is modulated by target epitope distance from the cell membrane. J Immunol. 2008;180:7028–38.
57. Wilkie S, Picco G, Foster J, et al. Retargeting of human T cells to tumor-associated MUC1: the evolution of a chimeric antigen receptor. J Immunol. 2008;180:4901–9.
58. Bridgeman JS, Hawkins RE, Bagley S, Blaylock M, Holland M, Gilham DE. The optimal antigen response of chimeric antigen receptors harboring the CD3zeta transmembrane domain is dependent upon incorporation of the receptor into the endogenous TCR/CD3 complex. J Immunol. 2010;184:6938–49.
59. Guedan S, Posey AD Jr, Shaw C, et al. Enhancing CAR T cell persistence through ICOS and 4-1BB costimulation. JCI Insight. 2018;3
60. Dotti G, Gottschalk S, Savoldo B, Brenner MK. Design and development of therapies using chimeric antigen receptor-expressing T cells. Immunol Rev. 2014;257:107–26.
61. Brocker T, Karjalainen K. Signals through T cell receptor-zeta chain alone are insufficient to prime resting T lymphocytes. J Exp Med. 1995;181:1653–9.
62. Sadelain M, Riviere I, Riddell S. Therapeutic T cell engineering. Nature. 2017;545:423–31.
63. Guedan S, Calderon H, Posey AD Jr, Maus MV. Engineering and design of chimeric antigen receptors. Mol Ther Methods Clin Dev. 2019;12:145–56.
64. Maude SL, Laetsch TW, Buechner J, et al. Tisagenlecleucel in children and young adults with B-cell lymphoblastic Leukemia. N Engl J Med. 2018;378:439–48.
65. Park JH, Riviere I, Gonen M, et al. Long-term follow-up of CD19 CAR therapy in acute lymphoblastic Leukemia. N Engl J Med. 2018;378:449–59.
66. Fraietta JA, Lacey SF, Orlando EJ, et al. Determinants of response and resistance to CD19 chimeric antigen receptor (CAR) T cell therapy of chronic lymphocytic leukemia. Nat Med. 2018;24:563–71.
67. Salter AI, Ivey RG, Kennedy JJ, et al. Phosphoproteomic analysis of chimeric antigen receptor signaling reveals kinetic and quantitative differences that affect cell function. Sci Signal. 2018;11

68. Kawalekar OU, RS OC, Fraietta JA, et al. Distinct signaling of coreceptors regulates specific metabolism pathways and impacts memory development in CAR T cells. Immunity. 2016;44:712.
69. Porter DL, Hwang WT, Frey NV, et al. Chimeric antigen receptor T cells persist and induce sustained remissions in relapsed refractory chronic lymphocytic leukemia. Sci Transl Med. 2015;7:303ra139.
70. van der Stegen SJ, Hamieh M, Sadelain M. The pharmacology of second-generation chimeric antigen receptors. Nat Rev Drug Discov. 2015;14:499–509.
71. Boroughs AC, Larson RC, Marjanovic ND, et al. A distinct transcriptional program in human CAR T cells bearing the 4-1BB Signaling domain revealed by scRNA-Seq. Mol Ther. 2020;28:2577–92.
72. Savoldo B, Ramos CA, Liu E, et al. CD28 costimulation improves expansion and persistence of chimeric antigen receptor-modified T cells in lymphoma patients. J Clin Invest. 2011;121:1822–6.
73. Ramos CA, Rouce R, Robertson CS, et al. In vivo fate and activity of second- versus third-generation CD19-specific CAR-T cells in B cell non-Hodgkin's lymphomas. Mol Ther. 2018;26:2727–37.
74. Hombach AA, Chmielewski M, Rappl G, Abken H. Adoptive immunotherapy with redirected T cells produces CCR7- cells that are trapped in the periphery and benefit from combined CD28-OX40 costimulation. Hum Gene Ther. 2013;24:259–69.
75. Hombach AA, Heiders J, Foppe M, Chmielewski M, Abken H. OX40 costimulation by a chimeric antigen receptor abrogates CD28 and IL-2 induced IL-10 secretion by redirected CD4(+) T cells. Onco Targets Ther. 2012;1:458–66.
76. Mata M, Gerken C, Nguyen P, Krenciute G, Spencer DM, Gottschalk S. Inducible activation of MyD88 and CD40 in CAR T cells results in controllable and potent antitumor activity in preclinical solid tumor models. Cancer Discov. 2017;7:1306–19.
77. Wang E, Wang LC, Tsai CY, et al. Generation of potent T-cell immunotherapy for cancer using DAP12-based, multichain, chimeric Immunoreceptors. Cancer Immunol Res. 2015;3:815–26.
78. Ramello MC, Benzaid I, Kuenzi BM, et al. An immunoproteomic approach to characterize the CAR interactome and signalosome. Sci Signal. 2019;12
79. Feucht J, Sun J, Eyquem J, et al. Calibration of CAR activation potential directs alternative T cell fates and therapeutic potency. Nat Med. 2019;25:82–8.
80. Ng YY, Tay JCK, Li Z, Wang J, Zhu J, Wang S. T cells expressing NKG2D CAR with a DAP12 Signaling domain stimulate lower cytokine production while effective in tumor eradication. Mol Ther. 2021;29:75–85.
81. Majzner RG, Mackall CL. Tumor antigen escape from CAR T-cell therapy. Cancer Discov. 2018;8:1219–26.
82. Rafiq S, Brentjens RJ. Tumors evading CARs-the chase is on. Nat Med. 2018;24:1492–3.
83. Xu X, Sun Q, Liang X, et al. Mechanisms of relapse after CD19 CAR T-cell therapy for acute lymphoblastic Leukemia and its prevention and treatment strategies. Front Immunol. 2019;10:2664.
84. Bielamowicz K, Fousek K, Byrd TT, et al. Trivalent CAR T cells overcome interpatient antigenic variability in glioblastoma. Neuro-Oncology. 2018;20:506–18.
85. Ruella M, Barrett DM, Kenderian SS, et al. Dual CD19 and CD123 targeting prevents antigen-loss relapses after CD19-directed immunotherapies. J Clin Invest. 2016;126:3814–26.
86. Huang L, Wang N, Li C, et al. Sequential infusion of anti-CD22 and anti-CD19 chimeric antigen receptor T cells for adult patients with refractory/relapsed B-cell acute lymphoblastic leukemia. Blood. 2017;130:846.
87. Yan Z, Cao J, Cheng H, et al. A combination of humanised anti-CD19 and anti-BCMA CAR T cells in patients with relapsed or refractory multiple myeloma: a single-arm, phase 2 trial. Lancet Haematol. 2019;6:e521–e9.
88. Wang N, Hu X, Cao W, et al. Efficacy and safety of CAR19/22 T-cell cocktail therapy in patients with refractory/relapsed B-cell malignancies. Blood. 2020;135:17–27.

89. Hegde M, Mukherjee M, Grada Z, et al. Tandem CAR T cells targeting HER2 and IL13Ralpha2 mitigate tumor antigen escape. J Clin Invest. 2016;126:3036–52.
90. Tong C, Zhang Y, Liu Y, et al. Optimized tandem CD19/CD20 CAR-engineered T cells in refractory/relapsed B-cell lymphoma. Blood. 2020;136:1632–44.
91. Ormhoj M, Scarfo I, Cabral ML, et al. Chimeric antigen receptor T cells targeting CD79b show efficacy in lymphoma with or without Cotargeting CD19. Clin Cancer Res. 2019;25:7046–57.
92. Zah E, Lin MY, Silva-Benedict A, Jensen MC, Chen YY. T cells expressing CD19/CD20 bispecific chimeric antigen receptors prevent antigen escape by malignant B cells. Cancer Immunol Res. 2016;4:498–508.
93. Qin H, Ramakrishna S, Nguyen S, et al. Preclinical development of bivalent chimeric antigen receptors targeting both CD19 and CD22. Mol Ther Oncolytics. 2018;11:127–37.
94. Kantarjian H, Stein A, Gokbuget N, et al. Blinatumomab versus chemotherapy for advanced acute lymphoblastic Leukemia. N Engl J Med. 2017;376:836–47.
95. Choi BD, Yu X, Castano AP, et al. CAR-T cells secreting BiTEs circumvent antigen escape without detectable toxicity. Nat Biotechnol. 2019;37:1049–58.
96. Cho JH, Collins JJ, Wong WW. Universal chimeric antigen receptors for multiplexed and logical control of T cell responses. Cell. 2018;173:1426–38. e11
97. Urbanska K, Lanitis E, Poussin M, et al. A universal strategy for adoptive immunotherapy of cancer through use of a novel T-cell antigen receptor. Cancer Res. 2012;72:1844–52.
98. Lohmueller JJ, Ham JD, Kvorjak M, Finn OJ. mSA2 affinity-enhanced biotin-binding CAR T cells for universal tumor targeting. Onco Targets Ther. 2017;7:e1368604.
99. Tamada K, Geng D, Sakoda Y, et al. Redirecting gene-modified T cells toward various cancer types using tagged antibodies. Clin Cancer Res. 2012;18:6436–45.
100. Kudo K, Imai C, Lorenzini P, et al. T lymphocytes expressing a CD16 signaling receptor exert antibody-dependent cancer cell killing. Cancer Res. 2014;74:93–103.
101. Lee YG, Chu H, Lu Y, et al. Regulation of CAR T cell-mediated cytokine release syndrome-like toxicity using low molecular weight adapters. Nat Commun. 2019;10:2681.
102. Rodgers DT, Mazagova M, Hampton EN, et al. Switch-mediated activation and retargeting of CAR-T cells for B-cell malignancies. Proc Natl Acad Sci U S A. 2016;113:E459–68.
103. Wu CY, Roybal KT, Puchner EM, Onuffer J, Lim WA. Remote control of therapeutic T cells through a small molecule-gated chimeric receptor. Science. 2015;350:aab4077.
104. Juillerat A, Tkach D, Busser BW, et al. Modulation of chimeric antigen receptor surface expression by a small molecule switch. BMC Biotechnol. 2019;19:44.
105. Jan M, Scarfo I, Larson RC, et al. Reversible ON- and OFF-switch chimeric antigen receptors controlled by lenalidomide. Sci Transl Med. 2021;13
106. Kloss CC, Condomines M, Cartellieri M, Bachmann M, Sadelain M. Combinatorial antigen recognition with balanced signaling promotes selective tumor eradication by engineered T cells. Nat Biotechnol. 2013;31:71–5.
107. Lanitis E, Poussin M, Klattenhoff AW, et al. Chimeric antigen receptor T cells with dissociated signaling domains exhibit focused antitumor activity with reduced potential for toxicity in vivo. Cancer Immunol Res. 2013;1:43–53.
108. Wilkie S, van Schalkwyk MC, Hobbs S, et al. Dual targeting of ErbB2 and MUC1 in breast cancer using chimeric antigen receptors engineered to provide complementary signaling. J Clin Immunol. 2012;32:1059–70.
109. Roybal KT, Williams JZ, Morsut L, et al. Engineering T cells with customized therapeutic response programs using synthetic notch receptors. Cell. 2016;167:419.
110. Roybal KT, Rupp LJ, Morsut L, et al. Precision tumor recognition by T cells with combinatorial antigen-sensing circuits. Cell. 2016;164:770–9.
111. Srivastava S, Salter AI, Liggitt D, et al. Logic-gated ROR1 chimeric antigen receptor expression rescues T cell-mediated toxicity to Normal tissues and enables selective tumor targeting. Cancer Cell. 2019;35:489–503. e8
112. Williams JZ, Allen GM, Shah D, et al. Precise T cell recognition programs designed by transcriptionally linking multiple receptors. Science. 2020;370:1099–104.

113. Fedorov VD, Themeli M, Sadelain M. PD-1- and CTLA-4-based inhibitory chimeric antigen receptors (iCARs) divert off-target immunotherapy responses. Sci Transl Med. 2013;5:215ra172.
114. Mestermann K, Giavridis T, Weber J, et al. The tyrosine kinase inhibitor dasatinib acts as a pharmacologic on/off switch for CAR T cells. Sci Transl Med. 2019;11
115. Griffioen M, van Egmond EH, Kester MG, Willemze R, Falkenburg JH, Heemskerk MH. Retroviral transfer of human CD20 as a suicide gene for adoptive T-cell therapy. Haematologica. 2009;94:1316–20.
116. Serafini M, Manganini M, Borleri G, et al. Characterization of CD20-transduced T lymphocytes as an alternative suicide gene therapy approach for the treatment of graft-versus-host disease. Hum Gene Ther. 2004;15:63–76.
117. Philip B, Kokalaki E, Mekkaoui L, et al. A highly compact epitope-based marker/suicide gene for easier and safer T-cell therapy. Blood. 2014;124:1277–87.
118. Wang X, Chang WC, Wong CW, et al. A transgene-encoded cell surface polypeptide for selection, in vivo tracking, and ablation of engineered cells. Blood. 2011;118:1255–63.
119. Di Stasi A, Tey SK, Dotti G, et al. Inducible apoptosis as a safety switch for adoptive cell therapy. N Engl J Med. 2011;365:1673–83.
120. Kloss CC, Lee J, Zhang A, et al. Dominant-negative TGF-beta receptor enhances PSMA-targeted human CAR T cell proliferation and augments prostate cancer eradication. Mol Ther. 2018;26:1855–66.
121. Chang ZL, Lorenzini MH, Chen X, Tran U, Bangayan NJ, Chen YY. Rewiring T-cell responses to soluble factors with chimeric antigen receptors. Nat Chem Biol. 2018;14:317–24.
122. Leen AM, Sukumaran S, Watanabe N, et al. Reversal of tumor immune inhibition using a chimeric cytokine receptor. Mol Ther. 2014;22:1211–20.
123. Mohammed S, Sukumaran S, Bajgain P, et al. Improving chimeric antigen receptor-modified T cell function by reversing the immunosuppressive tumor microenvironment of pancreatic cancer. Mol Ther. 2017;25:249–58.
124. Wilkie S, Burbridge SE, Chiapero-Stanke L, et al. Selective expansion of chimeric antigen receptor-targeted T-cells with potent effector function using interleukin-4. J Biol Chem. 2010;285:25538–44.
125. Moon EK, Wang LC, Dolfi DV, et al. Multifactorial T-cell hypofunction that is reversible can limit the efficacy of chimeric antigen receptor-transduced human T cells in solid tumors. Clin Cancer Res. 2014;20:4262–73.
126. Cherkassky L, Morello A, Villena-Vargas J, et al. Human CAR T cells with cell-intrinsic PD-1 checkpoint blockade resist tumor-mediated inhibition. J Clin Invest. 2016;126:3130–44.
127. Liu X, Ranganathan R, Jiang S, et al. A chimeric switch-receptor targeting PD1 augments the efficacy of second-generation CAR T cells in advanced solid Tumors. Cancer Res. 2016;76:1578–90.
128. Suarez ER, de Chang K, Sun J, et al. Chimeric antigen receptor T cells secreting anti-PD-L1 antibodies more effectively regress renal cell carcinoma in a humanized mouse model. Oncotarget. 2016;7:34341–55.
129. Li S, Siriwon N, Zhang X, et al. Enhanced cancer immunotherapy by chimeric antigen receptor-modified T cells engineered to secrete checkpoint inhibitors. Clin Cancer Res. 2017;23:6982–92.
130. Rafiq S, Yeku OO, Jackson HJ, et al. Targeted delivery of a PD-1-blocking scFv by CAR-T cells enhances anti-tumor efficacy in vivo. Nat Biotechnol. 2018;36:847–56.
131. Choi BD, Yu X, Castano AP, et al. CRISPR-Cas9 disruption of PD-1 enhances activity of universal EGFRvIII CAR T cells in a preclinical model of human glioblastoma. J Immunother Cancer. 2019;7:304.
132. Rupp LJ, Schumann K, Roybal KT, et al. CRISPR/Cas9-mediated PD-1 disruption enhances anti-tumor efficacy of human chimeric antigen receptor T cells. Sci Rep. 2017;7:737.
133. Curran KJ, Seinstra BA, Nikhamin Y, et al. Enhancing antitumor efficacy of chimeric antigen receptor T cells through constitutive CD40L expression. Mol Ther. 2015;23:769–78.

134. Kuhn NF, Purdon TJ, van Leeuwen DG, et al. CD40 ligand-modified chimeric antigen receptor T cells enhance antitumor function by eliciting an endogenous antitumor response. Cancer Cell. 2019;35:473–88. e6

135. Zhao Z, Condomines M, van der Stegen SJC, et al. Structural design of engineered costimulation determines tumor rejection kinetics and persistence of CAR T cells. Cancer Cell. 2015;28:415–28.

136. Batlevi CL, Palomba ML, Park J, et al. Phase I clinical trial of CD19-targeted 19-28Z/4-1BBL "ARMORED" car t cells in patients with relapsed or refractory NHL and CLL including RICHTER transformation. Hematol Oncol. 2019;37:166–7.

137. Chmielewski M, Hombach AA, Abken H. Of CARs and TRUCKs: chimeric antigen receptor (CAR) T cells engineered with an inducible cytokine to modulate the tumor stroma. Immunol Rev. 2014;257:83–90.

138. Yeku OO, Purdon TJ, Koneru M, Spriggs D, Brentjens RJ. Armored CAR T cells enhance antitumor efficacy and overcome the tumor microenvironment. Sci Rep. 2017;7:10541.

139. Koneru M, O'Cearbhaill R, Pendharkar S, Spriggs DR, Brentjens RJ. A phase I clinical trial of adoptive T cell therapy using IL-12 secreting MUC-16(ecto) directed chimeric antigen receptors for recurrent ovarian cancer. J Transl Med. 2015;13:102.

140. Hoyos V, Savoldo B, Quintarelli C, et al. Engineering CD19-specific T lymphocytes with interleukin-15 and a suicide gene to enhance their anti-lymphoma/leukemia effects and safety. Leukemia. 2010;24:1160–70.

141. Chen Y, Sun C, Landoni E, Metelitsa L, Dotti G, Savoldo B. Eradication of neuroblastoma by T cells redirected with an optimized GD2-specific chimeric antigen receptor and Interleukin-15. Clin Cancer Res. 2019;25:2915–24.

142. Krenciute G, Prinzing BL, Yi Z, et al. Transgenic expression of IL15 improves Antiglioma activity of IL13Ralpha2-CAR T cells but results in antigen loss variants. Cancer Immunol Res. 2017;5:571–81.

143. Hurton LV, Singh H, Najjar AM, et al. Tethered IL-15 augments antitumor activity and promotes a stem-cell memory subset in tumor-specific T cells. Proc Natl Acad Sci U S A. 2016;113:E7788–E97.

144. Chmielewski M, Abken H. CAR T Cells releasing IL-18 convert to T-bet(high) FoxO1(low) effectors that exhibit augmented activity against advanced solid Tumors. Cell Rep. 2017;21:3205–19.

145. Hu B, Ren J, Luo Y, et al. Augmentation of antitumor immunity by human and mouse CAR T cells secreting IL-18. Cell Rep. 2017;20:3025–33.

146. Garfall AL, Maus MV, Hwang WT, et al. Chimeric antigen receptor T cells against CD19 for multiple myeloma. N Engl J Med. 2015;373:1040–7.

147. Garfall AL, Stadtmauer EA, Hwang WT, et al. Anti-CD19 CAR T cells with high-dose melphalan and autologous stem cell transplantation for refractory multiple myeloma. JCI Insight. 2018;3

148. Jacobson CA, Maus MV. C(h)AR-ting a new course in incurable lymphomas: CAR T cells for mantle cell and follicular lymphomas. Blood Adv. 2020;4:5858–62.

149. Schneider D, Xiong Y, Wu D, et al. A tandem CD19/CD20 CAR lentiviral vector drives on-target and off-target antigen modulation in leukemia cell lines. J Immunother Cancer. 2017;5:42.

150. Shah NN, Zhu F, Schneider D, et al. Results of a phase I study of bispecific anti-CD19, anti-CD20 chimeric antigen receptor (CAR) modified T cells for relapsed, refractory, non-Hodgkin lymphoma. Am Soc Clin Oncol 2019

151. Schultz LM, Davis KL, Baggott C, et al. Phase 1 study of CD19/CD22 bispecific chimeric antigen receptor (CAR) therapy in children and young adults with B cell acute lymphoblastic leukemia (ALL). Am Soc Hematol. 2018.

152. Ormhoj M, Scarfo I, Cabral ML, et al. Chimeric antigen receptor T cells targeting CD79b show efficacy in lymphoma with or without Cotargeting CD19. Clin Cancer Res. 2019;25:7046.

153. Novak AJ, Darce JR, Arendt BK, et al. Expression of BCMA, TACI, and BAFF-R in multiple myeloma: a mechanism for growth and survival. Blood. 2004;103:689–94.
154. Berdeja JG, Lin Y, Raje N, et al. Durable clinical responses in heavily pretreated patients with relapsed/refractory multiple myeloma: updated results from a multicenter study of bb2121 Anti-Bcma CAR T cell therapy. Blood. 2017;130:740.
155. Raje N, Berdeja J, Lin Y, et al. Anti-BCMA CAR T-cell therapy bb2121 in relapsed or refractory multiple myeloma. N Engl J Med. 2019;380:1726–37.
156. Zhao WH, Liu J, Wang BY, et al. A phase 1, open-label study of LCAR-B38M, a chimeric antigen receptor T cell therapy directed against B cell maturation antigen, in patients with relapsed or refractory multiple myeloma. J Hematol Oncol. 2018;11:141.
157. Zudaire E, Madduri D, Usmani SZ, et al. Translational analysis from CARTITUDE-1, an ongoing phase 1b/2 study of JNJ-4528 BCMA-targeted CAR-T cell therapy in relapsed and/ or refractory multiple myeloma (R/R MM), indicates preferential expansion of CD8+ T cell central memory cell subset. Blood. 2019;134:928.
158. Brudno JN, Maric I, Hartman SD, et al. T cells genetically modified to express an anti-B-cell maturation antigen chimeric antigen receptor cause remissions of poor-prognosis relapsed multiple myeloma. J Clin Oncol. 2018;36:2267–80.
159. Cohen AD, Garfall AL, Stadtmauer EA, et al. Safety and efficacy of B-cell maturation antigen (BCMA)-specific chimeric antigen receptor T cells (CART-BCMA) with cyclophosphamide conditioning for refractory multiple myeloma (MM). Blood. 2017;130:505.
160. Lam N, Trinklein ND, Buelow B, Patterson GH, Ojha N, Kochenderfer JN. Anti-BCMA chimeric antigen receptors with fully human heavy-chain-only antigen recognition domains. Nat Commun. 2020;11:283.
161. Xu J, Chen LJ, Yang SS, et al. Exploratory trial of a biepitopic CAR T-targeting B cell maturation antigen in relapsed/refractory multiple myeloma. Proc Natl Acad Sci U S A. 2019;116:9543–51.
162. Mikkilineni L, Kochenderfer JN. CAR T cell therapies for patients with multiple myeloma. Nat Rev Clin Oncol. 2021;18:71–84.
163. Ding L, Hu Y, Huang H. Novel progresses of chimeric antigen receptor (CAR) T cell therapy in multiple myeloma. Stem Cell Investig. 2021;8:1.
164. Leick MB, Maus MV. CAR-T cells beyond CD19, UnCAR-ted territory. Am J Hematol. 2019;94:S34–41.
165. Smith EL, Harrington K, Staehr M, et al. GPRC5D is a target for the immunotherapy of multiple myeloma with rationally designed CAR T cells. Sci Transl Med. 2019;11:eaau7746.
166. Scarfo I, Ormhoj M, Frigault MJ, et al. Anti-CD37 chimeric antigen receptor T cells are active against B- and T-cell lymphomas. Blood. 2018;132:1495–506.
167. Warda W, Da Rocha MN, Trad R, et al. Overcoming target epitope masking resistance that can occur on low-antigen-expresser AML blasts after IL-1RAP chimeric antigen receptor T cell therapy using the inducible caspase 9 suicide gene safety switch. Cancer Gene Ther. 2021.
168. Gomes-Silva D, Atilla E, Atilla PA, et al. CD7 CAR T cells for the therapy of acute myeloid Leukemia. Mol Ther. 2019;27:272–80.
169. Perna F, Berman SH, Soni RK, et al. Integrating proteomics and transcriptomics for systematic combinatorial chimeric antigen receptor therapy of AML. Cancer Cell. 2017;32:506–19. e5
170. Petersdorf SH, Kopecky KJ, Slovak M, et al. A phase 3 study of gemtuzumab ozogamicin during induction and postconsolidation therapy in younger patients with acute myeloid leukemia. Blood. 2013;121:4854–60.
171. Wang QS, Wang Y, Lv HY, et al. Treatment of CD33-directed chimeric antigen receptor-modified T cells in one patient with relapsed and refractory acute myeloid leukemia. Mol Ther. 2015;23:184–91.
172. Kim MY, Yu KR, Kenderian SS, et al. Genetic inactivation of CD33 in hematopoietic stem cells to enable CAR T cell immunotherapy for acute myeloid Leukemia. Cell. 2018;173:1439–53. e19

173. Raikar SS, Fleischer LC, Moot R, et al. Development of chimeric antigen receptors targeting T-cell malignancies using two structurally different anti-CD5 antigen binding domains in NK and CRISPR-edited T cell lines. Onco Targets Ther. 2018;7:e1407898.
174. Gomes-Silva D, Srinivasan M, Sharma S, et al. CD7-edited T cells expressing a CD7-specific CAR for the therapy of T-cell malignancies. Blood. 2017;130:285–96.
175. Wagner J, Wickman E, DeRenzo C, Gottschalk S. CAR T Cell therapy for solid Tumors: bright future or dark reality? Mol Ther. 2020;28:2320–39.
176. Li G, Wong AJ. EGF receptor variant III as a target antigen for tumor immunotherapy. Expert Rev Vaccines. 2008;7:977–85.
177. O'Rourke DM, Nasrallah MP, Desai A, et al. A single dose of peripherally infused EGFRvIII-directed CAR T cells mediates antigen loss and induces adaptive resistance in patients with recurrent glioblastoma. Sci Transl Med. 2017;9:eaaa0984.
178. Goff SL, Morgan RA, Yang JC, et al. Pilot trial of adoptive transfer of chimeric antigen receptor-transduced T cells targeting EGFRvIII in patients with glioblastoma. J Immunother. 2019;42:126–35.
179. Mineo JF, Bordron A, Baroncini M, et al. Low HER2-expressing glioblastomas are more often secondary to anaplastic transformation of low-grade glioma. J Neuro-Oncol. 2007;85:281–7.
180. Ahmed N, Brawley V, Hegde M, et al. HER2-specific chimeric antigen receptor-modified virus-specific T cells for progressive glioblastoma: a phase 1 dose-escalation trial. JAMA Oncol. 2017;3:1094–101.
181. Jarboe JS, Johnson KR, Choi Y, Lonser RR, Park JK. Expression of interleukin-13 receptor alpha2 in glioblastoma multiforme: implications for targeted therapies. Cancer Res. 2007;67:7983–6.
182. Brown CE, Alizadeh D, Starr R, et al. Regression of glioblastoma after chimeric antigen receptor T-cell therapy. N Engl J Med. 2016;375:2561–9.
183. Morello A, Sadelain M, Adusumilli PS. Mesothelin-targeted CARs: driving T cells to solid Tumors. Cancer Discov. 2016;6:133–46.
184. Adusumilli PS, Zauderer MG, Rusch VW, et al. Abstract CT036: A phase I clinical trial of malignant pleural disease treated with regionally delivered autologous mesothelin-targeted CAR T cells: Safety and efficacy. Cancer Res. 2019;79:CT036-CT.
185. Haas AR, Tanyi JL, O'Hara MH, et al. Phase I study of lentiviral-transduced chimeric anti-gen receptor-modified T cells recognizing Mesothelin in advanced solid cancers. Mol Ther. 2019;27:1919–29.
186. Majzner RG, Theruvath JL, Nellan A, et al. CAR T cells targeting B7-H3, a pan-cancer anti-gen, demonstrate potent preclinical activity against Pediatric solid Tumors and brain Tumors. Clin Cancer Res. 2019;25:2560–74.
187. Du H, Hirabayashi K, Ahn S, et al. Antitumor responses in the absence of toxicity in solid Tumors by targeting B7-H3 via chimeric antigen receptor T cells. Cancer Cell. 2019;35:221–37. e8
188. Posey AD Jr, Schwab RD, Boesteanu AC, et al. Engineered CAR T cells targeting the cancer-associated Tn-Glycoform of the membrane mucin MUC1 control adenocarcinoma. Immunity. 2016;44:1444–54.
189. Gnjatic S, Nishikawa H, Jungbluth AA, et al. NY-ESO-1: review of an immunogenic tumor antigen. Adv Cancer Res. 2006;95:1–30.
190. Maus MV, Plotkin J, Jakka G, et al. An MHC-restricted antibody-based chimeric antigen receptor requires TCR-like affinity to maintain antigen specificity. Mol Ther Oncolytics. 2016;3:1–9,
191. Schuberth PC, Jakka G, Jensen SM, et al. Effector memory and central memory NY-ESO-1-specific re-directed T cells for treatment of multiple myeloma. Gene Ther. 2013;20:386–95.

Cell Types Used for CAR Generation

Carl DeSelm

Abstract The most common CAR T-cell product generated and infused into patients, today and in the past, is an unsorted, αβ T-cell derived directly from the cancer patient. Although this personalized autologous T-cell manufacturing method has many advantages and has resulted in outstanding clinical data in hematologic malignancies, a number of aspects require improvement for cell therapy to impact broader patient populations. The first aspect relates to the poor sustained anti-tumor response of CAR T-cells in solid tumors as well as a significant group of leukemia and lymphoma patients. Utilizing cells that naturally penetrate larger tumor masses better, kill through additional mechanisms, are less prone to antigen escape or intrinsic cytotoxic resistance, or that better establish and maintain an anti-tumor microenvironment, may overcome some of the deficiencies of CAR T-cells in poorly responsive tumors. Further, utilizing other cell types may lessen the tremendous cost of autologous manufacturing, the possibility of manufacturing failure in some patients, the length of time for manufacturing, and the side effect profile. This chapter will discuss alternative cellular sources developed to date, including allogeneic T-cells, Natural Killer (NK) cells, invariant NK T-cells (iNKT), induced pluripotent stem cells (iPSCs), T-cells of a defined CD4/CD8 ratio, T-cells of a defined memory phenotype, and myeloid cells modified with a CAR.

Keywords Allogeneic CAR T-cells · Off the shelf CAR T-cells · NK cells · Invariant NK T-cells (iNKT) · Macrophage · Neurophile · Induced pluripotent stem cells (iPSCs) · MHC-I and MHC-II · HLA-E · HLA-G · TCR α-chain (TRAC) · UCART19 · CRISPR/Cas9 · T effector (TE) · T memory phenotype (TM) · T central memory (TCM) · T effector memory (TEM) · T stem cell-like memory T cells (TSCM) · CD4+ · CD8+ · Antibody dependent cytotoxicity (ADCC) · Netosis

C. DeSelm (✉)
Department of Radiation Oncology, Center for Human Immunology and Immunotherapy Programs, Washington University School of Medicine, Saint Louis, MO, USA
e-mail: deselmc@wustl.edu

© Springer Nature Switzerland AG 2022
A. Ghobadi, J. F. DiPersio (eds.), *Gene and Cellular Immunotherapy for Cancer*, Cancer Drug Discovery and Development,
https://doi.org/10.1007/978-3-030-87849-8_4

57

Allogeneic CAR T-Cells

For hematologic malignancies treated with CAR T-cells for which efficacy is quite impressive, a current major limitation is patient access to the product, and the financial burden placed on the healthcare system due to the high cost of manufacturing a single product from a single patient using their own autologous T-cells [1]. The current list price for the approved CAR T-cell therapies is $373,000, and the process takes roughly 3 weeks to manufacture. These 3 weeks are a vulnerable time for patients; they have already progressed on the most effective known chemotherapy regimens so keeping their disease controlled can be a challenge, and progression of disease in this time sometimes renders them ineligible to receive the manufactured CAR T-cells. Even if they remain eligible, progression in this time may make the disease less controllable by the CAR T-cells. Allogeneic, or "off-the-shelf" CAR T-cells would provide a solution to these problems. Of course, the challenging question remains, can allogeneic CAR T-cells address these limitations while still providing the same level of efficacy as autologous CAR T-cells?

Theoretically, cancer patients who have anergic, exhausted, or senescent T-cells as a result of their cancer, their age, or their multiple prior lines of cytotoxic therapy [2], may enjoy improved disease response if given a CAR product from a healthy donor with optimally-functioning T-cells. However the inclination of the host immune system to reject the foreign T-cells tends to limit their efficacy, and the inclination of the foreign T-cells to reject the host's tissues or organs (i.e., graft-versus-host disease or GVHD) introduces the potential for additional toxicities with this strategy.

Overcoming these obstacles requires first understanding the mechanisms by which cells are rejected by either the host or the donor. Since GVHD is a major cause of death in allogeneic stem cell transplant, much research has been devoted to the subject, and $\alpha\beta$ T cells have been found to be central to its pathogenesis [3]. The $\alpha\beta$ TCR recognizes peptides presented by MHC molecules, which in humans are comprised of HLA proteins. HLA genes have more polymorphisms than any other human genes, leading to thousands of slightly different HLA protein variants. Of these many different variants, up to six MHC-I and six MHC-II variants are present in each individual. Through a process of negative selection in the thymus, T-cells are educated to not react against any self-MHC molecule, or even any self-MHC molecule loaded with a peptide derived from any of the thousands of proteins encoded in that individual's genome. However, a new peptide presented by a self-MHC, or a different MHC variant, may still be recognized and lead to alloreactivity. Further, amino acid differences in the peptide-binding region of a given MHC molecule determine the specific sequence of peptides that are capable of being presented, and thus simply changing the MHC results in a wide variety of different peptides presented that were not present in the thymus's negative selection process, even if the full proteins themselves are identical.

While it is nearly impossible to match all HLA variants among donors and recipients, matching HLA-A, HLA-B and HLA-DR is sufficient to reduce the incidence of allogeneic graft rejection. However, establishing a matched HLA CAR T-cell program would require a large bank from a wide range of donors, and would inevitably exclude a number of patients, especially ethnic minorities or those with less common HLA variants. Further, even though partially-matched CAR T-cells may not react strongly against the host, it is likely that these infused allogeneic CAR T-cells will be more rapidly eliminated by either host T-cells or antibodies recognizing remaining discordant peptide-MHC complexes, or other surface proteins.

Thus, achieving allogeneic CAR T-cell persistence is a major challenge. In addition to HLA matching, more intense lymphodepletion therapy may be required to further immunosuppress the host response against the infused CAR T-cells; however, this approach also compromises other aspects of host immunity, such as effective responses to infectious agents. Repeating intensive lymphodepletion for subsequent CAR T-cell administration carries additional risk and morbidity. A more specific, genetic approach to improving CAR T-cell persistence is to knock out (genetically delete) MHC-I, which is a potential major target of rejection of CAR T-cells by the host immune system. The most efficient way to do this is to delete β_2-microglobulin, which is essential for forming functional MHC-I molecules on the cell surface. MHC-II is also expressed on activated T-cells and may also likely be a target of host immune mediated rejection of allogeneic CAR T-cells. Therefore, knocking out or blocking MHC-II on CAR T-cells would also be necessary to maximize their persistence. A relatively efficient way of doing this is to knock out the master regulator of all MHC-II molecule expression, *CIITA*. Knocking both MHC-I and MHC-II molecules in CAR T-cells has been achieved in mouse studies [4].

Since MHC molecules are major inhibitors of NK cell cytotoxicity as they signify self, depleting MHC-I and MHC-II makes the CAR T-cells more susceptible to NK-mediated elimination. To circumvent this problem, the additional expression of non-classical HLA molecules (HLA-E or HLA-G), which can inhibit NK cells but are less common targets for T-cell rejection, can be added to the CAR vector [4, 5].

An option available to the relatively small number of patients who have previously had an allogeneic stem cell transplant and have subsequently relapsed is to generate CAR T-cells from the original stem cell donor. In this way, the host immune system, which has already been reconstituted with a different donor, will be genetically identical to the infused CAR-modified cells. In a series of 20 patients who underwent this strategy, eight had a response to CAR T-cells (six complete responses [CRs] and two partial responses [PRs]), and none developed new-onset GVHD after CAR T-cell infusion [6].

In addition to solving the problem of allogeneic CAR T-cell persistence, the problem of GVHD needs to be addressed. Beyond HLA matching, preventing GVHD can be successfully achieved through a variety of other means, such as knocking out the TCR from the infused cells, using a cell product with a restricted TCR profile (such as only those that recognize a viral antigen), or using cell types that naturally lack an αβ TCR. The TCR is a heterogeneous group of proteins consisting of either an α-chain and a β-chain (in αβ T cells) or a γ-chain and a δ-chain (in γδ T cells), as well as four separate CD3 transmembrane proteins (CD3δ, CD3γ, CD3ε and CD3ζ). The β-chain contains two possible constant regions, while the α-chain has one, making it logistically easier to abolish the αβ TCR by targeting the single α-chain (*TRAC*). Methods have progressed from successfully knocking out the *TRAC* in CAR T-cells [7], to knocking the CAR gene into the *TRAC* locus, putting the CAR under the natural transcriptional regulation of the TCRα and ameliorating some of the exhaustive effects of tonic signaling from constitutive high CAR expression [8]. TCR knockout CAR T-cells (UCART19) have shown feasibility in two clinical trials with relapsed B-cell leukemia, demonstrating a 67% CR, and a 6-month PFS of 27% [9]. In these studies, the UCART19 product has both the TCR and the mature lymphocyte marker CD52 knocked out, which allows for additional lymphodepletion but not CAR T-cell depletion using the monoclonal anti-CD52 antibody alemtuzumab. This strategy thus both prevents the CAR T-cells from recognizing the host through its TCR (deleted by CRISPR/Cas9), and reduces the host's ability to eliminate the CAR T-cells by depleting host lymphocytes (via infusion of alemtuzumab). How this approach will compare to autologous CAR T-cell efficacy remains to be seen in further studies.

While knocking out the TCR is an eloquent approach, it requires sophisticated and relatively expensive techniques. Another potential strategy, which still utilizes intact αβ T-cells, is to selectively employ memory T-cells that recognize a viral antigen for CAR transduction. Since the risk of GVHD is proportional to the diversity of the TCRs present, selecting for a smaller number of TCR clones against a known, non-human target should greatly reduce the risk. However, since TCRs are degenerate, the possibility remains that a particular antiviral TCR may still cross-react with a host tissue antigen. Additionally, since these are all T-cells that have previously encountered the viral antigen at least once, the baseline phenotype will be different; the effect of using this population of prior antigen-exposed cells is unknown. This approach has been demonstrated in glioblastoma patients targeting HER2 in a clinical trial, which showed feasibility and one partial response among 17 patients [9]. Whether this approach is will be effective against a more responsive tumor like ALL remains to be reported in clinical trials.

γδ T-Cells

Although αβ T-cells make up 95% of the T-cell population and have been most heavily studied over the years, the less common γδ T-cell has gained attraction as a CAR substrate for a variety of reasons. The γδ TCR does not utilize MHC molecules for antigen recognition, and is much less likely to cause GVHD if used in an allogeneic setting. γδ T-cells can naturally exert antitumor cytotoxicity without a CAR [10], demonstrating they have the appropriate machinery for tumor killing. They have a natural predilection for tissue residence, which may provide an advantage in tumors in which tissue infiltration by T-cells is a limitation, such as most solid tumors. CAR modified γδ T-cells can expand nearly 100-fold in the course of 2 weeks *in vitro*, and exert target-specific killing [11]. Clinical trials underway testing CAR γδ T-cells in solid tumors (NCT04107142) and liquid tumors (NCT02656147, NCT03885076) will provide insight into whether these types of CAR T-cells are safe and feasible, and may provide some insight into potential for efficacy in humans.

NK Cells

NK cells are the most common and successful non-T-cell source for CAR therapy to date. NK cells, like T-cells, exert potent cytotoxicity against target cells, making them an attractive candidate for CAR modification. Unlike T-cells, they do not have a TCR and do not exert significant GVHD, making them an attractive allogeneic product. NK cells recognize and kill their targets through a variety of mechanisms, including through activating receptors such as NKG2D, NKp44, NKp46, NKp30, and others, which can be triggered by a variety of ligands, many of which are upregulated by cellular stress and are thus often naturally found on tumor cells. Additionally, NK cells express the Fc receptor FcγRIIIa (CD16) and can recognize and kill cells coated with antibodies through antibody-dependent cellular cytotoxicity (ADCC). Thus, their ability to kill through multiple mechanisms in addition to the CAR may reduce the risk of tumor antigen escape. NK cells also possess inhibitory receptors, such as those that prevent killing of MHC-expressing self-cells, which may be useful in tumors that have downregulated MHC in order to escape endogenous T-cell recognition.

Unlike T-cells, NK cells do not undergo clonal expansion. While this can effectively limit toxicity of the therapy, it also makes transduction and generation of suitable numbers for treatment a challenge. However, also unlike T-cells, there is an NK cell line that is effective in cell killing (NK-92), which can be transduced with a CAR as a clinical-grade product and used in patients. A clinical trial of anti-CD33 CAR NK-92 cells expressing the 4-1BB costimulation domain treated three AML patients, one of whom experienced MRD+ remission for a short period [12]. Other sources for CAR NK cells that can be more readily expanded include cord blood, human embryonic stem cells, or induced pluripotent stem cells.

Additional strategies such as co-expressing IL-15 with the CAR have resulted in prolonged CAR NK survival [13, 14]. In 11 patients treated with IL-15 expressing CAR NK cells derived from HLA-mismatched cord blood, no GVHD or other major toxicity was observed, and 7 of the 11 patients had a CR (4 with lymphoma and 3 with CLL). Although NK cells generally survive an average of 2 weeks in humans, the cord blood-derived CAR NK cells utilized in this study expanded and persisted at low detectable levels for at least a year [14].

Like T-cells, NK cell activity can be modulated by a variety of cytokines. NK cells cultured with IL-12, IL-15, and IL-18 display enhanced effector function in response to further cytokines or tumor targets for weeks after the initial preactivation, developing a "memory-like" (ML) phenotype [15]. Modifying these ML NK cells with a CAR endows them with the capacity to specifically recognize tumor in an antigen-dependent manner, and to control lymphoma burden in mice [16]. Clinical trials using this strategy have yet to be performed.

Although many CAR NK studies utilize a traditional CAR design from a CAR T-cell, NK cells have different natural receptor requirements and the optimal costimulatory domain for NK cells may be different. Changing the costimulatory domain to the NK-cell-associated activating receptor 2B4, for example, results in increased engraftment and CAR NK persistence in mice [17]. Additional NK costimulatory CAR domains are under investigation and further improved combinations are likely to continue to emerge.

NKT and iNKT Cells

While NK cells can be easily distinguished from T-cells by the lack of a TCR, NKT cells have markers typical of NK cells, such as NK1.1, but also contain an $\alpha\beta$ TCR, and fall within the T-cell lineage. Unlike the $\alpha\beta$ TCR of conventional T-cells that recognize peptides displayed on MHC-I, the $\alpha\beta$ TCR of NKT cells recognizes glycolipid antigens presented on CD1d. Type I NKT cells (invariant or iNKT) possess a semi-invariant $V\alpha14$-$J\alpha18$ TCR in mice, and $V\alpha24$-$J\alpha18$ in humans paired with a limited repertoire of $V\beta$-chains making them an attractive choice for allogeneic cells. Type II NKT cells utilize a more diverse TCR repertoire, although still almost all exclusively recognize glycolipids presented on CD1d due to their positive selection process in the thymus. Rather than inducing GVHD like their conventional T-cell counterpart in allogeneic infusions, NKT cells are associated with protection from GVHD [18–21], further increasing their appeal for allogeneic therapy. CD1d is expressed on some tumors, allowing for additional killing through this receptor [22]. They also are reported to express CD40L, an activating molecule for macrophages and dendritic cells [23], which may help to favorably remodel the tumor microenvironment. Since NKT cells are a type of T-cell, they expand and persist much more readily than NK cells [24]. However, engineering sufficient numbers for therapy is still a challenge since they naturally make up <1% of peripheral T-cells. Ongoing clinical trials testing CAR NKT cells for GD2 (NCT03294954) and CD19 (NCT03774654) expressing malignancies are expected to offer more insight into their safety and feasibility in humans.

iPSC

An attractive source for theoretically unlimited CAR T-cells, or other immune cells, for allogeneic use is iPSCs. These cells could be genetically modified in numerous ways over time, unlike primary cells which are limited by the number of possible transductions before the must be used. For example, theoretically the TCR could be knocked out to prevent GVHD, MHC-I and MHC-II genes could be deleted to prevent T-cell rejection, non-classical HLA molecules (such as HLA-E or HLA-G) could be introduced to prevent NK cell rejection, additional inhibitory molecules such as PD1 could be removed, and/or they could be made to express stimulatory cytokines. Alternatively, a broad repository of HLA typed iPSCs could be utilized to create HLA-matched infusion products. Even without knocking out the TCR, since one clone can be used to generate all of the cells, the risk of GVHD would likely be very low. However, drawbacks of this approach are that iPSCs are difficult and expensive to culture in great quantities, and the process of differentiation into fully functional effector immune cells such as T-cells or NK cells after modification with a CAR is not a trivial process. However, iPSCs have been successfully used to generate CAR NK cells with functionality similar to CAR T-cells and less signs of GVHD in mice [25]. Human clinical trials with iPSC derived CARs are ongoing with results yet to be reported.

Defining the T-Cell Phenotype and CD4/CD8 Ratio

All of the clinical trials that led to initial FDA CAR T-cell approval used bulk T-cells derived from the peripheral blood of patients, without intentionally excluding or enriching a particular subset of T-cells for CAR modification or re-infusion. Subsequently, a CAR T-cell product has been approved by the FDA that consists of a defined 50:50 mixture of CD4:CD8 T-cells (lisocabtagene maraleucel). T-cells exist in a number of phenotypes, which depends on such things as whether they are in the throes of an antigen-specific response, have previously been strongly activated but have had some time to rest, or have never been activated at all. All T-cells start in a naïve state, and upon antigen encounter acquire an effector (T_E) or a memory phenotype (T_M), which can further be divided into central memory (T_{CM}) and effector memory (T_{EM}) compartments. An additional group of stem cell-like memory T cells (T_{SCM}) have been identified as a long-lived human memory T cell population with an enhanced capacity for self-renewal [26]. In addition to these phenotypes, T-cells are either CD8 or CD4 positive. CD8+ T-cells are traditionally thought of as the cytotoxic T-cells which are responsible for killing, while CD4+ T-cells perform a helper function, by secreting cytokines to improve CD8+ T-cell proliferation and function. However, after modification with a CAR, CD4 T-cells can effectively kill similarly to CD8+ T-cells. Amidst all of these complexities, it is not inherently obvious whether particular subsets, or combinations of subsets, may provide greater efficacy against tumor.

To begin to answer this question, mouse studies were performed in which puri-fied individual CD8+ and CD4+ T-cell subsets were CAR modified and then injected into tumor-bearing mice [27]. First, pure CD4+ CAR T-cells generated from naïve or T_{CM} precursors significantly improved survival compared with T_{EM} CD4+ CAR T cells. Among the purified CD8+ CAR T-cell subsets, T_{CM} cells were slightly better than naïve, which were slightly better than T_{EM}. Additionally, combining CD8+ T_{CM} CAR T-cells with CD4+ naïve or CD4+ T_{CM} CAR T-cells significantly improved survival relative to pure CD8+ T_{CM} cells alone [27].

These findings inspired clinical trials utilizing defined T-cell subsets. A phase I-II study of CAR T-cells targeting CD19 using a 1:1 ratio of CD4:CD8 was per-formed in ALL patients, in which the CD8 T-cells were enriched for a T_{CM} pheno-type. Patients achieved a 93% remission rate by flow cytometry and 86% MRD-negative CR rate, which compared favorably with other trials using bulk T-cells [28, 29]. CD19 CAR-T cells have also been administered in a 1:1 CD4+:CD8+ ratio, in which the CD8 T-cells were enriched for a T_{CM} phenotype, to relapsed and/or refractory B cell non-Hodgkin lymphoma patients [30]. The CR in patients treated with Cy/Flu at the maximally tolerated dose was 64%, with a low incidence of serious toxicity.

Since patients exhibit a wide range of dominant T-cell phenotypes at baseline, which is reflective of their antigen-exposure history, treatment history, and numer-ous other factors, informative correlations have been drawn from those who respond well to CAR T-cells versus those who do not. In single cell RNAseq analysis of CD19 CAR T-cells isolated from the infusion bag of large cell lymphoma patients, the CD8 T-cell phenotype most associated with achieving a CR was a T_{CM} pheno-type. The frequency of these cells were also low in patients with high-stage disease (III and IV) and high international prognostic index (IPI 3–4), suggesting clinical factors prior to leukapheresis may influence the transcriptional state of CAR T cells [31]. Similarly, transcriptomic profiling revealed that CAR T cells from complete-responding patients with CLL were enriched in memory-related genes prior to infu-sion [32].

It is still unclear whether enriching for a particular phenotype prior to infusion, or whether attempting to induce a favorable phenotype during the CAR modifica-tion process such as through culture with IL-7 and IL-15, will lead to improved result in patients. However, the preclinical and phase I human data suggest these approaches may confer advantages, especially for more difficult to treat tumors, and warrant further investigation.

Macrophages

Macrophages, being completely unrelated to T-cells on the hematologic family tree, have a plethora of different functions that make them attractive candidates for CAR modification in cases where T-cells encounter changes. For example, while T-cells poorly infiltrate solid tumors, macrophages are often summoned to them by cytokines released by the tumor; the actively migrate into the tumor against a pressure gradient while T-cells largely lack this capacity. While T-cells kill primarily through inducing apoptosis by granzyme and perforin secretion, to which tumor cells have variably levels of innate and acquired resistance, macrophages can theoretically dispose of their targets by direct phagocytosis. Additionally, they have been known to exert cytotoxic effects through antibody dependent cytotoxicity (ADCC). Unfortunately, macrophages are usually drawn to the tumor microenvironment to provide a "healing" role; they sense destruction and arrive to reduce inflammation and promote recovery. This role generally has the effect of promoting tumor growth, spread, and metastasis. Since they are highly plastic, they can change from this reparative, pro-tumor role to an inflammatory, anti-tumor role and back again, depending on their stimuli.

Engineering macrophages with a CAR is an appealing way to genetically instruct them to maintain an inflammatory anti-tumor phenotype, as well as to infiltrate and phagocytose tumor. Macrophages modified with a CAR containing a signaling domain from Megf10 or FcRγ have both been found to achieve target-specific phagocytosis [33]. A CAR macrophage targeting the extracellular matrix protein CD147 successfully reduced tumor collagen deposition and improved T-cell infiltration [34]. CAR macrophages expressing a CD3z-based CAR phagocytosed tumor *in vitro* and reduced tumor burden *in vivo*, expressed proinflammatory cytokines and chemokines, converted bystander M2 macrophages to M1, resisted the effects of immunosuppressive cytokines, and activated anti-tumor T-cells [35]. Challenges to macrophage therapy include genetically modifying the cells in large numbers, and potentially finding ways to increase the magnitude of their direct anti-tumor efficacy *in vivo,* as studies thus far have shown tumor reduction but not elimination. Given the number of T-cell supportive functions CAR macrophages have, they may function synergistically with CAR T-cells; however, these studies have yet to be reported. One Phase I clinical trial is currently open utilizing CAR macrophages for HER2 expressing tumors (NCT04660929).

Neutrophils

Neutrophils, like macrophages, often have pro-tumor functions, however they are relatively less well characterized in the tumor microenvironment. Their ability to kill through alternative mechanisms, such as netosis, is conceptually appealing. Before CAR T-cells had gained significant momentum, a report in 1998 of neutrophils being modified with a CAR (then called a CIR, for chimeric immune receptor) containing a CD3z intracellular domain showed antigen-specific tumor lysis [36]. However, no CAR neutrophil reports have been generated since. Whether these cells may someday play a more central role in CAR therapies remains to be seen (Fig. 1).

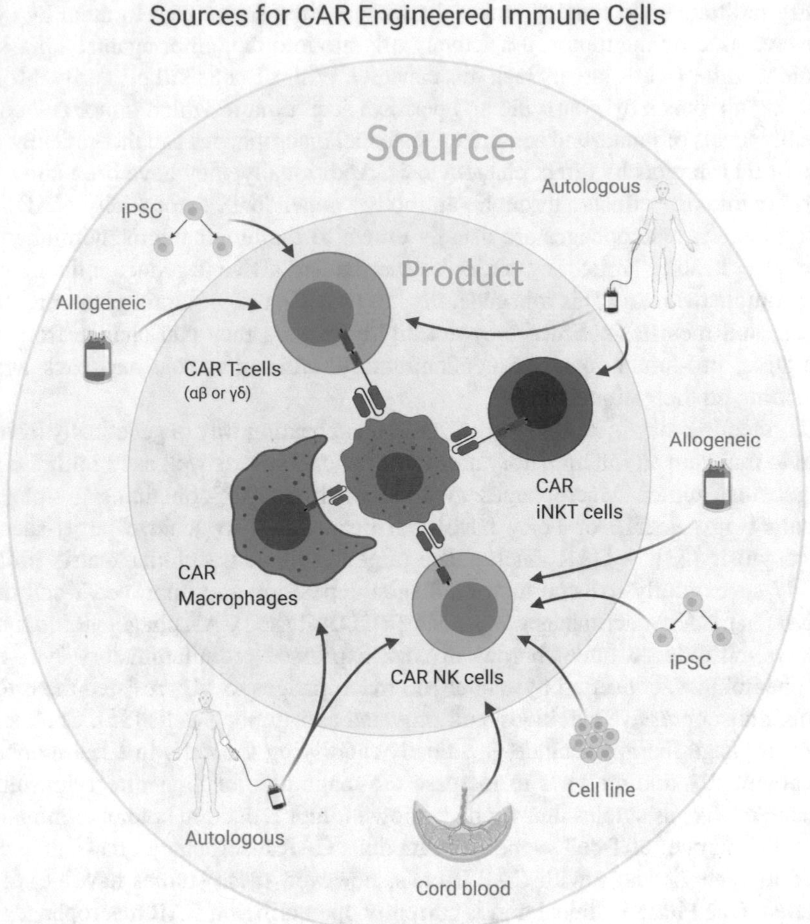

Fig. 1 **Sources of CAR Engineered Immune Cells**. The most common source of CAR-modified cells is autologous peripheral blood. However, allogeneic sources are being used and further developed, as are cord blood cells, induced pluripotent stem cell (iPSCs), or even cell lines in the case of CAR NK cells

References

1. Lin JK, Muffly LS, Spinner MA, Barnes JI, Owens DK, Goldhaber-Fiebert JD. Cost effectiveness of chimeric antigen receptor T-cell therapy in multiply relapsed or refractory adult large B-cell lymphoma. J Clin Oncol. 2019;37:2105–19.
2. Thommen DS, Schumacher TN. T cell dysfunction in cancer. Cancer Cell. 2018;33:547–62.
3. Zeiser R, Blazar BR. Acute graft-versus-host disease—biologic process, prevention, and therapy. N Engl J Med. 2017;377:2167–79.
4. Kagoya Y, Guo T, Yeung B, et al. Genetic ablation of HLA class I, class II, and the T-cell receptor enables allogeneic T cells to be used for adoptive T-cell therapy. Cancer Immunol Res. 2020;8:926–36.

5. Gornalusse GG, Hirata RK, Funk SE, et al. HLA-E-expressing pluripotent stem cells escape allogeneic responses and lysis by NK cells. Nat Biotechnol. 2017;35:765–72.
6. Brudno JN, Somerville RP, Shi V, et al. Allogeneic T cells that express an anti-CD19 chimeric antigen receptor induce remissions of B-cell malignancies that Progress after allogeneic hematopoietic stem-cell transplantation without causing graft-versus-host disease. J Clin Oncol. 2016;34:1112–21.
7. Torikai H, Reik A, Liu PQ, et al. A foundation for universal T-cell based immunotherapy: T cells engineered to express a CD19-specific chimeric-antigen-receptor and eliminate expression of endogenous TCR. Blood. 2012;119:5697–705.
8. Eyquem J, Mansilla-Soto J, Giavridis T, et al. Targeting a CAR to the TRAC locus with CRISPR/Cas9 enhances tumour rejection. Nature. 2017;543:113–7.
9. Benjamin R, Graham C, Yallop D, et al. Genome-edited, donor-derived allogeneic anti-CD19 chimeric antigen receptor T cells in paediatric and adult B-cell acute lymphoblastic leukaemia: results of two phase 1 studies. Lancet. 2020;396:1885–94.
10. Kato Y, Tanaka Y, Miyagawa F, Yamashita S, Minato N. Targeting of tumor cells for human gammadelta T cells by nonpeptide antigens. J Immunol. 2001;167:5092–8.
11. Capsomidis A, Benthall G, Van Acker HH, et al. Chimeric antigen receptor-engineered human Gamma Delta T cells: enhanced cytotoxicity with retention of cross presentation. Mol Ther. 2018;26:354–65.
12. Tang X, Yang L, Li Z, et al. Erratum: first-in-man clinical trial of CAR NK-92 cells: safety test of CD33-CAR NK-92 cells in patients with relapsed and refractory acute myeloid leukemia. Am J Cancer Res. 2018;8:1899.
13. Liu E, Tong Y, Dotti G, et al. Cord blood NK cells engineered to express IL-15 and a CD19-targeted CAR show long-term persistence and potent antitumor activity. Leukemia. 2018;32:520–31.
14. Liu E, Marin D, Banerjee P, et al. Use of CAR-transduced natural killer cells in CD19-positive lymphoid tumors. N Engl J Med. 2020;382:545–53.
15. Wagner JA, Berrien-Elliott MM, Rosario M, et al. Cytokine-induced memory-like differentiation enhances unlicensed natural killer cell Antileukemia and FcgammaRIIIa-triggered responses. Biol Blood Marrow Transplant. 2017;23:398–404.
16. Gang M, Marin ND, Wong P, et al. CAR-modified memory-like NK cells exhibit potent responses to NK-resistant lymphomas. Blood. 2020;136:2308–18.
17. Xu Y, Liu Q, Zhong M, et al. 2B4 costimulatory domain enhancing cytotoxic ability of anti-CD5 chimeric antigen receptor engineered natural killer cells against T cell malignancies. J Hematol Oncol. 2019;12:49.
18. Chaidos A, Patterson S, Szydlo R, et al. Graft invariant natural killer T-cell dose predicts risk of acute graft-versus-host disease in allogeneic hematopoietic stem cell transplantation. Blood. 2012;119:5030–6.
19. Leveson-Gower DB, Olson JA, Sega EI, et al. Low doses of natural killer T cells provide protection from acute graft-versus-host disease via an IL-4-dependent mechanism. Blood. 2011;117:3220–9.
20. Rubio MT, Bouillie M, Bouazza N, et al. Pre-transplant donor CD4(−) invariant NKT cell expansion capacity predicts the occurrence of acute graft-versus-host disease. Leukemia. 2017;31:903–12.
21. Schneidawind D, Pierini A, Alvarez M, et al. CD4+ invariant natural killer T cells protect from murine GVHD lethality through expansion of donor CD4+CD25+FoxP3+ regulatory T cells. Blood. 2014;124:3320–8.
22. Rotolo A, Caputo VS, Holubova M, et al. Enhanced anti-lymphoma activity of CAR19-iNKT cells underpinned by dual CD19 and CD1d targeting. Cancer Cell. 2018;34:596–610. e11
23. Gottschalk C, Mettke E, Kurts C. The role of invariant natural killer T cells in dendritic cell licensing, cross-priming, and memory CD8(+) T cell generation. Front Immunol. 2015;6:379.
24. Heczey A, Liu D, Tian G, et al. Invariant NKT cells with chimeric antigen receptor provide a novel platform for safe and effective cancer immunotherapy. Blood. 2014;124:2824–33.

25. Li Y, Hermanson DL, Moriarity BS, Kaufman DS. Human iPSC-derived natural killer cells engineered with chimeric antigen receptors enhance anti-tumor activity. Cell Stem Cell. 2018;23:181–92. e5
26. Gattinoni L, Lugli E, Ji Y, et al. A human memory T cell subset with stem cell-like properties. Nat Med. 2011;17:1290–7.
27. Sommermeyer D, Hudecek M, Kosasih PL, et al. Chimeric antigen receptor-modified T cells derived from defined CD8+ and CD4+ subsets confer superior antitumor reactivity in vivo. Leukemia. 2016;30:492–500.
28. Turtle CJ, Hanafi LA, Berger C, et al. CD19 CAR-T cells of defined CD4+:CD8+ composition in adult B cell ALL patients. J Clin Invest. 2016;126:2123–38.
29. Abramson JS, Palomba ML, Gordon LI, et al. Lisocabtagene maraleucel for patients with relapsed or refractory large B-cell lymphomas (TRANSCEND NHL 001): a multicentre seamless design study. Lancet. 2020;396:839–52.
30. Turtle CJ, Hanafi LA, Berger C, et al. Immunotherapy of non-Hodgkin's lymphoma with a defined ratio of CD8+ and CD4+ CD19-specific chimeric antigen receptor-modified T cells. Sci Transl Med. 2016;8:355ra116.
31. Deng Q, Han G, Puebla-Osorio N, et al. Characteristics of anti-CD19 CAR T cell infusion products associated with efficacy and toxicity in patients with large B cell lymphomas. Nat Med. 2020;26:1878–87.
32. Fraietta JA, Lacey SF, Orlando EJ, et al. Determinants of response and resistance to CD19 chimeric antigen receptor (CAR) T cell therapy of chronic lymphocytic leukemia. Nat Med. 2018;24:563–71.
33. Morrissey MA, Williamson AP, Steinbach AM, et al. Chimeric antigen receptors that trigger phagocytosis. elife. 2018;7:e36688.
34. Zhang W, Liu L, Su H, et al. Chimeric antigen receptor macrophage therapy for breast tumours mediated by targeting the tumour extracellular matrix. Br J Cancer. 2019;121:837–45.
35. Klichinsky M, Ruella M, Shestova O, et al. Human chimeric antigen receptor macrophages for cancer immunotherapy. Nat Biotechnol. 2020;38:947–53.
36. Roberts MR, Cooke KS, Tran AC, et al. Antigen-specific cytolysis by neutrophils and NK cells expressing chimeric immune receptors bearing zeta or gamma signaling domains. J Immunol. 1998;161:375–84.

Combination Therapeutics with CAR-T Cell Therapy

Mohamad M. Adada, Elizabeth L. Siegler, and Saad S. Kenderian

Abstract Adoptive cellular immunotherapy, specifically chimeric antigen receptor T-cell (CAR-T) therapy, has recently emerged as a breakthrough treatment for multiple hematological malignancies with potential for long term cure. However, multiple hurdles remain to be overcome. Some issues are inherent to CAR-T cells, such as suboptimal expansion, rapid exhaustion, or rejection. Other problems are related to the immunosuppressive tumor microenvironment, which dampens CAR-T activity. Additionally, CAR-T cell treatment is associated with significant toxicities relating to activation of the immune system, most notably cytokine release syndrome (CRS) and immune effector cell-associated neurotoxicity syndrome (ICANS). Multiple strategies are currently underway to increase CAR-T efficacy and decrease toxicity. Some of those strategies involve creating optimized stand-alone CAR-T cell products, while other strategies involve combining existing CAR-T therapies with other treatment modalities. In this chapter, we will focus on combination

M. M. Adada
T cell Engineering, Mayo Clinic, Rochester, MN, USA

Division of Hematology, Mayo Clinic, Rochester, MN, USA

Division of Oncology, Mayo Clinic, Rochester, MN, USA

E. L. Siegler
T cell Engineering, Mayo Clinic, Rochester, MN, USA

Division of Hematology, Mayo Clinic, Rochester, MN, USA

S. S. Kenderian (✉)
T cell Engineering, Mayo Clinic, Rochester, MN, USA

Division of Hematology, Mayo Clinic, Rochester, MN, USA

Department of Immunology, Mayo Clinic, Rochester, MN, USA

Department of Molecular Medicine, Mayo Clinic, Rochester, MN, USA
e-mail: Kenderian.Saad@mayo.edu

© Springer Nature Switzerland AG 2022
A. Ghobadi, J. F. DiPersio (eds.), *Gene and Cellular Immunotherapy for Cancer*, Cancer Drug Discovery and Development,
https://doi.org/10.1007/978-3-030-87849-8_5

strategies that are currently being used and/or are under exploration. We will first discuss strategies used to increase CAR-T effectiveness through combination with immunomodulatory agents, cancer-directed therapies, tumor antigen expression enhancers, or HCT. We will then discuss strategies aimed at decreasing CAR-T toxicity through combination with other immunomodulatory agents. All current clinical trials exploring these strategies will also be discussed.

Keywords Chimeric antigen receptor T cells · Cellular immunotherapy · CAR-T combination therapy · Immunomodulation · Solid tumors · Oncolytic viral therapy · Cytotoxic therapy · Radiation · Hematopoietic cell transplantation · Tocilizumab · GM-CSF

Introduction

Cellular immunotherapy has increasingly been used alongside or as an alternative to the traditional cancer treatments of surgery, chemotherapy, and radiation [1]. Chimeric antigen receptor T (CAR-T) cells are modified with an artificial receptor composed of an extracellular antibody-derived antigen-binding domain and intracellular T cell signaling and costimulatory domains [2]. CAR-T cells are MHC-independent and recognize tumor-associated antigens expressed on the cell surface. CAR-T cell therapy has displayed impressive clinical results in certain hematological malignancies, and outcomes from pivotal trials have led to the FDA approval of four different CD19-targeted CAR-T (CAR-T19) and one BCMA-targeted CAR-T cell products to date [3–5]. CAR-T cells display potent antitumor effects and high initial responses, but relapse within 1 year of treatment is common, often as a result of antigen escape or limited CAR-T persistence [6]. Additionally, CAR-T cell therapy is largely ineffective in solid tumors, due in part to the surrounding tumor microenvironment, which includes suppressive immune cells such as regulator T cells and myeloid-derived suppressor cells [7]. CAR-T cell therapy is often accompanied by severe toxicities. CAR-T cells can cause cytokine release syndrome (CRS) by prompting a massive release of inflammatory cytokines. CRS has been reported to be as high as 100% in some CAR-T19 clinical trials. CAR-T cell therapy also often results in immune effector cell-associated neurotoxicity syndrome (ICANS), which occurs in up to two-thirds of patients treated in CAR-T19 clinical trials [8].

CAR-T cell therapy is promising, but several significant hurdles must be overcome: achieving durable responses, demonstrating clinically significant activity in solid tumors, and mitigating toxicities such as CRS and ICANS. Researchers have sought to improve CAR-T cell therapy through combination therapies of CAR-T cells and additional agents such as monoclonal antibodies, small molecule inhibitors, and chemotherapeutic drugs (Table 1). These combinations are aimed to improve efficacy in hematological malignancies and in solid tumors as well as to reduce toxicity, are increasingly used in clinical trials (Table 2), and will likely play a role in the future of CAR-T cell therapy.

Table 1 Summary of CAR-T cell therapy combinations with different agents

Main Goal	Agent	Rationale	References
Increase CAR-T efficacy	Lenalidomide	– Shift Th2 to Th1 – Inhibit regulatory T cells	[12–15]
	Ibrutinib	– Irreversibly inhibit BTK – Immunomodulator – Shift Th2 to Th1	[16, 17, 19–23]
	Immune checkpoint inhibitors (pembrolizumab)	– Block the exhaustion marker, PD-1, expressed on CAR-T cells	[24–31, 93]
	Anti-4-1BB antibody	– Bind and activate the 4-1BB co-stimulatory domain on CAR-T cells	[32, 33]
	Oncolytic viruses	– Induce cancer cell lysis, thus exposing antigens to activate CAR-T cells – Use as a vehicle to carry antigens, antibodies, chemokines to the tumor cells to enhance CAR-T-specific functions	[35–38]
	PI3K inhibitors (idelalisib, bb007)	– Reduce CAR-T differentiation – Decrease rapid exhaustion	[40–47]
	Long-acting interleukin-7 agonist, NT-I7 (efineptakin alpha)	– Enhance UCAR T19 proliferation, persistence and tumor killing	[48]
	Anti-CD20 antibody (rituximab)	– Enhance synergistic cytotoxicity against tumors co-expressing CD19 and CD20 (B-NHL)	[49]
	Venetoclax	– Antagonize anti-apoptotic Bcl-2 family of proteins – Pre-sensitize cancer cells to CAR-T	[52]
	Radiation	– Sensitize CAR-T cells against tumor cells – Expose tumor antigens	[53, 54]
	Small molecule g-secretase inhibitors	– Reduce soluble BCMA shedding – Increase BCMA antigen expression on MM cells	
	Bryostatin 1	– Modulate PKC activity – Increase CD22 expression – Enrich effector and memory CAR-T cells	[55]
	HCT	– Use CAR-T as a bridge to induce remission prior to HCT consolidative treatment – Use CAR-T as a rescue following HCT relapse	[2, 56, 94]

(continued)

Table 1 (continued)

Main Goal	Agent	Rationale	References
Decrease CAR-T toxicity	IL-6 or IL-6R inhibitors (tocilizumab, siltuximab)	– Target IL-6, an essential cytokine in CRS development – Reduce CRS manifestations	[50, 71]
	GM-CSF blockers (lenzilumab)	– Block GM-CSF to suppress myeloid cells, a significant source of pro-inflammatory cytokines	[70, 77]
	IL-1 inhibitors (anakinra)	– Block pro-inflammatory cytokine IL-1, which in turn reduces IL-6 during CRS, to lessen CRS and ICANS manifestations	[78]
	JAK/STAT inhibitors (ruxolitinib, itacitinib)	– Decrease levels of inflammatory cytokines	[79, 81]
	CAR-T inhibitors (dasatinib)	– Reversibly suppress T cell activity by inhibiting T cell signaling kinases (Src, Fyn,Lck) – Decrease cytokine and chemokine levels	[82, 83]
	Defibrotide	– Protect endothelial cells from excessive cytokines, which may play a role in endothelial damage and ICANS	[84]
	TNF-a inhibitors (etanercept)	– Block the effect of the proinflammatory mediator TNFa	[85–87]
	Steroids	– Systemically suppress the immune system – Inhibit white blood cell and cytokine production	[88–90]
	PI3K inhibitors (duvelisib)	– Decrease the secretion of IL-6 – No effect on CAR-T19 functions	[91]

Table 2 Current clinical trials examining different combination therapeutics with CAR-T cell therapy

Agent	Agent function	Clinical trial identifier	CAR-T target	Cancer type
Lenalidomide	Immunomodulatory drug	NCT03070327	EGFRt/ BCMA-41BBz-CAR-T	MM
		NCT04287660	BCMA-CAR-T	MM
Ibrutinib	BTK inhibitor	NCT03960840	CD19-CAR-T (YTB323)	CLL SLL DLBCL ALL
		NCT04234061	CD19-CAR-T (tisagenlecleucel)	MCL
		NCT03331198	CD19-CAR-T (JCAR017)	CLL SLL

(continued)

Table 2 (continued)

Agent	Agent function	Clinical trial identifier	CAR-T target	Cancer type
Durvalumab	Anti-PD-L1 antibody	NCT02706405	Autologous CD19–4-1BB-CD3zeta-EGFRt-expressing CD4+/CD8+ Central Memory T-lymphocytes JCAR014	DLBCL Primary Mediastinal Large B-Cell Lymphoma High Grade B-Cell Lymphoma
		NCT03310619	CD19-CAR-T (JCAR017)	NHL DLBCL FL
Atezolizumab	Anti-PD-L1 antibody	NCT02926833	KTE-C19	DLBCL
Pembrolizumab	Anti-PD-1 antibody	NCT03287817	CD19/CD22-CAR-T (AUTO3)	DLBCL
		NCT02650999	CD19-CAR-T (CTL019)	DLBCL FL MCL
Utomilumab	4-1BB/CD137 agonist antibody	NCT03704298	CD19-CAR-T (axicabtagene ciloleucel)	Large B-cell Lymphoma
CAdVEC	Oncolytic adenovirus	NCT03740256	HER2-CAR-T	Bladder Cancer Head and Neck Squamous Cell Carcinoma Cancer of the Salivary Gland Lung Cancer Breast Cancer Gastric Cancer Esophageal Colorectal cancer Pancreatic cancer
bb007	PI3K inhibitor	NCT03274219	BCMA-CAR-T (bb21217)	MM
Rituximab	Anti-CD20 antibody	NCT00799136	CD19-CAR-T	AIDS-related lymphoma

(continued)

Table 2 (continued) M. M. Adada et al.

Agent	Agent function	Clinical trial identifier	CAR-T target	Cancer type
Venetoclax	BH3 mimetic	NCT04640909	CD19-CAR-T	CLL
Radiation		NCT04473937	CD19-CAR-T	B-cell Lymphoma
		NCT04726787	CD19-CAR-T	DLCBL
		NCT03392545	CAR-T cells	High Grade Glioma. Glioblastoma
LY3039478 (JSMD194)	Small molecule g-secretase inhibitor	NCT03502577	BCMA-CAR-T	MM
Lenzilumab	Anti-GM-CSF antibody	NCT04314843	CD19-CAR-T (axicabtagene ciloleucel)	Large B-cell Lymphoma
Anakinra	Anti-IL1 receptor antibody	NCT04148430	CAR-T cells	ALL B-Cell lymphoma NHL
		NCT04359784	CD19-CAR-T (axicabtagene ciloleucel)	NHL
		NCT04432506	CD19-CAR-T (axicabtagene ciloleucel)	DLBCL Primary Mediastinal Large B-Cell Lymphoma High Grade B-Cell Lymphoma
		NCT04150913	CD19-CAR-T (axicabtagene ciloleucel)	NHL
		NCT04205838	CD19-CAR-T (axicabtagene ciloleucel)	DLBCL Primary Mediastinal Large B-Cell Lymphoma High Grade B-Cell Lymphoma
		NCT03430011	BCMA-CAR-T (JCARH125)	MM
Itacitinib	JAK1-specific inhibitor	NCT04071366	CD19-CAR-T	Any approved hematologic indication
Dasatinib	Tyrosine kinase inhibitor	NCT04603872	CD19-CAR-T and BCMA-CAR-T	MM ALL NHL
Defibrotide	Endothelial cell protector	NCT03954106	CD19-CAR-T	DLBCL

MM multiple myeloma, *DLBCL* Diffuse large B-cell lymphoma, *FL* Follicular lymphoma, *NHL* Non-Hodgkin Lymphoma, *MCL* Mantle Cell Lymphoma, *ALL* Acute lymphocytic leukemia, *CLL* chronic lymphocytic leukemia, *SLL* small lymphocytic lymphoma, *Th* T helper

Combinations that Increase CAR-T Efficacy

CAR-T Combination with Immunomodulatory Agents

Lenalidomide

Lenalidomide (LEN) is currently approved for the treatment of multiple myeloma (MM) and mantle cell lymphoma (MCL) [9, 10]. LEN acts by inducing the degradation of transcription factors (such as Ikaros and Aiolos) [11]. This leads to modification of T cell responses by increasing IL-2 production, shifting the T helper 2 (Th2) response to Th1, and inhibiting the expansion of regulatory T cells (Treg). LEN was shown to increase the efficacy of CD19- and CD20-targeted CAR-T cells by increasing IFNg production and CD69 activation marker *in vitro* [12]. It also resulted in increased antitumor activity in various murine models of B-cell non-Hodgkin lymphoma (B-NHL) [12]. Similarly, LEN enhanced the immune functions of CAR-T cells targeting CS1 [13] or B-cell maturation antigen (BCMA) [14] for the treatment of MM by improving cytotoxicity, Th1 cytokine production, and immune synapse formation. Importantly, LEN maintained CAR-T activity in repeated stimulation assays, suggesting a possible role in curbing T cell exhaustion [14]. Multiple clinical trials evaluating the effectiveness of CAR-T combination with LEN are currently underway. Among these are a phase 1 study of EGFRt/BCMA-CAR-T cells in patients with MM with or without LEN (NCT03070327) and a phase 3 trial that is evaluating the safety and efficacy of BiRd regimen (clarithromycin, LEN, dexamethasone and BCMA-CAR-T cells in MM patients (NCT04287660). The effect of LEN in promoting CAR-T cell activity against solid tumors was also recently tested in preclinical studies. CAR-T cells directed against CD133 and HER2 expressed in glioma and breast cancer exhibited superior killing of target cells, and enhanced CAR-T proliferation and cytokine secretion [15]. However, these effects were only tested on human cancer cell lines *in vitro* and not *in vivo* in solid cancer models.

Ibrutinib

Ibrutinib is an irreversible inhibitor of Bruton's tyrosine kinase (BTK) that is currently being used for the treatment of several types of B-cell lymphoma, Waldenstrom's macroglobulinemia, and chronic graft versus host disease. Several reports have demonstrated the immune-modulatory properties of ibrutinib on CAR-T cells. It was noted that patients with chronic lymphocytic leukemia (CLL) who were receiving ibrutinib for more than 1 year at the time of apheresis to generate CD19-targeted CAR-T cells (CAR-T19) had improved CAR-T expansion *ex vivo* and enhanced engraftment and positive clinical response following treatment [16]. This also correlated with decreased expression of exhaustion markers such as PD-1 and CD200. These results were also verified in xenograft mouse models of acute lymphoblastic leukemia (ALL) in which concurrent therapy with ibrutinib and CAR-T19 resulted in enhanced T cell expansion and decreased tumor burden

[16]. Similar results were obtained *in vitro* and in *in vivo* mouse models of MCL [17]. This combination has been hypothesized to induce complete remission in patients with high-risk CLL with TP53 aberrations that failed prior Bcl-2 inhibitor therapy, and to act as an excellent bridge for hematopoietic stem cell transplantation [18]. Given the promising results of these preclinical experiments, the first clinical trial assessing the safety and feasibility of administering ibrutinib concurrently with CAR-T19 in patients with CLL was completed and published in 2020 [19]. Out of the 19 patients enrolled, 15 patients responded, with 11 patients achieving undetectable minimal residual disease in bone marrow. Although CRS severity was lower with the addition of ibrutinib, progression-free survival was unchanged [19]. Furthermore, ibrutinib has recently been shown to improve CAR-T19 production from patients with CLL, with increased cell viability and expansion, and enrichment in less-differentiated naïve-like CAR-T cells (CD45RA + CCR7+) with decreased expression of exhaustion markers such as PD-1, TIM-3 and LAG-3 [20]. Finally, emerging evidence suggest that this combination can be applied to other types of B-cell lymphomas [21]. It remains unclear how or when ibrutinib should be used to enhance CAR-T cell therapy. One study treated patients with CAR-T19 after they achieved partial or minimal residual disease positive response with ibrutinib while another study used CAR-T19 in patients progressing/failing ibrutinib [22, 23].

PD-1 Blockade

(a) Hematologic malignancies

CAR-T19 cell therapy has been shown to induce complete remission in more than 90% of patients with ALL with durable remission rates of 50–60%; however, only 20–30% of CLL patients achieve sustained remission following CAR-T cell therapy [24]. Transcriptomic analyses revealed that T cells obtained from non-responder CLL patients have upregulated pathways involved in exhaustion and apoptosis with increased expression of co-inhibitory receptors such as PD-1, TIM-3 and LAG-3. Pediatric patients with ALL who had failed previous CAR-T19 therapy displayed improved outcomes and better CAR-T persistence when the anti-PD-1 antibody pembrolizumab was added to the treatment regimen [25]. These outcomes were similar to two other reports that evaluated the role of combining CAR-T19 cells with another anti-PD1 antibody, nivolumab, in 11 patients with refractory/relapsed B-NHL [26] and refractory follicular lymphoma [27]. Multiple clinical trials are currently exploring the role of immune checkpoint blockade with CAR-T cell therapy in diffuse large B cell lymphoma (DLBCL) (NCT02706405, NCT02926833, NCT03287817), aggressive B-NHL (NCT03310619), and MCL (NCT02650999).

(b) Solid tumors

The application of CAR-T cell therapy to solid tumors has proven to be more challenging due to antigen sequestration in organ tissues (discussed below) and the immunosuppressive tumor microenvironment. The combination of immune checkpoint inhibition (ICI) with CAR-T cell therapy has proven to be beneficial in Her-2 transgenic mice models where anti-PD-1 antibody improved CAR-T proliferation and antitumor efficacy [28]. Similar findings were also observed in an orthotopic mouse model of pleural mesothelioma, where anti-PD-1 antibody rescued the effector functions of exhausted CAR-T cells [29]. Blocking PD-1 on liver myeloid-derived suppressor cells (L-MDSC) proved beneficial in a murine model of carcinoembryonic antigen+ liver metastases, where L-MDSCs are thought to suppress CAR-T function [30]. On the other hand, not all trials yielded a clear benefit of adding PD-1 blockade to CAR-T cell therapy. In particular, one clinical trial investigated the efficacy of combining ICI with CAR-T cell therapy in patients with relapsed or refractory neuroblastoma. While lymphodepletion with fludarabine and cyclophosphamide increased CAR-T cell expansion and persistence, the addition of pembrolizumab did not yield additional benefit [31]. This trial was conducted on 11 patients; therefore, larger trials are needed.

Agonistic Anti-Costimulatory Receptor Antibodies

Third-generation CAR constructs contain two co-stimulatory domains: CD28 and 4-1BB. Initially, these had been developed to improve the efficacy and decrease rapid exhaustion of second-generation CARs, which only had one co-stimulatory domain; however, they did not show superiority over second-generation CARs, and it is unclear whether including more than two co-stimulatory signals adds any benefits to CAR-T cell function. Alternatively, stimulatory monoclonal antibodies against 4-1BB have been developed and used in combination with second-generation CARs [32]. Anti-4-1BB enhanced the anti-tumor efficacy of CAR-T cells directed against Her2 in a Her-2 transgenic mouse model [33]. Surprisingly, this not only resulted in increased IFNg secretion, but also reduced the levels of Tregs and MDSCs, thus decreasing immunosuppression [33]. This could prove to be a safer approach for using CAR-T cells, as it would allow for dose reduction and overcoming the immunosuppressive tumor environment. Zuma-11 (NCT03704298) is currently underway to evaluate the safety of CAR-T19 in combination with utomilumab (a human monoclonal antibody that is a 4-1BB/CD137 agonist [34]) in patients with refractory large B-cell lymphoma.

Oncolytic Viral Therapy

Oncolytic viruses (OV) have emerged as encouraging agents for the treatment of solid tumors. They are currently being engineered to specifically target cancer cells, which they infect, undergo replication, and induce lysis. OVs are also used as a vehicle to carry genes encoding cytokines, chemokines, enzymes, or antibodies to further bolster their therapeutic potential. The recent approval of talimogene laheparepvec (T-VEC), human herpes simplex virus carrying recombinant granulo-cyte macrophage colony-stimulating factor (GM-CSF) for the treatment of mela-noma, has increased the interest in the field and resulted in a boom of clinical trials assessing the use of OV therapy in a myriad of tumors. OV therapy is able to release tumor antigens that were previously hidden from the immune system, promote a strong anti-tumor response, and debulk solid tumors. This provided a strong ratio-nale to combine OVs with CAR-T cell therapy, and several strategies have been employed. One study aimed to use OV as an approach to overcome the failure of T cells to migrate to the highly immunosuppressive tumor milieu of neuroblastoma. The oncolytic adenovirus Ad5d24 was engineered to express IL-15 and RANTES, which are known in inducing T cell migration and survival. When combined with CAR-T cells directed against the tumor antigen GD2, the apoptosis of cancer cells was accelerated and the intratumoral concentration of CAR-T cells was increased. This led to an increase in the survival of tumor-bearing mice [35]. Further studies assessed the possibility of blocking inhibitory immune checkpoints such as PD-L1 by local production of anti-PD-L1 mini-antibodies to improve CAR-T efficacy. The co-administration of the OV expressing PD-L1-blocking mini-antibody, CAd-VECPDL1, with CAR-T cells directed against HER2 in a prostate cancer xenograft mouse model led enhanced antitumor activity compared to the administration of each element as a monotherapy [36]. This strategy was further optimized by allow-ing the OV to co-express the PD-L1 mini-antibody and IL-12p70 to prevent the loss of CAR-T cells from the tumor site in a head and neck squamous cell carcinoma xenograft mouse model [37]. This proved to be superior to Cad-VECPDL1, with substantial improvement in overall survival [37]. Surprisingly, this result was not reproduced by coadministration of CAR-T cells and systemic infusion of anti-PD-L1 antibody [36]. A different approach engineered OV to express the same tumor antigens targeted by the CAR-T cells as a strategy to re-stimulate the CAR-T cells and enhance their functions [38]. These promising strategies opened the door to a myriad of other opportunities that can be exploited by combining OVs which act as a local source of multiple proteins to enhance CAR-T effectiveness. In addition to delivering immunostimulatory cytokines and ICIs, we can envision other tactics such as using OVs to deliver immune co-stimulatory molecules, molecules targeting immunosuppressive cells or metabolic pathways, pro-apoptotic molecules, or mol-ecules that are able to alter the structure of the tumor microenvironment such matrix metalloproteinases.

Inhibitors of the PI3K Pathway

The PI3K-AkT-mTOR-c-myc pathway is essential for T cell activation, prolifera-tion, and differentiation [39]. It was suggested that inhibiting this pathway might halt T cell differentiation during *ex vivo* T cell expansion and thus shift the CAR-T phenotype into a less differentiated state that is less prone to rapid exhaustion. IL-15 has been reported to reduce mTOR activity, and its supplementation to CAR-T cell culture resulted in less differentiated CAR-T cells [40]. Similarly, inhibition of AkT yielded analogous results [41]. Importantly, the treatment of T cells with the B cell receptor and PI3K delta inhibitor, idelalisib (which is currently approved for the treatment of CLL and follicular lymphoma), led to the production of less differentiated CAR-T cells with improved antitumor activity against CD19+ [42], CD33+ [43], and mesothelin+ target cells [44]. The simultaneous treatment of CAR-T cells with vasoactive intestinal peptide and PI3K antagonists lead to the inhibition of anti-CD5 CAR-T cell differentiation during *ex vivo* expansion, which lead to increased persistence in DLBCL mouse models [45]. These results have led to the development of bb21217, which is an anti-BCMA CAR-T cell therapy that adds the PI3K inhibitor, bb007, during *ex vivo* expansion to enrich memory-like T cells. Clinical trial NCT03274219 (CRB-402) is currently underway to assess the safety, efficacy and duration of bb21217 therapy in patients with relapsed refractory multiple myeloma. Preliminary results published in 2019 were encouraging, with 83% of patients demonstrating clinical response and long term persistence of CAR-T cells [46]. Updated results presented at the ASH annual meeting in 2020 showed similar trends. Other possible modulators of this pathway include B cell adaptor for PI3K [47] and c-myc [47], which have been shown to decrease CAR-T differentiation and improve CAR-T persistence and antitumor activity upon inhibition. Therefore, the inhibition of the PI3K/AkT axis represents a generalizable strategy that can generate large numbers of CAR-T cells with superior cytotoxic abilities and an early memory phenotype.

Long-Acting Interleukin-7 Agonist (NT-I7)

IL-7 is pro-lymphoid growth factor that promotes T cell growth. Its efficacy in promoting CAR-T functions was tested using its long-acting form of recombinant human ilterleukin-7 that is fused with hybrid Fc and is known as NT-I7 or efineptakin alpha [48]. Mice treated with Universal CAR-T19 (UCAT19) and who received 3 infusions of NT-I7 had improved survival compared to those that did not receive interleukin 7 products. In addition, there was a better tumor control with enhanced UCAR T19 proliferation and persistence [48]. This combination has recently received FDA clearance to initiate phase 1b clinical trial for patients with relapsed/refractory large B-cell lymphoma.

Combination with Cancer Directed Therapies

Rituximab

Rituximab is an anti-CD20 antibody that is used in a vast array of B cell lymphomas with variable success. The development of CAR-T cells targeting CD19 or CD38 on B-NHL cells has shown clinical benefit. It was previously shown that the combination of CAR-T19 and/or anti-CD38 CAR-T with rituximab confers an enhanced synergistic cytotoxicity against B-NHL in xenograft models [49]. In addition, this combination increased tumor suppressing activity for over 2 months [49]. Antigen escape was a common resistance mechanism that was observed in patients who relapsed or failed CAR-T19 therapy in the landmark Zuma-1 trial that led to CAR-T19 approval in adults with NHL [50]. Currently, ZUMA-14 (NCT04002401) is a clinical trial that is evaluating the combination of CAR-T19 with either rituximab or lenalidomide in refractory large B cell lymphoma [51].

Venetoclax

The anti-apoptotic Bcl-2 family of proteins is overexpressed in CLL and NHL. Compounds such as venetoclax are BH3 mimetics and antagonize these proteins. They have demonstrated significant efficacy in clinical trials and are currently used in the clinic. The combination of venetoclax with CAR-T19 was studied under three different conditions: pre-treatment with venetoclax prior to CAR-T19 administration, simultaneous therapy, or the injection of CAR-T19 cells following venetoclax treatment [52]. It was shown that only the pre-sensitization of the cancer cells with venetoclax enhanced CAR-T cells cytotoxicity and persistence by upregulating the CD19 antigen and pro-apoptotic proteins [52]. On the other hand, venetoclax administration with or following CAR-T cell administration decreased CAR-T proliferation and led to inferior outcomes [52]. A new cohort of the TRANSCEND 004 clinical trial is investigating the combination of venetoclax with the CAR-T19 product lisocabtagene maraleucel in the treatment of CLL.

Radiation

Radiation is emerging as an attractive tool to sensitize CAR-T cells against tumor cells. Exposing pancreatic cancer cells to low dose radiation increased the efficacy of CAR-T cells in killing sialyl Lewis-A (sLeA) + cells. Surprisingly, it also increased CAR-T efficacy in killing sLeA- cells, providing a novel approach to preventing CAR-T resistance upon antigen escape [53]. Similarly, radiation increased CAR-T cell efficacy, persistence, and activity in an orthotopic glioblastoma mouse model [54].

Combination to Modulate Tumor Antigen Expression

Small Molecule g-Secretase (GS) Inhibitors

BCMA is a tumor necrosis factor receptor superfamily member that binds B-cell activating factor to promote differentiation of B cells and survival of malignant MM. However, most patients relapse following treatment. Failures has been attributed to decreased levels of BCMA expression on the MM cell surface due to cleavage by the GS complex, thus limiting CAR-T cell recognition. In addition, following cleavage, there is release of soluble BCMA, which in turn is capable of inhibiting CAR-T cell functions. GS inhibitors that were initially studied for Alzheimer's disease have been tested to see if they can reduce soluble BCMA shedding and thus restore CAR-T functions. Indeed, administration of GS inhibitors increased the density of BCMA on MM cells in mice and in patients. A clinical trial is currently underway to test the efficacy of combining GS inhibitors and anti-BCMA CAR-T in MM patients (NCT03502577) (36).

Bryostatin 1

Anti-CD22-CAR-T cell therapy has been proven to induce rapid remission in the majority of patients with ALL. Unfortunately, most patients relapse due to antigen escape manifested by decreased CD22 expression on malignant cells. Bryostatin 1, a natural product that is used in humans and shown to modulate protein kinase C, is known to upregulate CD22 expression. Bryostatin 1 pretreatment of both B-ALL and DLCBL cell lines enhanced CD22 CAR-T cytotoxicity and cytokine production. Mice that received leukemic cells that were pretreated with bryostatin 1 showed enrichment in effector and memory CAR-T cell populations. In addition, the administration of bryostatin 1 following CAR-T injection resulted in increased CAR-T persistence and lengthening of the remission time [55].

Combination with Hematopoietic Cell Transplantation

The role of CAR-T cell therapy in the context of hematopoietic cell transplantation (HCT) has been studied with different orders of administration. HCT remains an important option in multiple hematologic malignancies as it offers considerable cure rates. However, it comes with significant morbidity and mortality, and relapses are not uncommon. Several studies have shown that CAR-T cells can induce remissions as a bridge to HCT; This is especially true in patients with B-ALL. In multiple trials, children and young adults with ALL who received CAR-T19 constructed with the CD28 co-stimulatory domains showed improved survival among those who proceeded with allo-HCT [56, 57]. This was not the case in another study performed at the University of Pennsylvania Children's hospital of Philadelphia, where the ELIANA trial showed that proceeding with allo-HCT following CAR-T19 does not confer a survival benefit [58–61]. This trial differed from the previous as it used CAR-T19 cells constructed with the 4-1BB costimulatory domain, which showed superior persistence. However, these results did not hold in multiple subsequent studies done in the United States and outside, where bridging to allo-HCT seemed to provide better outcomes [62–65]. In summary, until further randomized trials are conducted, the decision to proceed with allo-HCT following CAR-T19 administration should be individualized according to the tumor involved, patients' characteristics and prior treatment. In general, young patients with B-ALL that received CD28-based CAR-T19 should proceed to allo-HCT due to lack of persistence. Those who received 4-1BB-based CAR-T 19 (such as tisagenlecluecel) may not need transplantation given sustained remissions. However, it is prudent to prepare all these patients for possible transplant given unpredictability of CAR-T19 persistence in this population. On the other hand, unlike B-ALL, current trials data does not support consolidative transplantation for Non Hodgkin Lymphoma patients, and who responded to CAR-T19 [66].

Combinations that Decrease CAR-T Toxicity

Despite the remarkable efficacy of CAR-T cell therapy, treatment-associated toxicities remain a huge barrier, with considerable morbidity and mortality. The two most common CAR-T-associated toxicities are CRS and ICANS, which will be described in detail later in this book [67]. In short, these events are caused by the secretion of high levels of pro-inflammatory cytokines, particularly IL-6 and GM-CSF, by activated T cells and myeloid cells and are characterized by fever, hypotension, pulmonary insufficiency and altered mental status. Currently, the mainstays of treatment of CAR-T cell toxicities include tocilizumab and steroids. While tocilizumab is effective in reversing CRS, it does not reduce the severity or rates of ICANS [68, 69]. The use of steroids has been shown to ameliorate the severity of ICANS in cohort 4 of the Zuma-1 clinical trial, but its role in the management of ICANS remains controversial, and concerns exist regarding the impact of steroids on CAR-T cell efficacy.

In this section, we will be describing several therapeutic agents that are given alongside or shortly after CAR-T injection to manage CAR-T-associated toxicities.

IL-6 or IL-6R Inhibition (Tocilizumab, Siltuxumab)

The inflammatory cytokine IL-6 has been shown to play an essential part in the development of CRS [70]. Monoclonal antibodies targeting IL-6R (tocilizumab) or IL-6 (siltuxumab) are currently the main stay of treatment for CRS [50, 71]. Tocilizumab, originally used for the treatment of rheumatoid arthritis, has been more commonly used than siltuxumab, and usually results in the resolution of CRS symptoms within hours [72]. It has proven to be compatible with CAR-T cell therapy as it does not appear to affect therapeutic outcomes [50, 71]. Combination of CAR-T19 with the IL-6 receptor blockade tocilizumab has been investigated as a strategy to prevent CAR-T cell toxicity. Results from the PLAT-02 study, which was originally designed to study the safety and efficacy of CAR-T19 cell therapy in patients with ALL, showed that giving tocilizumab early in the course of mild CRS decreased the transition into severe CRS with no negative effects on therapeutic efficacy of CAR-T cells [73]. Similar results were seen in the safety expansion cohort of the Zuma-1 trial evaluating CAR-T19 cell therapy in patients with NHL [74]. Tocilizumab administration on day 2 reduced the incidence of severe CRS but had no effect on ICANS [74].

GM-CSF Depletion (Lenzilumab)

Multiple recent studies have suggested that myeloid cells are considered an essential source for the production of proinflammatory cytokines that are involved in CRS and ICANS [75, 76]. Therefore, GM-CSF, an important growth factor involved in myeloid cell stimulation, evolved as a possible target for the treatment of CAR-T-associated toxicities. Indeed, the neutralization of GM-CSF with lenzilumab significantly reduced markers of CRS and ICANS (weight loss, neuroinflammation, inflammatory cytokines) when administered with CAR-T cells in a patient-derived ALL xenograft model [77]. GM-CSF neutralization also enhanced CAR-T19 therapeutic efficacy. Given the dual benefit of improved CAR-T efficacy and reduced toxicity, a phase I/II clinical trial (NCT04314843) is currently under way to evaluate the safety and efficacy of sequenced therapy with CAR-T19 and lenzilumab in patients with relapsed or refractory large-B-cell lymphoma [70].

IL-1 Inhibition (Anakinra)

The failure of tocilizumab to ameliorate ICANS has led to the investigation of the role of other cytokines in ICANS development. IL-1 has been shown to precede IL-6 secretion in CAR-T-associated toxicities. Anakinra, an IL-1 receptor-blocking antibody used in the treatment of rheumatoid arthritis, abolished both CRS and ICANS in a humanized leukemia mouse model [78]. This led to a substantial increase in survival and paved the way for two clinical trials (NCT04148430, NCT04150913) currently underway for the evaluation of anakinra as a strategy to prevent ICANS during the infusion of CAR-T19 in patients with NHL.

JAK/STAT Inhibition (Ruxolitinib, Itacitinib)

Ruxolitinib, a JAK/STAT pathway inhibitor, has been shown to be efficacious in decreasing the levels of inflammatory cytokines in myelofibrosis, polycythemia vera and hemophagocytic lymphohistiocytosis in multiple clinical studies. In an acute myeloid leukemia xenograft model, mice that were co-treated with CD23-targeted CAR-T cells and ruxolitinib exhibited a decrease in the levels of IFN-g and TNF-a, with less severe CRS manifestations than mice treated with CAR-T alone. In addition, CAR-T anti leukemic efficacy was not affected, and survival was improved [79]. The inhibition of the JAK/STAT pathway was further studied with the JAK1-specific inhibitor itacitinib [79] [80],. Using NSG mice bearing CD19-expressing NAMALWA human lymphoma cells, itacitinib significantly reduced CRS-associated cytokine levels without affecting the antitumor activity of CAR-T19 cells [81]. Interestingly, the inhibition of cytokine release was more substantial than that seen with the current standard of care, tocilizumab. This has led to a clinical trial (NCT04071366) that is currently evaluating the role of itacitinib in the prevention of CRS.

Reversible CAR-T Inhibition (Dasatinib)

Dasatinib is a tyrosine kinase inhibitor that is FDA-approved for the treatment of chronic myelogenous leukemia and ALL. It suppresses the activity of T cells by inhibiting signaling kinases (Src, Fyn, Lck) which are downstream of the T cell receptor. Dasatinib has also been shown to decrease the levels of multiple cytokines and chemokines; as such, it has subsequently been explored in preventing CAR-T-associated toxicities. Treatment with dasatinib caused a rapid and reversible inhibition of antigen-dependent activation of CAR-T cells with decreased proliferation, killing and cytokine production in a xenograft model [82]. Interestingly, dasatinib-treated CAR-T cells regained their full anti-tumor capacity once dasatinib was removed. Similar results were described in another publication, which also showed that a short course treatment with this kinase inhibitor was protective against CRS in a xenograft mouse model [83].

Endothelial Cell Protection (Defibrotide)

Defibrotide is a mixture of single-stranded oligonucleotides and is used in the treatment of veno-occlusive disease by protecting endothelial cells and inhibiting clotting. ICANS has been suggested to be caused by endothelial cell damage from excessive cytokine release [84]. There are currently no preclinical studies assessing the combination of CAR-T19 and defibrotide; however, a clinical trial (NCT03954106) is currently under way to evaluate the safety and efficacy of defibrotide in the prevention of ICANS in patients with relapsed or refractory DLBCL receiving CAR-T cell therapy.

TNF-a Inhibition (Etanercept)

Etanercept, soluble TNF-a receptor, is widely used in the treatment of CRS in clinical trials conducted in China [85, 86]. However, its efficacy is not well studied, and results have been controversial. One ALL patient who was treated with CAR-T19 and developed severe CRS responded very well to a combination treatment of etanercept and tocilizumab without affecting CAR-T expansion [87]. In another study involving ALL as well, one patient developed severe and ultimately fatal CRS that was unresponsive to this combination treatment [87]. Further larger scale studies are needed to evaluate the benefit of TNF-a blockade in the treatment of CAR-T-associated toxicities.

Systemic Immune System Suppression (Steroids)

Steroids have long been used to suppress an overly active immune system in the context of auto-immune disease. Steroids are commonly used in the treatment of CAR-T-associated CRS and ICANS in addition to currently approved therapies such as tocilizumab. Earlier reports have suggested that corticosteroids are associated with CAR-T cell exhaustion and decreased efficacy [88]. Recent studies are more controversial. One study has shown no difference in patients who received steroids versus those that received tocilizumab in patients with B-cell ALL [89]. On the other hand, a more recent report that was presented at ASH in 2021 showed that corticosteroids used at higher dosages, or at earlier stages with prolonged use, have been associated with shorter progression-free and overall survival in patients with large B-cell lymphoma [90].

PI3K Inhibition

Finally, duvelisib, a selective dual PI3K-δ,γ that is approved for the treatment of relapsed/refractory CLL and follicular lymphoma, has been shown to decrease CRS while maintaining CAR-T19 functions [91]. This has been shown by measuring the levels of IL-6, as a surrogate marker for CRS. Although duvelisib resulted in significant reductions of IL-6 levels in vitro and in-vivo, there was a statistically insignificant decrease of CAR-T19 efficacy (~20%) [92]. Further preclinical and clinical studies are needed to confirm the role of PI3K inhibition on CRS prevention.

The use of novel molecular inhibitors or antibodies to modulate the toxicities of CAR-T cell therapy is promising yet still in its beginning. There is a fine balance between decreasing toxic amounts of proinflammatory cytokines induced by CAR-T cells while still maintaining their antitumor efficacy. While current modalities focus on treating CAR-T side effects, there is emerging evidence which suggests that treatment with these molecules prior to CAR-T administration could be more beneficial. Additional studies are needed to weigh the benefits of preventative, preemptive, vs reactive treatment with respect to CAR-T cell efficacy.

Conclusion

CAR-T cell therapy has demonstrated remarkable clinical outcomes in certain blood cancers, but lack of long-term efficacy, inactivity in solid tumors, and serious toxicities present challenges to its widespread adoption. As the mechanisms behind each of these shortcomings become untangled, researchers have applied additional agents in CAR-T cell therapy to improve safety and efficacy. Immunomodulatory agents, including small molecule inhibitors, monoclonal antibodies, and oncolytic viruses, have been shown to improve CAR-T cell function in hematological malignancies and in solid tumors. Combination with existing chemotherapeutic drugs or radiation has demonstrated increased tumor suppression and CAR-T persistence. Small molecule drugs have been employed to prevent antigen escape, which remains one of the most common reasons for CAR-T failure. Progress has been made on the toxicity front as well, with small molecule drugs and monoclonal antibodies displaying improved outcomes regarding CRS and ICANS incidence and severity. Clinical trials of such combination therapies are nascent but promising and need close follow up as new results emerge. Additional patient data and clinical experience is needed to bring these therapies into mainstream medicine. The current studies outlined in this chapter offer potential solutions to removing medical, geographical, and financial barriers to CAR-T cell therapy through improving therapeutic efficacy and expanding applications to solid tumors, lowering safety risks to allow the adoption of CAR-T cell therapy outside select large medical facilities, and reducing costs through the simplification of patient care.

Acknowledgments This work was supported through K12CA090628 (SSK), Mayo Clinic K2R Career Development Program (SSK), the Mayo Clinic Center for Individualized Medicine (SSK).

Disclosures SSK is an inventor on patents in the field of CAR immunotherapy that are licensed to Novartis (through an agreement between Mayo Clinic, University of Pennsylvania, and Novartis). SSK is an inventor on patents in the field of CAR immunotherapy that are licensed to Humanigen (through Mayo Clinic). SSK is an inventor on patents in the field of CAR immunotherapy that are licensed to Mettaforge (through Mayo Clinic). SSK receives research funding from Kite, Gilead, Juno, Celgene, Novartis, Humanigen, MorphoSys, Leahlabs, Tolero, Sunesis, and Lentigen. SSK has participated in advisory meetings of Juno, Celegene, Kite, Gilead and Humanigen. SSK has participated in data safety monitoring boards of Humanigen.

Author Contributions SSK formulated the initial concept and outline of the manuscript. MMA, ELS and SSK wrote the manuscript. All authors edited and approved the final version of the book chapter.

References

1. Ruella M, Kenderian SS. Next-generation chimeric antigen receptor T-cell therapy: going off the shelf. BioDrugs. 2017;31:473–81.
2. Porter DL, Levine BL, Kalos M, Bagg A, June CH. Chimeric antigen receptor-modified T cells in chronic lymphoid leukemia. N Engl J Med. 2011;365:725–33.
3. Han D, Xu Z, Zhuang Y, Ye Z, Qian Q. Current progress in CAR-T cell therapy for hematological malignancies. J Cancer. 2021;12:326–34.
4. Vitale C, Strati P. CAR T-cell therapy for B-cell non-Hodgkin lymphoma and chronic lymphocytic Leukemia: clinical trials and real-world experiences. Front Oncol. 2020;10:849.
5. Yu B, Jiang T, Liu D. BCMA-targeted immunotherapy for multiple myeloma. J Hematol Oncol. 2020;13:125.
6. Cox MJ, Lucien F, Sakemura R, et al. Leukemic extracellular vesicles induce chimeric antigen receptor T cell dysfunction in chronic lymphocytic leukemia. Mol Ther. 2021;29:1529.
7. Rodriguez-Garcia A, Palazon A, Noguera-Ortega E, Powell DJ Jr, Guedan S. CAR-T cells hit the tumor microenvironment: strategies to overcome tumor escape. Front Immunol. 2020;11:1109.
8. Ruff MW, Siegler EL, Kenderian SS. A concise review of neurologic complications associated with chimeric antigen receptor T-cell immunotherapy. Neurol Clin. 2020;38:953–63.

9. Raza S, Safyan RA, Lentzsch S. Immunomodulatory drugs (IMiDs) in multiple myeloma. Curr Cancer Drug Targets. 2017;17:846–57.
10. Skarbnik AP, Goy AH. Lenalidomide for mantle cell lymphoma. Expert Rev Hematol. 2015;8:257–64.
11. Yamshon S, Ruan J. IMiDs new and old. Curr Hematol Malig Rep. 2019;14:414–25.
12. Otáhal P, Průková D, Král V, et al. Lenalidomide enhances antitumor functions of chimeric antigen receptor modified T cells. Onco Targets Ther. 2016;5:e1115940.
13. Wang X, Walter M, Urak R, et al. Lenalidomide enhances the function of CS1 chimeric antigen receptor-redirected T cells against multiple myeloma. Clin Cancer Res. 2018;24:106–19.
14. Works M, Soni N, Hauskins C, et al. Anti-B-cell maturation antigen chimeric antigen receptor T cell function against multiple myeloma is enhanced in the presence of Lenalidomide. Mol Cancer Ther. 2019;18:2246–57.
15. Wang Z, Zhou G, Risu N, et al. Lenalidomide enhances CAR-T cell activity against solid tumor cells. Cell Transplant. 2020;29:963689720920825.
16. Fraietta JA, Beckwith KA, Patel PR, et al. Ibrutinib enhances chimeric antigen receptor T-cell engraftment and efficacy in leukemia. Blood. 2016;127:1117–27.
17. Ruella M, Kenderian SS, Shestova O, et al. The addition of the BTK inhibitor Ibrutinib to anti-CD19 chimeric antigen receptor T cells (CART19) improves responses against mantle cell lymphoma. Clin Cancer Res. 2016;22:2684–96.
18. Gong JJ, Yin QS, Li MJ, et al. Ibrutinib combined with CAR-T cells in the treatment of del (17p) chronic lymphocytic leukemia with BCL-2 inhibitor resistance: a case report and literature review. Zhonghua Xue Ye Xue Za Zhi. 2019;40:750–4.
19. Gauthier J, Hirayama AV, Purushe J, et al. Feasibility and efficacy of CD19-targeted CAR T cells with concurrent ibrutinib for CLL after ibrutinib failure. Blood. 2020;135:1650–60.
20. Fan F, Yoo HJ, Stock S, et al. Ibrutinib for improved chimeric antigen receptor T-cell production for chronic lymphocytic leukemia patients. Int J Cancer. 2021;148:419–28.
21. Liu M, Wang X, Li Z, et al. Synergistic effect of ibrutinib and CD19 CAR-T cells on Raji cells in vivo and in vitro. Cancer Sci. 2020;111:4051–60.
22. Gill SI, Vides V, Frey NV, et al. Prospective Clinical Trial of Anti-CD19 CAR T Cells in Combination with Ibrutinib for the Treatment of Chronic Lymphocytic Leukemia Shows a High Response Rate. Blood. 2018;132:298.
23. Wierda WG, Dorritie KA, Munoz J, et al. Transcend CLL 004: phase 1 cohort of lisocabtagene Maraleucel (liso-cel) in combination with Ibrutinib for patients with relapsed/refractory (R/R) chronic lymphocytic leukemia/small lymphocytic lymphoma (CLL/SLL). Blood. 2020;136:39–40.
24. Fraietta JA, Nobles CL, Sammons MA, et al. Disruption of TET2 promotes the therapeutic efficacy of CD19-targeted T cells. Nature. 2018;558:307–12.
25. Li AM, Hucks GE, Dinofia AM, et al. Checkpoint inhibitors augment CD19-directed chimeric antigen receptor (CAR) T cell therapy in relapsed B-cell acute lymphoblastic leukemia. Blood. 2018;132:556.
26. Cao Y, Lu W, Sun R, et al. Anti-CD19 chimeric antigen receptor T cells in combination with nivolumab are safe and effective against relapsed/refractory B-cell non-hodgkin lymphoma. Front Oncol. 2019;9:767.
27. Wang J, Deng Q, Jiang YY, et al. CAR-T 19 combined with reduced-dose PD-1 blockade therapy for treatment of refractory follicular lymphoma: a case report. Oncol Lett. 2019;18:4415–20.
28. John LB, Devaud C, Duong CP, et al. Anti-PD-1 antibody therapy potently enhances the eradication of established tumors by gene modified T cells. Clin Cancer Res. 2013;19:5636–46.
29. Cherkassky L, Morello A, Villena-Vargas J, et al. Human CAR T cells with cell-intrinsic PD-1 checkpoint blockade resist tumor-mediated inhibition. J Clin Invest. 2016;126:3130–44.
30. Burga RA, Thorn M, Point GR, et al. Liver myeloid-derived suppressor cells expand in response to liver metastases in mice and inhibit the anti-tumor efficacy of anti-CEA CAR-T. Cancer Immunol Immunother. 2015;64:817–29.
31. Heczey A, Louis CU, Savoldo B, et al. CAR T cells administered in combination with Lymphodepletion and PD-1 inhibition to patients with neuroblastoma. Mol Ther. 2017;25:2214–24.

32. May KF Jr, Chen L, Zheng P, Liu Y. Anti-4-1BB monoclonal antibody enhances rejection of large tumor burden by promoting survival but not clonal expansion of tumor-specific CD8+ T cells. Cancer Res. 2002;62:3459–65.

33. Mardiana S, John LB, Henderson MA, et al. A multifunctional role for adjuvant anti-4-1BB therapy in augmenting antitumor response by chimeric antigen receptor T cells. Cancer Res. 2017;77:1296–309.

34. Segal NH, He AR, Doi T, et al. Phase I study of single-agent Utomilumab (PF-05082566), a 4-1BB/CD137 agonist, in patients with advanced cancer. Clin Cancer Res. 2018;24:1816–23.

35. Nishio N, Diaconu I, Liu H, et al. Armed oncolytic virus enhances immune functions of chimeric antigen receptor-modified T cells in solid tumors. Cancer Res. 2014;74:5195–205.

36. Tanoue K, Rosewell Shaw A, Watanabe N, et al. Armed oncolytic adenovirus-expressing PD-L1 mini-body enhances antitumor effects of chimeric antigen receptor T cells in solid tumors. Cancer Res. 2017;77:2040–51.

37. Rosewell Shaw A, Porter CE, Watanabe N, et al. Adenovirotherapy delivering cytokine and checkpoint inhibitor augments CAR T cells against metastatic head and neck cancer. Mol Ther. 2017;25:2440–51.

38. Sakemura R, Eckert EC, Crotts SB, et al. Vesicular stomatitis virus (VSV) engineered to express CD19 stimulates anti-CD19 chimeric antigen receptor modified T cells and promotes their anti-tumor effects. Blood. 2020;136:30–1.

39. Kim EH, Suresh M. Role of PI3K/Akt signaling in memory CD8 T cell differentiation. Front Immunol. 2013;4:20.

40. Alizadeh D, Wong RA, Yang X, et al. IL15 enhances CAR-T cell antitumor activity by reducing mTORC1 activity and preserving their stem cell memory phenotype. Cancer Immunol Res. 2019;7:759–72.

41. Klebanoff CA, Crompton JG, Leonardi AJ, et al. Inhibition of AKT signaling uncouples T cell differentiation from expansion for receptor-engineered adoptive immunotherapy. JCI Insight. 2017;2

42. Stock S, Übelhart R, Schubert ML, et al. Idelalisib for optimized CD19-specific chimeric antigen receptor T cells in chronic lymphocytic leukemia patients. Int J Cancer. 2019;145:1312–24.

43. Zheng W, O'Hear CE, Alli R, et al. PI3K orchestration of the in vivo persistence of chimeric antigen receptor-modified T cells. Leukemia. 2018;32:1157–67.

44. Bowers JS, Majchrzak K, Nelson MH, et al. PI3Kδ inhibition enhances the antitumor fitness of adoptively transferred CD8(+) T cells. Front Immunol. 2017;8:1221.

45. Petersen CT, Hassan M, Morris AB, et al. Improving T-cell expansion and function for adoptive T-cell therapy using ex vivo treatment with PI3Kδ inhibitors and VIP antagonists. Blood Adv. 2018;2:210–23.

46. Berdeja JG, Alsina M, Shah ND, et al. Updated results from an ongoing phase 1 clinical study of bb21217 anti-Bcma CAR T cell therapy. Blood. 2019;134:927.

47. Singh MD, Ni M, Sullivan JM, Hamerman JA, Campbell DJ. B cell adaptor for PI3-kinase (BCAP) modulates CD8(+) effector and memory T cell differentiation. J Exp Med. 2018;215:2429–43.

48. Cooper ML, Staser KW, Ritchey J, et al. A long-acting pharmacological grade interleukin-7 molecule logarithmically accelerates ucart proliferation, differentiation, and tumor killing. Blood. 2018;132:2199.

49. Mihara K, Yanagihara K, Takigahira M, et al. Synergistic and persistent effect of T-cell immunotherapy with anti-CD19 or anti-CD38 chimeric receptor in conjunction with rituximab on B-cell non-Hodgkin lymphoma. Br J Haematol. 2010;151:37–46.

50. Neelapu SS, Locke FL, Bartlett NL, et al. Axicabtagene Ciloleucel CAR T-cell therapy in refractory large B-cell lymphoma. N Engl J Med. 2017;377:2531–44.

51. Neelapu SS, Kharfan-Dabaja MA, Oluwole OO, et al. A phase 2, open-label, multicenter study evaluating the safety and efficacy of axicabtagene ciloleucel in combination with either rituximab or lenalidomide in patients with refractory large B-cell lymphoma (ZUMA-14). Blood. 2019;134:4093.

52. Yang M, Wang L, Ni M, et al. Pre-sensitization of malignant B cells through venetoclax significantly improves the cytotoxic efficacy of CD19.CAR-T cells. Front Immunol. 2020;11:608167.
53. DeSelm C, Palomba ML, Yahalom J, et al. Low-dose radiation conditioning enables CAR T cells to mitigate antigen escape. Mol Ther. 2018;26:2542–52.
54. Weiss T, Weller M, Guckenberger M, Sentman CL, Roth P. NKG2D-based CAR T cells and radiotherapy exert synergistic efficacy in glioblastoma. Cancer Res. 2018;78:1031–43.
55. Ramakrishna S, Highfill SL, Walsh Z, et al. Modulation of target antigen density improves CAR T-cell functionality and persistence. Clin Cancer Res. 2019;25:5329–41.
56. Lee DW, Kochenderfer JN, Stetler-Stevenson M, et al. T cells expressing CD19 chimeric antigen receptors for acute lymphoblastic leukaemia in children and young adults: a phase 1 dose-escalation trial. Lancet. 2015;385:517–28.
57. Lee DW III, Stetler-Stevenson M, Yuan CM, et al. Long-term outcomes following CD19 CAR T cell therapy for B-ALL are superior in patients receiving a fludarabine/cyclophosphamide preparative regimen and post-CAR hematopoietic stem cell transplantation. Washington, DC: American Society of Hematology; 2016.
58. Maude SL, Frey N, Shaw PA, et al. Chimeric antigen receptor T cells for sustained remissions in leukemia. N Engl J Med. 2014;371:1507–17.
59. Maude SL, Laetsch TW, Buechner J, et al. Tisagenlecleucel in children and young adults with B-cell lymphoblastic leukemia. N Engl J Med. 2018;378:439–48.
60. Grupp SA, Maude SL, Rives S, et al. Tisagenlecleucel for the treatment of pediatric and young adult patients with relapsed/refractory acute lymphoblastic leukemia: updated analysis of the ELIANA clinical trial. Biol Blood Marrow Transplant. 2019;25:S126–S7.
61. Pulsipher MA, Are CAR. T cells better than antibody or HCT therapy in B-ALL? Hematology. 2018;2018:16–24.
62. Gardner RA, Finney O, Annesley C, et al. Intent-to-treat leukemia remission by CD19 CAR T cells of defined formulation and dose in children and young adults. Blood. 2017;129:3322–31.
63. Pan J, Yang J, Deng B, et al. High efficacy and safety of low-dose CD19-directed CAR-T cell therapy in 51 refractory or relapsed B acute lymphoblastic leukemia patients. Leukemia. 2017;31:2587–93.
64. Jiang H, Li C, Yin P, et al. Anti-CD19 chimeric antigen receptor-modified T-cell therapy bridging to allogeneic hematopoietic stem cell transplantation for relapsed/refractory B-cell acute lymphoblastic leukemia: an open-label pragmatic clinical trial. Am J Hematol. 2019;94:1113–22.
65. Summers C, Annesley C, Bleakley M, Dahlberg A, Jensen MC, Gardner R. Long term follow-up after SCRI-CAR19v1 reveals late recurrences as well as a survival advantage to consolidation with HCT after CAR T cell induced remission. Blood. 2018;132:967.
66. Goldsmith SR, Ghobadi A, DiPersio JF. Hematopoeitic cell transplantation and CAR T-cell therapy: complements or competitors? Front Oncol. 2020;10:608916.
67. Zahid A, Siegler EL, Kenderian SS. CART cell toxicities: new insight into mechanisms and management. Clin Hematol Int. 2020;2:149–55.
68. Brudno JN, Kochenderfer JN. Toxicities of chimeric antigen receptor T cells: recognition and management. Blood. 2016;127:3321–30.
69. Hay KA. Cytokine release syndrome and neurotoxicity after CD19 chimeric antigen receptor-modified (CAR-) T cell therapy. Br J Haematol. 2018;183:364–74.
70. Siegler EL, Kenderian SS. Neurotoxicity and cytokine release syndrome after chimeric antigen receptor T cell therapy: insights into mechanisms and novel therapies. Front Immunol. 2020;11:1973.
71. Maude SL, Laetsch TW, Buechner J, et al. Tisagenlecleucel in children and young adults with B-cell lymphoblastic leukemia. N Engl J Med. 2018;378:439–48.
72. Mahmoudjafari Z, Hawks KG, Hsieh AA, Plesca D, Gatwood KS, Culos KA. American Society for Blood and Marrow Transplantation Pharmacy Special Interest Group Survey on chimeric antigen receptor T cell therapy administrative, logistic, and toxicity management practices in the United States. Biol Blood Marrow Transplant. 2019;25:26–33.

73. Gardner RA, Ceppi F, Rivers J, et al. Preemptive mitigation of CD19 CAR T-cell cytokine release syndrome without attenuation of antileukemic efficacy. Blood. 2019;134:2149–58.
74. Locke FL, Neelapu SS, Bartlett NL, et al. Preliminary results of prophylactic tocilizumab after axicabtageneciloleucel (axi-cel; KTE-C19) treatment for patients with refractory,aggressive non-Hodgkin Lymphoma (NHL). Blood. 2017;130:1547.
75. Giavridis T, van der Stegen SJC, Eyquem J, Hamieh M, Piersigilli A, Sadelain M. CAR T cell-induced cytokine release syndrome is mediated by macrophages and abated by IL-1 blockade. Nat Med. 2018;24:731–8.
76. Liu D, Zhao J. Cytokine release syndrome: grading, modeling, and new therapy. J Hematol Oncol. 2018;11:121.
77. Sterner RM, Sakemura R, Cox MJ, et al. GM-CSF inhibition reduces cytokine release syndrome and neuroinflammation but enhances CAR-T cell function in xenografts. Blood. 2019;133:697–709.
78. Norelli M, Camisa B, Barbiera G, et al. Monocyte-derived IL-1 and IL-6 are differentially required for cytokine-release syndrome and neurotoxicity due to CAR T cells. Nat Med. 2018;24:739–48.
79. Kenderian SS, Ruella M, Shestova O, et al. Ruxolitinib prevents cytokine release syndrome after CART cell therapy without impairing the anti-tumor effect in a Xenograft Model. Blood. 2016;128:652.
80. Huarte E, O'Connor RS, Peel MT, et al. Itacitinib (INCB039110), a JAK1 inhibitor, reduces cytokines associated with cytokine release syndrome induced by CAR T-cell therapy. Clin Cancer Res. 2020;26:6299–309.
81. Huarte E, O'Connor RS, Parker M, Huang T, Milone MC, Smith P. Prophylactic Itacitinib (INCB039110) for the prevention of cytokine release syndrome induced by chimeric antigen receptor T-cells (CAR-T-cells) therapy. Blood. 2019;134:1934.
82. Weber EW, Lynn RC, Sotillo E, Lattin J, Xu P, Mackall CL. Pharmacologic control of CAR-T cell function using dasatinib. Blood Adv. 2019;3:711–7.
83. Mestermann K, Giavridis T, Weber J, et al. The tyrosine kinase inhibitor dasatinib acts as a pharmacologic on/off switch for CAR T cells. Sci Transl Med. 2019;11
84. Mackall CL, Miklos DB. CNS endothelial cell activation emerges as a driver of CAR T cell-associated neurotoxicity. Cancer Discov. 2017;7:1371–3.
85. Dong L, Chang L-J, Gao Z, et al. Chimeric antigen receptor 4SCAR19-modified T cells in acute lymphoid leukemia: a phase II multi-center clinical trial in China. Washington, DC: American Society of Hematology; 2015.
86. Zhang JP, Zhang R, Tsao ST, et al. Sequential allogeneic and autologous CAR-T-cell therapy to treat an immune-compromised leukemic patient. Blood Adv. 2018;2:1691–5.
87. Turtle CJ, Hanafi LA, Berger C, et al. CD19 CAR-T cells of defined CD4+:CD8+ composition in adult B cell ALL patients. J Clin Invest. 2016;126:2123–38.
88. Davila ML, Riviere I, Wang X, et al. Efficacy and toxicity management of 19-28z CAR T cell therapy in B cell acute lymphoblastic leukemia. Sci Transl Med. 2014;6:224ra25.
89. Liu S, Deng B, Yin Z, et al. Corticosteroids do not influence the efficacy and kinetics of CAR-T cells for B-cell acute lymphoblastic leukemia. Blood Cancer J. 2020;10:15.
90. Strati P, Ahmed S, Furqan F, et al. Prognostic Impact of Corticosteroids on Efficacy of Chimeric Antigen Receptor T-cell Therapy in Large B-cell Lymphoma. Blood. 2021;137:3272.
91. Amatya PN, Carter AJ, Ritchey JK, et al. The dual PI3Kδγ inhibitor Duvelisib potently inhibits IL-6 production and cytokine release syndrome (CRS) while maintaining CAR-T function in vitro and in vivo. Blood. 2020;136:1–2.
92. Amatya PN, Carter AJ, Ritchey JK, et al. The Dual PI3K delta gamma Inhibitor Duvelisib Potently Inhibits IL-6 Production and Cytokine Release Syndrome (CRS) While Maintaining CAR-T Function in Vitro and In Vivo. BLOOD; 2020: AMER SOC HEMATOLOGY 2021 L ST NW, SUITE 900, WASHINGTON, DC 20036 USA.
93. Zou W, Wolchok JD, Chen L. PD-L1 (B7-H1) and PD-1 pathway blockade for cancer therapy: Mechanisms, response biomarkers, and combinations. Sci Transl Med. 2016;8:328rv4-rv4.
94. Grupp SA, Maude SL, Shaw PA, et al. Durable remissions in children with relapsed/refractory all treated with t cells engineered with a CD19-targeted chimeric antigen receptor (CTL019). Washington, DC: American Society of Hematology; 2015.

Safety Switches Used for Cellular Therapies

Lauren Smith and Antonio Di Stasi

Abstract Gene and cellular immunotherapy is rapidly changing the way we treat cancer. But, unfortunately, these promising therapies can result in serious, sometimes fatal complications. Safety switches are increasingly used to manage serious side effects associated with these advanced cellular therapies. In this chapter, we review safety switches categorized in three classes: (a) metabolic (gene-directed enzyme prodrug therapy, GDEPT), (b) dimerization-induced apoptosis, and (c) monoclonal antibody-mediated cytotoxicity.

Keywords Suicide gene · Safety · Cellular therapy · T cells · Immune effector cells · iCasp9 suicide gene · HSV-TK suicide gene · Gene-directed enzyme prodrug therapy (GDEPT) · CD19 · CRS · Neurotoxicity · GVHD

Introduction

Cellular therapies represent one of the important components in the current management of cancer [1], from the infusion of hematopoietic stem cells (HSC) to ensure hematopoietic reconstitution, to the infusion of mature donor lymphocytes (DLI) to boost adoptive immunity [2], or to the treatment with genetically redirected T cells via T cell receptor (TCR) or chimeric antigen receptor (CAR) gene transfer [3]. Cellular therapies also pose a risk of serious adverse events. Donor T cells within the HSC product or infused post-transplant as DLI have been associated with potentially fatal graft-versus-host-disease (GVHD). Administration of engineered T cells has also resulted in toxicity, related to on/off-target effects as well as serious cytokine release syndrome (CRS) and neurotoxicity [4]. Additionally,

L. Smith · A. Di Stasi (✉)
Department of Medicine, Division of Hematology-Oncology, Bone Marrow Transplantation and Cellular Therapy Unit, The University of Alabama at Birmingham, Birmingham, AL, USA
e-mail: adistasi@uabmc.edu

© Springer Nature Switzerland AG 2022
A. Ghobadi, J. F. DiPersio (eds.), *Gene and Cellular Immunotherapy for Cancer*, Cancer Drug Discovery and Development,
https://doi.org/10.1007/978-3-030-87849-8_6

vector-induced insertional mutagenesis following HSC transduction can result in neoplastic transformation [5, 6]. Overall, these issues prompted the Recombinant DNA Advisory Committee of the National Institute of Health to make some clinical recommendations, including implementing careful dose-escalation plans and co-expressing a suicide gene for switching off or controlling unpredicted or long-term toxicities [7].

Genetic modification of cells with a suicide gene enables the selective ablation of gene-modified cells with potential amelioration of the associated adverse event [8, 9]. A suicide gene can be applied for the safety of therapies employing hemato-poietic stem cells, inducible pluripotent stem cells and progeny, or immune effector cells. (Table 1). Suicide gene technologies can be broadly classified based upon their mechanism of action in (a) metabolic (gene-directed enzyme prodrug therapy, GDEPT), (b) dimerization-induced apoptosis, and (c) monoclonal antibody-mediated cytotoxicity. Examples of GDEPT include the Herpes simplex virus thy-midine kinase (HSV-TK) activated by the prodrug ganciclovir. The iCasp9 suicide gene is a chimeric protein composed of a drug-binding domain linked in frame with a component of the apoptotic pathway, allowing conditional dimerization and apop-tosis of the transduced cells after administration of a non-therapeutic small mole-cule dimerizer [10–13] (Table 2, Fig. 1). Genetic modification of cells with a protein expressed in the plasma membrane [14] enables cell removal after administration of a specific monoclonal antibody. Examples of this class of suicide genes include: CD20 [15–17], the compact suicide gene (RQR8) combining epitopes from CD34 and CD20 enabling CD34 selection, cell tracking, and deletion [18], epidermal growth factor receptor (EGFR) [19], and the incorporation of a myc-tag sequence within the transgenic construct [20].

The ideal inducing agent for suicide gene activation should be biologically inert with adequate bio-availability and bio-distribution. These strategies should permit flexibility in which the cell therapy could be either downregulated to control moder-ate toxicities while preserving the therapeutic effect, or eliminated completely in the case of severe toxicities for which the presence of residual cells after suicide gene

Table 1 Suicide gene applications for the safety of cellular products

Cell type	Major toxicity risk	Desirable suicide gene strategy
T cells	GVHD	All cells must harbor suicide gene
Gene redirected T cells (CAR, TCR)	Cytokine release syndrome, neurotoxicity,	All transduced cells must harbor suicide gene
Gene corrected stem cells	Malignant transformation	All transduced cells must harbor suicide gene
Pluripotent cells (PC)	Malignant transformation Excessive proliferation	Expression only in PC: Pluripotent cell-specific promoter, but progeny cells can still give adverse events (transformation, reversion to pluripotency, or damage from excess proliferation) Bystander effect (killing of surrounding cells) can be desirable in case of solid tumor formation.

GVHD graft versus host disease, *CAR* chimeric artificial receptors, *TCR* T cell receptor

Table 2 Comparison of suicide genes for cell therapies

Category	Technology	Source	Activating Agent	Mechanism(s)	Pros	Cons	References
Metabolic	HSV-TK	Viral derived	GCV	1. Phosphorylated nucleotide disrupts DNA with cell death; 2. Apoptosis	– Gradual onset – Eliminates alloreactive cells	– Immunogenic in immunocompetent patients – Unwanted elimination of modified T cells with use of GCV	[33–35, 37–39, 41]
Dimerization inducing	iCasp9	Human derived	Dimerizing agent	Dimerization and induction of apoptosis	– Rapid onset – Eliminates alloreactive cells – Non immunogenic – Use non-therapeutic agent Titratable	Spare only a fraction (≥90%) of cells	[21–23, 31, 68]
Therapeutic mAb mediated	CD20, RQR8, c-myc, EGFR	Human derived	mAb	Complement dependent/ antibody dependent cellular cytotoxicity	– Rapid onset – Non immunogenic – No additional selectable marker required	On-target toxicity from mAb	[15–20]

HSV-TK Herpes simplex virus thymidine kinase, *GCV* ganciclovir, *iCasp9* inducible Caspase9, *mAb* monoclonal antibody

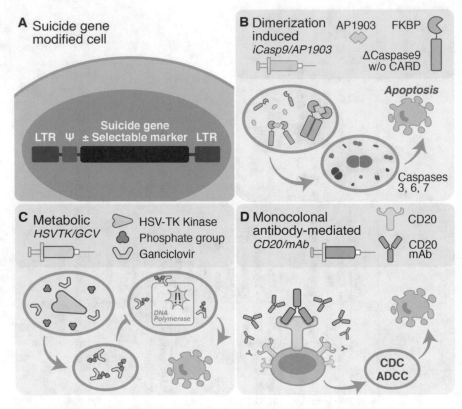

Fig. 1 Mechanism of action of the different suicide gene technologies. (**a**) Suicide gene modification of cells of interest to allow conditional elimination in case of serious adverse events. Surface marker suicide genes, e.g., CD20, can also function as a selectable markers. (**b**) Dimerization-induced, e.g., iCasp9 protein with FKBP12-F36V binding domain joined to human caspase-9. Administration of AP1903 leads to dimerization of iCasp9, activating the intrinsic mitochondrial apoptotic pathway. (**c**) Metabolic, e.g., HSV-TK leads to phosphorylation of ganciclovir, and its triphosphate form (also phosphorylated through cellular kinases) incorporates into DNA with chain termination. (**d**) Monoclonal antibody (mAb)-mediated, e.g., CD20 overexpression allows elimination after exposure to CD20 mAb through complement/antibody dependent cellular cytotoxicity (CDC/ADCC). *LTR: long terminal repeat, psi: retroviral packaging element, iCasp9: inducible Caspase9, CARD: Caspase recruitment domain, HSV-TK: Herpes simplex virus thymidine kinase, GCV: ganciclovir, mAb: monoclonal antibody.* Reproduced from [8]

activation is unwanted. In this chapter, we present an overview and update [8] of available suicide gene therapy strategies. We will analyze the clinical results of the inducible Caspase 9 (iCasp9), and the Herpes simplex virus thymidine kinase (HSV-TK) clinically investigated safety switch systems in the setting of allogeneic hematopoietic transplant, and present the state-of-the-art of suicide gene applications for other immune effector cell therapies.

Suicide Genes for Control of GVHD

Two suicide genes have been validated in the clinic for control of GVHD from the administration of donor T cells after allogeneic hematopoietic stem cell transplant (HSCT) to enhance immune recovery and maximize graft-versus-tumor: the iCasp9 and the HSV-TK suicide genes. Clinical results are summarized in Table 3.

iCasp9 Suicide Gene

The iCasp9 suicide gene is a chimeric protein composed of a drug-binding domain linked in frame with a component of the apoptotic pathway, allowing conditional dimerization and apoptosis of the transduced cells after administration of a non-therapeutic small molecule dimerizer [9–13]. In a Phase 1 clinical trial, the inducible Caspase9 (iCasp9) suicide gene [21, 22] was used in concert with the small molecule dimerizer AP1903. Seminal experiments performed by Spencer et al. [21, 23] and Clackson et al. [8]· demonstrated the ability to control signaling pathways through administration of lipid-permeable synthetic ligands, inducing conditional dimerization of intracellular proteins. They generated an inducible Casp9 suicide gene consisting of a *FKBP12-F36V* domain linked, via a flexible *Ser-Gly-Gly-Gly-Ser* linker, to *Δcaspase 9*, which is caspase 9 without its physiological dimerization domain, or caspase recruitment domain (*CARD*) [13]. *FKBP12-F36V* consists of an *FKBP* domain with a substitution at residue 36 of phenylalanine for valine, binding the synthetic dimeric ligand, such as AP1903 [24], with high selectivity and sub-nanomolar affinity. Straathof et al. [13] and Tey et al. [25] validated the *iCasp9* construct for T cell applications, demonstrating optimal transduction efficiency, expansion, and elimination of iCasp9 T cells with strong expression of the transgene [13, 22, 25]. *iCasp9* was cloned in-frame, using a *2A*-like sequence from Thosea asigna insect virus [26, 27], with a truncated CD19 domain (*ΔCD19*) serving as a selectable marker to ensure ≥90% purity (Table 4) [25, 28, 29].

Administration of Allo-Depleted iCasp9 T Cells

Brenner and collaborators reported their early results of a phase I clinical trial using the iCasp9 system [22]. Recipients of CD34-selected haplo-HSCT for hematological malignancies received escalating doses (1×10^6–1×10^7 cells/kg) [25, 30] of iCasp9-modified allo-depleted T cells from day 30 onwards. [45; 50] The iCasp9-modified T cells expanded and were detected in the peripheral blood as early as 7 days after infusion and persisted for at least 2 years in surviving patients. The engrafted iCasp9-modified T cells included both CD4+ and CD8+ T cells and pre-dominantly had an effector-memory or central-memory phenotype. Four patients

Table 3 Suicide gene modified donor T cells after HSCT for hematologic malignancies

References	Graft	N.	Disease status pre(N)	T cell infused and dose	T cell infusion day	Disease status post (N)	aGVHD	aGVHD Response (N)	cGVHD	Reported outcome
[22, 31]	**CD34 selected 5/10 Haplo**	10	CR (9), AD (1)	RV: iCasp9 allodepleted (1 × 10^6–1 × 10^7/kg)	30–124 (P2,7,9,10 had second infusion day 248–368)	Rel.: (4)	P1:G2 skin, liver; P2,4,5;G1 skin	CR (4) in 24 hrs.	None	5/10 alive disease free at 1016 days (835–1440)
[68]	**CD34 selected 5/10 Haplo**	12	CR (9) AD (2) HLH (1)	RV: iCasp9 not allodepleted (1 × 10^4–5 × 10^6/kg)	31–82 (P7 had 2 second infusion on day 116)	Rel.: (2 PD: (4)	P6: skin/gut G1 P8: skin G2 P9: skin G2, liver G2 P12:? CNS	CR (3) in 6–48 hrs.	None	6/12 alive at a median 476 days post-transplant (278–674)
[37]	**Not reported**	8	NR. Rel. or EBV-PTLD pre T cells	RV: TK: 0.5–38.6 × 10^6/kg	6–276 weeks	CR (3), PR (2), NR (2), NE (1)	P1: G2/3 skin; P2: G3 liver	CR (2) 24 h After	P8: G1 (oral, lung, skin);PR with GCV	CR (3); PR (2); NR (2); NE (1)
[38]	**MRD** Female donor to male recipient	12	AD (5), CR (3), CP (4)	RV: TK: 2 × 10^5/kg	Day 0	CR (4), rel. (2), Non-rel. Death (6)	P1,6: G2 skin; P3: G3 skin, liver; P12: G1 NA	CR within 1 week of GCV treatment (3patients; 1 CR + steroids).	P9 (extensive skin) (CR)	4/12 alive at 29–38 months

[34]	MRD (N:25) MMRD (N:5)	30	All at rel. Pre T cells	RV: TK: 1×10^5–1×10^8/kg; 23 had T cells	Variable: <1 week –270 weeks; monthly infusion	CR: (6)	P1,22: skin; P2: liver	CR (2 treated patients, P1 only topical treatment)	P8: extensive lung & skin improved after GCV	6/17 evaluable patients had CR after TK-DLI, 5/17 (PR), 6/17 (PD)
[33]	CD34 selected 5/10 Haplo	50	AD (20), CR (30)	RV:TK:1×10^6–1×10^7 cells/kg (1–4 infusions) 28 had T cells	Day 28, then monthly	Rel. (17), CR (33)	P6: G1 skin; P5,16,20,25,43,47,50, G2 skin; P8: G4 liver, gut P38: G3 skin	CR (9 post GCV, one untreated): 3–84 days after. –4 patients + steroids -P8 + CysA	P44: Extensive (CR post GCV and low dose MMF)	3 years NRM: 40%; median survival (patients with AD): 177 days; OS (de-novo AML in CR): 49%. CR (5), CCR 11)

HLA human leukocyte antigens, *NHL* non Hodgkin lymphoma, *GVHD* graft-versus-host-disease, *a* acute, *c* chronic, *5/10 haplo* 5/10 HLA matched haploidentical, *CR* complete remission, *AD* active disease, *Rel.* relapse, *RV* retrovirus, *P* patient, *DL* dose level, *G* grade, *hrs.* Hours, *EBV-PTLD* Epstein-Barr virus post-transplant lymphoproliferative disease, *(HSV)-TK* (Herpes simplex virus) thymidine kinase, *NR* not reported, *GCV* ganciclovir, *(M)MRD* (mis)matched related donor. *CP* chronic phase, *NR* no response, *NE* non-evaluable, *NA* not available, *CySA* cyclosporine A, *MMF* mycophenolate mofetil

Table 4 Suicide gene-modified chimeric antigen T-cell clinical trials

Clinical Trial	Study sponsor	Description	Suicide gene/ activating drug	Diagnosis
NCT03696784	UNC Lineberger Comprehensive Cancer Center	Phase I: Autologous activated CD 19 CAR-T cells.	iC9; AP1903	Relapsed/refractory B cell lymphoma
NCT03016377	UNC Lineberger Comprehensive Cancer Center	Phase I/II: Autologous CD19 CAR T cells	iC9; AP1903	Relapsed/refractory Acute Lymphoblastic leukemia
NCT01822652	Baylor College of Medicine	Phase I: Autologous activated GD-2 CAR-T cells	iC9; AP1903	Relapsed or refractory Neuroblastoma
NCT01953900	Baylor College of Medicine	Phase I: Autologous VZV-specific GD2 CAR-T cells	iC9; AP1903	Relapsed or refractory Osteosarcoma or Neuroblastoma
NCT03190278	Cellectis S.A.	Phase I: Allogeneic engineered CD123 CAR T-cells	RQR8; rituximab	Relapsed/Refractory Acute Myeloid Leukemia

out of ten developed acute GVHD (aGVHD) grade 1–2 of the liver and/or skin. Administration of a single dose of 0.4 mg/kg AP1903 resulted in apoptosis of ≥90% of iCasp9-modified T cells within 30 minutes, followed by a rapid (within 24 hours) and permanent abrogation of GVHD. Remarkably, residual iCasp9-modified T cells were able to re-expand, contained pathogen-specific precursors, and had a poly-clonal T cell receptor repertoire. The cell counts and composition of T cell subsets of patients who developed GVHD and were treated with AP1903 were similar to those who did not require the administration of the drug. Although they found that T cells recognizing tumor-associated antigens can be reactivated *ex vivo* from the peripheral blood both before and after AP1903 infusion, three of the four patients receiving AP1903 for control of GVHD subsequently relapsed, compared to only one of six patients who were not treated. One patient who relapsed without prior GVHD was subsequently salvaged with a second allograft, while another patient died of complications secondary to autoimmune hemolytic anemia. Overall, five patients were alive and in ongoing remission at a median follow-up of 1016 days after transplant (range 835–1440 days) [31].

Given this success, several ongoing clinical trials have replaced the time-consuming *in vitro* allo-depletion step with *in vivo* allo-depletion using AP1903 for those developing GVHD in the haploidentical (Clinicaltrials.gov identifier NCT01494103; NCT02065869; NCT01744223, NCT03459170) and matched related setting (Clinicaltrials.gov identifier NCT01875237, NCT02849886, NCT03459170). Some studies also included non-malignant diseases (NCT03733249, NCT03639844). An additional advantage of infusing suicide gene-modified T-lymphocytes is the omission of immune-suppressive agents associated with organ dysfunction and dampened immune responses.

Administration of Alloreplete iCasp9 T Cells

Zhou et al. investigated whether the *iCasp9* activation alone is sufficient to produce both rapid and long-term control of GVHD caused by alloreplete haploidentical donor T cells in 12 patients. This new method greatly shortened the manufacturing time to less than 2 weeks. In this subsequent clinical trial, alloreplete iCasp9-T cells were also able to engraft when given at doses of 1×10^5/kg or higher, persisted for at least 2 years, provided effective antiviral immunity, and enabled more rapid immune reconstitution than reported after haplo-HSCT without adoptive T cell transfer. The absolute count of endogenous $CD3^+$ T cells was greater than 500 cells per µl at 4 months after iCasp9 T cell infusion (approximately 5.5 months post-transplantation), while similar T cell counts are reached only between 9–12 months after haplo-HSCT if patients do not receive T lymphocyte add-back. Four patients required activation of the suicide gene for GVHD, with the elimination of 85–95% gene-modified cells, amelioration of GVHD without recurrence within 90 days. One patient in this study who received multiple doses of the drug had mild and transient pancytopenia (Grade 2) that was present immediately after each administration of AP1903 and resolved within 72 hrs. The mechanism underlying this idiosyncratic reaction is unclear, but it is likely not attributable to direct myelotoxicity. In one patient, acute GVHD became associated with cytokine release syndrome (CRS), as manifested by hyperpyrexia and a high level of circulating cytokines. Within 2 h of AP1903 administration and in the absence of additional therapy, the patient's temperature normalized, skin rash dramatically improved, and the elevated plasma cytokine levels declined. From these seminal studies, there is evidence that AP1903 can effectively deplete iCasp9 T cells in the CNS as well as in the skin, gut, and liver if these organs are affected by GVHD. Thus, iCasp9 *in vivo* allodepletion can be achieved by a single dose of AP1903 dimerizer administration, with the resolution of associated signs and symptoms of GVHD within 6–48 h. Importantly, there was no recurrence of GVHD associated with the gradual recovery of iCasp9 T cells following AP1903 administration.

It remains to be determined if mitigation of GVHD with AP1903 impacts the graft-versus-leukemia (GVL) effect of donor T cells. In the clinical trial described above, the suicide gene is activated only in patients whose GvHD is unresponsive to standard treatments. An alternative approach would be a regulated elimination of the allo-reactive cells by titrating the dose of the dimerizing agent using a continuous reassessment method.

HSV-TK Suicide Gene

Gene-directed enzyme prodrug therapy (GDEPT) [32] converts a nontoxic drug to a toxic drug in gene-modified cells, as with HSV-TK [33, 34]. HSV-TK phosphory-lates nucleoside analogs, including acyclovir and ganciclovir (GCV), resulting in their triphosphate forms being incorporated into DNA via the action of DNA poly-merase, leading to chain termination and cell death [35]. Unlike the mammalian thymidine kinase, HSV-TK is characterized by 1000 fold higher affinity to specific nucleoside analogs [36], including GCV, making it suitable for use as a suicide gene in mammalian cells. A report in *Science* in 1997 by Bonini et al. demonstrated the efficacy of HSV-TK suicide gene-modified T cells in controlling aGVHD resulting from donor T cell infusion after HSCT for disease relapse or treatment of EBV post-transplant lymphoproliferative disease (PTLD). A GVL effect was demonstrated in five patients receiving donor lymphocyte infusions (DLI). Of the three patients that developed aGVHD post-DLI, two patients had a rapid (<24 h) resolution following treatment with GCV. Additionally, the single patient who developed chronic GVHD (cGVHD) achieved a partial response with GCV [37]. Subsequently, the French group led by Tiberghien investigated 12 patients with hematologic malignancies who underwent HLA-matched related donor allogeneic HSCT [38]. These patients were treated with HSV-TK gene-modified T cells on the day of transplantation. Three patients developed aGVHD of at least grade 2, and one patient developed cGVHD. Treatment with GCV alone resulted in complete remission (CR) in two of the three patients with aGVHD and CR was achieved with the addition of steroids in the third. GCV treatment also resulted in CR for the patient with cGVHD [38].

The anti-tumor effects of HSV-TK-engineered donor lymphocytes were studied in 23 patients with hematologic malignancies who relapsed after matched related allo-HSCT. 65% of the patients had clinical benefit, with either a CR or partial response (PR) consequent to the administration of donor T cells. Seven patients developed antibodies against HSV-TK, but this did not preclude a GVL effect. Interestingly, the patients who achieved complete remission remained in remission after administration of ganciclovir or development of an anti-HSV-TK immune response. The authors postulated it was likely due to the eradication of disease and survival of a low numbers of alloreactive T cells after GCV treatment, resulting in continued and effective immune-surveillance. Three patients developed aGVHD (grade 1–3 skin/liver) that was controlled by GCV in all but one patient, while one patient with cGVHD also had a clinical benefit after GCV treatment [34]. Of note, infused T cells persisted *in vivo* up to 14 years after infusion [39]. Another long term follow-up study in haploidentical and matched transplant recipients demonstrated persistence of these cells for up to 2 years post-infusion [40].

The largest study of suicide gene engineered DLI after haploidentical HSCT was published in 2009 by the Milan group [33]. This phase I/II study enrolled 50 patients with high-risk hematologic malignancies, and 28 were eligible for HSV-TK DLI. Infusions started at day 28 after transplant and continued monthly up to a total of four infusions, with doses ranging from 0.9 to 40 x 10^6 cells/kg. After HSV-TK

DLI, no GVHD prophylaxis was given. Ten out of 22 immune-reconstituted patients developed aGVHD, and one had cGVHD. Nine patients were treated with GCV at 5 mg/kg twice daily for 2 weeks and attained complete resolution of GVHD. Some patients required transient courses of other immune-suppressive agents including steroids, cyclosporine, and mycophenolate mofetil for treatment of GVHD. There were no cases of GCV resistance, progression from acute to chronic GVHD or GVHD-associated deaths in this study. For patients with primary acute leukemia transplanted in remission, the non-relapse mortality was 19% at 3 years. All patients in remission 3 years after transplant remained in remission (longest follow up 9 years) [33, 39]. Indirect evidence suggesting a GVL effect was the finding of *de novo* loss of mismatched HLA expression on leukemic blasts in one haploidentical transplant recipient at the time of relapse [41].

In contrast to the iCasp9 suicide gene, the HSV-TK transgene proved immunogenic as measured by development of TK-specific CD8$^+$ T cells in immune-competent patients with limited persistence of HSV-TK cells [42]. Additionally, GCV-resistant truncated HSV-TK forms have been observed in some patients [43]. In both the HSV-TK and iCasp9 studies, infusion of suicide gene-modified cells aided non-gene modified T cell immune reconstitution [22, 33, 44], possibly as a consequence of interleukin-7 secretion by gene-modified cells [45]. The lack of further acute GVHD in these studies might suggest either complete elimination of alloreactive cells or development of peripheral tolerance. Additionally, the incidence of chronic GVHD was low in the HSV-TK T cell studies, and absent in the iCasp9 trial [22, 31]. Finally, no skewing of the T cell-repertoire was observed with either suicide gene platforms [22, 46].

Suicide Gene Application with Gene-Redirected T Cells

T Cell Receptor (TCR)- or Chimeric Antigen Receptor (CAR)-redirected T cells have now been used widely for the treatment of hematologic and solid tumor malignancies. Autoimmune phenomena due to infusion of TCR-redirected T cells may be due to expression of the target antigens on normal tissues [47–51] or cross-reactive phenomena [52]. In theory, mispairing of alpha or beta TCR chains with the endogenous TCR could generate TCR of autoreactive specificities. However, this has not been observed in clinical trials (Table 4) [53].

Toxicities observed in CAR T cell clinical trials include cytokine release syndrome (CRS), neurotoxicity, and tumor lysis syndrome [54–62], organ damage including fatal acute lung injury [63], liver toxicity [64, 65], hypogammaglobulinemia from depletion of normal host CD19 expressing B cells [54], and anaphylactic reactions due to the development of antibodies to the mouse sequences in CAR constructs [66].

Since toxicities resulting from these living drugs cannot be reduced by stopping the offending agent as is the case with pharmacologic agents, suicide gene modification of gene redirected T cells is an appealing strategy. CRS is an inflammatory response arising from CAR stimulation. Clinical manifestations include fever, nausea, headache, tachycardia, hypotension, hypoxia, as well as cardiac [56, 59], toxicities. Although no standard treatment exists, CRS has been managed with steroids and the interleukin-6 monoclonal antibody tocilizumab [67]. It is unclear whether activation of a suicide gene would abate CAR-T cell-mediated CRS when already clinically evident. Trials of iCasp9 suicide gene-modified T cells infused after haploidentical hematopoietic stem cell transplantation showed that administration of the AP1903 resulted in defervescence and reduction of inflammatory cytokines, including serum interleukin-6. Additionally, some indirect preliminary evidence suggested a reduction in iCasp9-T cells in the CNS following dimerizer administration [68].

Pre-clinical experiments in which iCasp9 is expressed in conjunction with CAR CD19/CD20 in genetically modified T cells support the feasibility of such an approach [69–71]. Clinical trials combining CAR CD19 and the iCasp9 are ongoing both in lymphoma (NCT03696784) and acute leukemia (NCT03016377). Additionally, phase 1 clinical trials in patients with sarcoma or neuroblastoma receiving iCasp9 T cells co-expressing a CAR against the disialoganglioside GD2 molecule are ongoing (Clinicaltrials.gov identifier NCT01822652, NCT01953900, respectively).

Finally, in an approach targeting CD123 for AML (NCT03190278), the gene-modified T cells harbor the RQR8 compact suicide gene. RQR8 is a highly compact epitope-based construct that acts as both a suicide gene as well as a selective marker. It is a CD20 mimotope that renders T cells susceptible to lysis by CD20 monoclonal antibody, Rituximab in combination with the QBend10 epitope of CD34 which is recognized by anti-CD34 antibody used in the Miltenyi CliniMACS CD34 selection system. [18]

Insertional Mutagenesis Risks of Gene-Modified Cellular Products

Examples of insertional mutagenesis and malignant transformation were reported in the setting of gene-modified hematopoietic stem cells using gamma retroviral vectors in clinical trials for severe combined immune deficiency (SCID) [72–74], X-linked chronic granulomatous disease [75], and Wiskott-Aldrich syndrome [76]. Clonal dominance has also been reported from a clinical trial in beta-thalassemia using a lentiviral vector [77, 78]. Modifications of the lentiviral vector (incorporation of insulator sequences) have overcome this complication and this approach is currently under clinical investigation in patients with hemoglobinopathies (NCT01745120 and NCT02140554). Although newer self-inactivating lentiviral vectors are being used for hematopoietic stem cell gene therapy, no serious adverse mutagenic events had been reported in T cells using retroviral vectors, despite the identification of integration hotspots in some patients, likely due to safer packaging systems or the inability to transform T cells vs. stem cells.

With the broader application of gene-modified cellular products, costs and accessibility need to be taken into account. Some experts are suggesting waiving the costly testing for replication-competent retroviral/lentiviral particles, in view of demonstrated safety over several decades. In fact, a recent commentary [79] summarized the negative results reported in the literature for replication-competent retroviral/lentiviral testing of 188 vector products, 2797 genetically-modified T cell products, and 3861 patient follow-up samples. In 2011, the National Gene Vector Biorepository similarly reported that 16 lentiviral vector products manufactured for clinical trial use had no evidence of replication-competent lentiviruses [79].

Fascinating reports on the mapping of retroviral integration sites have been published from both studies employing the HSV-TK or the iCasp9 suicide gene system. Those studies reported an absence of substantial genotoxic risks and selection bias. Consistently, retroviral vectors display an integration pattern distinct from lentiviral vectors. Cattoglio et al. [80] reported a selective post-infusion loss of cells harboring proviruses in direct transcriptional orientation within introns or exons. A study from Chang et al. [81] involved extensive characterization of vector integration sites using epigenetic and promoter-level atlas, reporting that elimination of iCasp9 T cells is determined by a minimum expression threshold of the transgene, which is dependent on T cell receptor activation state of the T cells, as well as cis-acting influences by host promoters on the proviral transgene. Viral integration studies highlighting safety have also been performed in the context of CAR-T cells [82].

Conclusions

Potent immune effector cell therapies have entered clinical practice. Such therapies require attention from regulatory agencies to provide guidelines and accreditation for the safe delivery of therapeutic products to the patients. The advent of such novel forms of treatment have been associated with the emergence of novel toxicities. Patients and staff education are crucial for recognizing, scoring, and prompt initiation of the most appropriate available treatment for these toxicities. Successful clinical validation of suicide gene strategies to control GVHD after allogeneic HSCT or to reduce toxicities associated with infusion of genetically modified stem cells and T cells are currently underway. In vivo elimination of therapeutic cellular products via suicide gene therapy or other forms of cellular switches may be essential to eliminate or mitigate many of their expected toxicities while maintaining their therapeutic benefits. Effective safety switches could aid in broader applicability of emerging complex cellular therapeutics for cancer or regenerative medicine.

Conflict of Interests The authors declare no competing conflict of interests.

Authors and Contributors All the authors contributed to conception, acquisition, analysis of data, participated in the manuscript draft preparation, revision, and approved and revised the final version.

References

1. Copelan EA. Hematopoietic stem-cell transplantation. N Engl J Med. 2006;354:1813–26.
2. Bar M, Sandmaier BM, Inamoto Y, et al. Donor lymphocyte infusion for relapsed hematological malignancies after allogeneic hematopoietic cell transplantation: prognostic relevance of the initial CD3+ T cell dose. Biol Blood Marrow Transpl. 2013;19:949–57.
3. Minagawa K, Zhou X, Mineishi S, Di Stasi A. Seatbelts in CAR therapy: how safe are CARS? Pharmaceuticals (Basel, Switzerland). 2015;8:230–49.
4. Tey S-K. Adoptive T-cell therapy: adverse events and safety switches. Clin Transl Immunol. 2014;3:e17.
5. Mukherjee S, Thrasher AJ. Gene therapy for PIDs: progress, pitfalls and prospects. Gene. 2013;525:174–81.
6. Narsinh K, Narsinh KH, Wu JC. Derivation of human induced pluripotent stem cells for cardiovascular disease modeling. Circ Res. 2011;108:1146–56.
7. Ertl HCJ, Zaia J, Rosenberg SA, et al. Considerations for the clinical application of chimeric antigen receptor T cells: observations from a recombinant DNA advisory committee symposium held June 15, 2010. Cancer Res. 2011;71:3175–81.
8. Jones BS, Lamb LS, Goldman F, Di Stasi A. Improving the safety of cell therapy products by suicide gene transfer. Front Pharmacol. 2014;5:254.
9. Falcon C, Al-Obaidi M, Di Stasi A. Exploiting cell death pathways for inducible cell elimination to modulate graft-versus-host-disease. Biomedicine. 2017;5:30.
10. Spencer DM, Belshaw PJ, Chen L, et al. Functional analysis of Fas signaling in vivo using synthetic inducers of dimerization. Curr Biol: CB. 1996;6:839–47.
11. Belshaw PJ, Spencer DM, Crabtree GR, Schreiber SL. Controlling programmed cell death with a cyclophilin-cyclosporin-based chemical inducer of dimerization. Chem Biol. 1996;3:731–8.
12. MacCorkle RA, Freeman KW, Spencer DM. Synthetic activation of caspases: artificial death switches. Proc Natl Acad Sci U S A. 1998;95:3655–60.
13. Straathof KC, Pule MA, Yotnda P, et al. An inducible caspase 9 safety switch for T-cell therapy. Blood. 2005;105:4247–54.
14. Hewitt Z, Priddle H, Thomson AJ, Wojtacha D, McWhir J. Ablation of undifferentiated human embryonic stem cells: exploiting innate immunity against the gal alpha1-3Galbeta1-4GlcNAc-R (alpha-gal) epitope. Stem Cells (Dayton, Ohio). 2007;25:10–8.
15. Griffioen M, van Egmond EH, Kester MG, Willemze R, Falkenburg JH, Heemskerk MH. Retroviral transfer of human CD20 as a suicide gene for adoptive T-cell therapy. Haematologica. 2009;94:1316–20.
16. Introna M, Barbui AM, Bambacioni F, et al. Genetic modification of human T cells with CD20: a strategy to purify and lyse transduced cells with anti-CD20 antibodies. Hum Gene Ther. 2000;11:611–20.
17. Serafini M, Manganini M, Borleri G, et al. Characterization of CD20-transduced T lymphocytes as an alternative suicide gene therapy approach for the treatment of graft-versus-host disease. Hum Gene Ther. 2004;15:63–76.
18. Philip B, Kokalaki E, Mekkaoui L, et al. A highly compact epitope-based marker/suicide gene for easier and safer T-cell therapy. Blood. 2014;124:1277–87.
19. Wang X, Chang WC, Wong CW, et al. A transgene-encoded cell surface polypeptide for selection, in vivo tracking, and ablation of engineered cells. Blood. 2011;118:1255–63.
20. Kieback E, Charo J, Sommermeyer D, Blankenstein T, Uckert W. A safeguard eliminates T cell receptor gene-modified autoreactive T cells after adoptive transfer. Proc Natl Acad Sci U S A. 2008;105:623–8.
21. Clackson T, Yang W, Rozamus LW, et al. Redesigning an FKBP-ligand interface to generate chemical dimerizers with novel specificity. Proc Natl Acad Sci U S A. 1998;95:10437–42.
22. Di Stasi A, Tey SK, Dotti G, et al. Inducible apoptosis as a safety switch for adoptive cell therapy. N Engl J Med. 2011;365:1673–83.

23. Spencer DM, Wandless TJ, Schreiber SL, Crabtree GR. Controlling signal transduction with synthetic ligands. Science. 1993;262:1019–24.
24. Iuliucci JD, Oliver SD, Morley S, et al. Intravenous safety and pharmacokinetics of a novel dimerizer drug, AP1903, in healthy volunteers. J Clin Pharmacol. 2001;41:870–9.
25. Tey SK, Dotti G, Rooney CM, Heslop HE, Brenner MK. Inducible caspase 9 suicide gene to improve the safety of allodepleted T cells after haploidentical stem cell transplantation. Biol Blood Marrow Transplant. 2007;13:913–24.
26. Donnelly MLL, Hughes LE, Luke G, et al. The 'cleavage' activities of foot-and-mouth disease virus 2A site-directed mutants and naturally occurring '2A-like' sequences. J Gen Virol. 2001;82:1027–41.
27. Donnelly MLL, Luke G, Mehrotra A, et al. Analysis of the aphthovirus 2A/2B polyprotein 'cleavage' mechanism indicates not a proteolytic reaction, but a novel translational effect: a putative ribosomal 'skip'. J Gen Virol. 2001;82:1013–25.
28. Zhou LJ, Ord DC, Hughes AL, Tedder TF. Structure and domain organization of the CD19 antigen of human, mouse, and Guinea pig B lymphocytes. Conservation of the extensive cytoplasmic domain. J Immunol. 1991;147:1424–32.
29. Fujimoto M, Poe JC, Inaoki M, Tedder TF. CD19 regulates B lymphocyte responses to transmembrane signals. Semin Immunol. 1998;10:267–77.
30. Amrolia PJ, Muccioli-Casadei G, Huls H, et al. Adoptive immunotherapy with allodepleted donor T-cells improves immune reconstitution after haploidentical stem cell transplantation. Blood. 2006;108:1797–808.
31. Zhou X, Di Stasi A, Tey SK, et al. Long-term outcome after haploidentical stem cell transplant and infusion of T cells expressing the inducible caspase 9 safety transgene. Blood. 2014;123:3895–905.
32. Springer CJ, Niculescu-Duvaz I. Prodrug-activating systems in suicide gene therapy. J Clin Invest. 2000;105:1161–7.
33. Ciceri F, Bonini C, Stanghellini MT, et al. Infusion of suicide-gene-engineered donor lymphocytes after family haploidentical haemopoietic stem-cell transplantation for leukaemia (the TK007 trial): a non-randomised phase I-II study. Lancet Oncol. 2009;10:489–500.
34. Ciceri F, Bonini C, Marktel S, et al. Antitumor effects of HSV-TK-engineered donor lymphocytes after allogeneic stem-cell transplantation. Blood. 2007;109:4698–707.
35. Moolten FL. Tumor chemosensitivity conferred by inserted herpes thymidine kinase genes: paradigm for a prospective cancer control strategy. Cancer Res. 1986;46:5276–81.
36. Elion GB, Furman PA, Fyfe JA, de Miranda P, Beauchamp L, Schaeffer HJ. Selectivity of action of an antiherpetic agent, 9-(2-hydroxyethoxymethyl) guanine. Proc Natl Acad Sci U S A. 1977;74:5716–20.
37. Bonini C, Ferrari G, Verzeletti S, et al. HSV-TK gene transfer into donor lymphocytes for control of allogeneic graft-versus-leukemia. Science. 1997;276:1719–24.
38. Tiberghien P, Ferrand C, Lioure B, et al. Administration of herpes simplex-thymidine kinase-expressing donor T cells with a T-cell-depleted allogeneic marrow graft. Blood. 2001;97:63–72.
39. Oliveira G, Greco R, Lupo-Stanghellini MT, Vago L, Bonini C. Use of TK-cells in haploidentical hematopoietic stem cell transplantation. Curr Opin Hematol. 2012;19:427–33.
40. Weissinger EM, Borchers S, Silvani A, et al. Long term follow up of patients after allogeneic stem cell transplantation and transfusion of HSV-TK transduced T-cells. Front Pharmacol. 2015;6:76.
41. Vago L, Perna SK, Zanussi M, et al. Loss of mismatched HLA in leukemia after stem-cell transplantation. N Engl J Med. 2009;361:478–88.
42. Traversari C, Marktel S, Magnani Z, et al. The potential immunogenicity of the TK suicide gene does not prevent full clinical benefit associated with the use of TK-transduced donor lymphocytes in HSCT for hematologic malignancies. Blood. 2007;109:4708–15.
43. Garin MI, Garrett E, Tiberghien P, et al. Molecular mechanism for ganciclovir resistance in human T lymphocytes transduced with retroviral vectors carrying the herpes simplex virus thymidine kinase gene. Blood. 2001;97:122–9.

44. Bondanza A, Hambach L, Aghai Z, et al. IL-7 receptor expression identifies suicide gene-modified allospecific CD8+ T cells capable of self-renewal and differentiation into antileukemia effectors. Blood. 117:6469–78.
45. Vago L, Oliveira G, Bondanza A, et al. T-cell suicide gene therapy prompts thymic renewal in adults after hematopoietic stem cell transplantation. Blood. 2012;120:1820–30.
46. Borchers S, Provasi E, Silvani A, et al. Genetically modified donor leukocyte transfusion and graft-versus-leukemia effect after allogeneic stem cell transplantation. Hum Gene Ther. 2011;22:829–41.
47. Dudley ME, Wunderlich JR, Robbins PF, et al. Cancer regression and autoimmunity in patients after clonal repopulation with antitumor lymphocytes. Science (New York, NY). 2002;298:850–4.
48. Yee C, Thompson JA, Roche P, et al. Melanocyte destruction after antigen-specific immunotherapy of melanoma: direct evidence of t cell-mediated vitiligo. J Exp Med. 2000;192:1637–44.
49. Johnson LA, Morgan RA, Dudley ME, et al. Gene therapy with human and mouse T-cell receptors mediates cancer regression and targets normal tissues expressing cognate antigen. Blood. 2009;114:535–46.
50. Parkhurst MR, Yang JC, Langan RC, et al. T cells targeting carcinoembryonic antigen can mediate regression of metastatic colorectal cancer but induce severe transient colitis. Mol Ther. 2011;19:620–6.
51. Morgan RA, Chinnasamy N, Abate-Daga D, et al. Cancer regression and neurological toxicity following anti-MAGE-A3 TCR gene therapy. J Immunother (Hagerstown, Md: 1997). 2013;36:133–51.
52. Linette GP, Stadtmauer EA, Maus MV, et al. Cardiovascular toxicity and titin cross-reactivity of affinity-enhanced T cells in myeloma and melanoma. Blood. 2013;122:863–71.
53. Rosenberg SA. Of mice, not men: no evidence for graft-versus-host disease in humans receiving T-cell receptor-transduced autologous T cells. Mol Ther. 2010;18:1744–5.
54. Kochenderfer JN, Dudley ME, Feldman SA, et al. B-cell depletion and remissions of malignancy along with cytokine-associated toxicity in a clinical trial of anti-CD19 chimeric-antigen-receptor-transduced T cells. Blood. 2012;119:2709–20.
55. Brentjens R, Yeh R, Bernal Y, Riviere I, Sadelain M. Treatment of chronic lymphocytic leukemia with genetically targeted autologous T cells: case report of an unforeseen adverse event in a phase I clinical trial. Mol Ther. 2010;18:666–8.
56. Kalos M, Levine BL, Porter DL, et al. T cells with chimeric antigen receptors have potent antitumor effects and can establish memory in patients with advanced leukemia. Sci Transl Med. 2011;3:95ra73.
57. Grupp SA, Kalos M, Barrett D, et al. Chimeric antigen receptor-modified T cells for acute lymphoid leukemia. N Engl J Med. 2013;368:1509–18.
58. Brentjens RJ, Davila ML, Riviere I, et al. CD19-targeted T cells rapidly induce molecular remissions in adults with chemotherapy-refractory acute lymphoblastic leukemia. Sci Transl Med. 2013;5:177ra38.
59. Brentjens RJ, Riviere I, Park JH, et al. Safety and persistence of adoptively transferred autologous CD19-targeted T cells in patients with relapsed or chemotherapy refractory B-cell leukemias. Blood. 2011;118:4817–28.
60. Kochenderfer JN, Wilson WH, Janik JE, et al. Eradication of B-lineage cells and regression of lymphoma in a patient treated with autologous T cells genetically engineered to recognize CD19. Blood. 2010;116:4099–102.
61. Brentjens RJ, Davila ML, Riviere I, et al. CD19-targeted T cells rapidly induce molecular remissions in adults with chemotherapy-refractory acute lymphoblastic leukemia. Sci Transl Med. 2013;5:177.
62. Porter DL, Levine BL, Kalos M, Bagg A, June CH. Chimeric antigen receptor-modified T cells in chronic lymphoid leukemia. N Engl J Med. 2011;365:725–33.
63. Morgan RA, Yang JC, Kitano M, Dudley ME, Laurencot CM, Rosenberg SA. Case report of a serious adverse event following the administration of T cells transduced with a chimeric antigen receptor recognizing ERBB2. Mol Ther. 2010;18:843–51.

64. Lamers CH, Sleijfer S, van Steenbergen S, et al. Treatment of metastatic renal cell carcinoma with CAIX CAR-engineered T cells: clinical evaluation and management of on-target toxicity. Mol Ther. 2013;21:904–12.
65. Lamers CH, Sleijfer S, Vulto AG, et al. Treatment of metastatic renal cell carcinoma with autologous T-lymphocytes genetically retargeted against carbonic anhydrase IX: first clinical experience. J Clin Oncol. 2006;24:e20–2.
66. Maus MV, Haas AR, Beatty GL, et al. T cells expressing chimeric antigen receptors can cause anaphylaxis in humans. Cancer Immunol Res. 2013;1:26–31.
67. Maude SL, Frey N, Shaw PA, et al. Chimeric antigen receptor T cells for sustained remissions in leukemia. N Engl J Med. 2014;371:1507–17.
68. Zhou X, Dotti G, Krance RA, et al. Inducible caspase-9 suicide gene controls adverse effects from alloreplete T cells after haploidentical stem cell transplantation. Blood. 2015;125:4103–13.
69. Hoyos V, Savoldo B, Quintarelli C, et al. Engineering CD19-specific T lymphocytes with interleukin-15 and a suicide gene to enhance their anti-lymphoma/leukemia effects and safety. Leukemia. 2010;24:1160–70.
70. Budde LE, Berger C, Lin Y, et al. Combining a CD20 chimeric antigen receptor and an inducible caspase 9 suicide switch to improve the efficacy and safety of T cell adoptive immunotherapy for lymphoma. PLoS One. 2013;8:e82742.
71. Diaconu I, Ballard B, Zhang M, et al. Inducible Caspase-9 selectively modulates the toxicities of CD19-specific chimeric antigen receptor-modified T cells. Mol Ther. 2017;25:580–92.
72. Hacein-Bey-Abina S, Hauer J, Lim A, et al. Efficacy of gene therapy for X-linked severe combined immunodeficiency. N Engl J Med. 2010;363:355–64.
73. Hacein-Bey-Abina S, Garrigue A, Wang GP, et al. Insertional oncogenesis in 4 patients after retrovirus-mediated gene therapy of SCID-X1. J Clin Invest. 2008;118:3132–42.
74. Boztug K, Schmidt M, Schwarzer A, et al. Stem-cell gene therapy for the Wiskott-Aldrich syndrome. N Engl J Med. 2010;363:1918–27.
75. Ott MG, Schmidt M, Schwarzwaelder K, et al. Correction of X-linked chronic granulomatous disease by gene therapy, augmented by insertional activation of MDS1-EVI1, PRDM16 or SETBP1. Nat Med. 2006;12:401–9.
76. Braun CJ, Boztug K, Paruzynski A, et al. Gene therapy for Wiskott-Aldrich syndrome--long-term efficacy and genotoxicity. Sci Transl Med. 2014;6:227ra33.
77. Cavazzana-Calvo M, Payen E, Negre O, et al. Transfusion independence and HMGA2 activation after gene therapy of human beta-thalassaemia. Nature. 2010;467:318–22.
78. Uchida N, Evans ME, Hsieh MM, et al. Integration-specific in vitro evaluation of Lentivirally transduced rhesus CD34(+) cells correlates with in vivo vector copy number. Mol Ther Nucleic Acids. 2013;2:e122.
79. Heslop HE, Brenner MK. Seek and you will not find: ending the hunt for replication-competent retroviruses during human gene therapy. Mol Ther. 2018;26:1–2.
80. Cattoglio C, Maruggi G, Bartholomae C, et al. High-definition mapping of retroviral integration sites defines the fate of allogeneic T cells after donor lymphocyte infusion. PLoS One. 2010;5:e15688.
81. Chang EC, Liu H, West JA, et al. Clonal dynamics in vivo of virus integration sites of T cells expressing a safety switch. Mol Ther. 2016;24:736–45.
82. Scholler J, Brady TL, Binder-Scholl G, et al. Decade-long safety and function of retroviral-modified chimeric antigen receptor T cells. Sci Transl Med. 2012;4:132ra53.

Off-the-Shelf CAR-T

Matthew L. Cooper, Giorgio Ottaviano, John F. DiPersio, and Waseem Qasim

Abstract The FDA has approved CAR-T cell therapy for the treatment of B cell malignancies. Despite the clinical success of CD19 targeted CAR-T, several barriers limit the wider adoption of CAR-based therapies as viable long-term cancer therapies. Many of the barriers that limit the routine use of CAR-T cell therapies stem from utilizing autologous patient T cells as the starting material to generate CAR-T. Here we will describe the limitations of autologous CAR-T, the advantages and hurdles of allogeneic donor CAR-T, the learnings from clinical trials using allogeneic CART19 and discuss the future direction of the field.

Keywords Off the shelf CAR-T · Universal CAR-T · Allogeneic cellular therapy · Allogeneic CAR-T · Genetically edited donor derived CAR-T · CAR-T · TCRab deleted T cells · UCART19 · UCART7 · UCART123 · TALEN · CRISPR/Cas9 · TRAC · β2-microglobulin (B2M)

Autologous Donor CAR-T

Limitation of Autologous Donor CAR-T

Currently approved CAR-T cell therapeutics are generated using autologous T cells derived from the patient. In general, a single therapeutic dose is manufactured from a single apheresis. As with any personalized medicine, CAR-T represent a great financial burden. The cost of currently approved therapies ranges from

M. L. Cooper (✉) · J. F. DiPersio
Division of Oncology, Washington University School of Medicine, St. Louis, MO, USA
e-mail: matthewcooper@wustl.edu

G. Ottaviano · W. Qasim
Molecular and Cellular Immunology Unit, University College London (UCL)
Great Ormond Street Institute of Child Health, London, UK

© Springer Nature Switzerland AG 2022
A. Ghobadi, J. F. DiPersio (eds.), *Gene and Cellular Immunotherapy for Cancer*, Cancer Drug Discovery and Development,
https://doi.org/10.1007/978-3-030-87849-8_7

$373 K–$475 K per product. CAR-T manufacture is time-consuming and labor intensive and the number of patients that can be treated is limited by the capacity of external manufacturing sites, presenting logistical hurdles for scheduling personalized manufacturing runs. Additionally, failure of CAR-T cell manufacturing, reported in as many as 13% of patients has been observed [1], primarily due to low T cell numbers in patient derived apheresis products; a common occurrence in patients with hematological malignancy undergoing chemotherapy. As a result, CAR-T clinical trials often exclude patients with low absolute lymphocyte counts. Unfortunately, a number of patients fail to survive the length of time required for CAR-T manufacturing (~3–6 weeks) and never receive the final product [1]. The use of allogeneic donors as a cell source is an attractive solution to the limitations of autologous cellular therapies.

Allogeneic Cellular Therapy

For allogeneic cellular therapies to be successful, they must exhibit certain criteria. First and foremost, they must be safe and not induce undue toxicity resulting from their unrelated, mismatched donor source. They must overcome immunological rejection and persist long enough to demonstrate sufficient efficacy and may need to be amenable to repeat dosing regimens. Additionally, allogeneic cell therapies must maintain consistent efficacy and safety profiles accounting for donor-to-donor variability.

There are essentially two different strategies for developing 'off-the-shelf' allogeneic cellular therapies. The first is to use an innate donor cell type that is generally safe to transplant into HLA disparate patients without the risk of inducing Graft Versus Host Disease (GvHD), a potentially life-threatening condition in which the donor T cells recognize the recipient as foreign, leading to immunological reactions against the patient. Suitable innate cell types deficient at inducing GvHD include gamma delta T cells, in which activation occurs primarily in an MHC independent manner [2]; invariant natural killer T cells (iNKT), which express restricted T cell receptors unable to recognize allo-antigens [3, 4]; and NK cells which express germline encoded receptors of the innate immune system which do not induce GvHD [5]. The second option is an engineered approach in which donor Alpha Beta T cells, capable of adaptive immunity, are modified to inhibit alloreactivity.

Genetically Edited Allogeneic Donor Derived CAR-T

Allogeneic donor derived CAR-T risk inducing life threatening GvHD, providing the greatest barrier to the safe use of universal donor T cells. Fortuitously, the advent and evolution or genome editing strategies coincided with the early development of CAR-T. Furthermore, the ex vivo manipulation of CAR-T provides an opportune

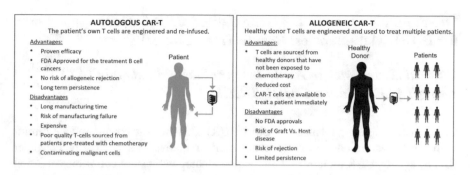

Fig. 1 Advantages and disadvantages of autologous and allogeneic CAR-T

environment in which to implement gene-editing strategies clinically. Efficient genetic deletion of the T cell receptor (TCR) allows for the generation of CAR-T cells from healthy donors without risk of these T cells causing severe and life-threatening GvHD. Disruption of the TRAC gene, encoding the TCRα chain was initially targeted for this purpose [6]; similarly, deletion of TCRβ or CD3ε will result in the failure of the TCR to complex and present on the cell surface [7–10]. Additionally, mechanical cell selection strategies, such as anti-TCRαβ magnetic bead-based depletion, are currently required to remove residual TCR+ T cells that escaped gene editing [9]. This ensures the fraction of TCR+ T cells contained in the final product is below the threshold required to induce GvHD.

TCR deficient or "universal" CAR-T offer several other advantages over autologous CAR-T (Fig. 1). Multiple patients (perhaps 50–200) can be treated with CAR-T manufactured from a single apheresis product, which in turn, substantially reduces production costs. Additionally, patients could be infused with CAR-T sooner after diagnosis since the product can be generated and frozen in advance, eliminating the risk of patients succumbing to disease before receiving CAR-T due to manufacturing issues. Allogeneic CAR-T are manufactured from healthy donor T cells and thus, eligibility for CAR-T cell therapy is not dependent on patient lymphocyte counts allowing patients that have received multiple rounds of chemotherapy to receive CAR-T.

While TCRαβ deleted T cells may improve the safety of CAR-T cells, allogeneic T cells may themselves be subject to immunological rejection by the recipient, which may be antibody or cell mediated. Strategies being adopted clinically to prevent CAR-T rejection will be discussed in subsequent sections in the context of UCART19.

Off-the-Shelf "Universal" Gene-Edited CAR-T Cells for B-Cell Malignancies: Results from Clinical Trials

Clinical Experience in Acute Lymphoblastic Leukemia (ALL) Using TALEN-Edited CAR19 T Cells

Children experiencing relapse/refractory (R/R) ALL are now considered for immunotherapy interventions including monoclonal antibodies, bi-specific T cell engager (BiTE) agents, CAR therapy and allogenic hematopoietic stem cell transplantation for a chance of cure [11, 12]. The success of autologous CAR-T cells in seminal clinical trials led to approval by health authorities in U.S. and Europe of Tisagenlecleucel (autologous lentiviral transduced CAR19 T cells) for treatment of pediatric ALL, and since 2017, immunotherapy using adoptive T cells has become a licensed therapy [13, 14]. However, the high demand of so called "salvage" strategies for patients refractory to first and second line of treatments, has highlighted challenges of manufacturing, timing, logistics and costs for the generation of a highly personalized treatment, such as autologous CAR-T. Pre-manufactured CAR T cells from non-HLA matched donors have been in development but have had to overcome above mentioned key barriers. These include addressing host mediated rejection and cell driven graft versus host disease (GvHD), while preserving antileukemic effects. In 2015, the highly attractive potential of this approach was evaluated in the first clinical experience of genome edited off-the-shelf CAR-T cell therapy used to treat two infants with R/R B-ALL [9]. Here, 'universal' CAR19 T cells (UCART19) from a non-HLA matched donor were manufactured by TALEN mediated editing of lentiviral modified T cells. Genome editing disrupted the expression of CD52, allowing evasion of the depleting antibody alemtuzumab by the UCART19s, and simultaneously knocked out the TRAC gene in order to limit occurrence of GvHD. Cells were infused in a single dose in both infants, after lymphodepletion comprising fludarabine, cyclophosphamide and alemtuzumab and mediated molecular remissions within 28 days, allowing consolidation with allogeneic stem cell transplantation (SCT). Phase 1 trials were subsequently conducted in both children ("PALL trial") and adults ("CALM trial")(Table 1) [15] Results from 21 patients treated revealed a response rate of 67%, comparable to autologous CAR T cells. Allogenic CAR-T cells actively expanded in the first weeks after infusion and treatment response was correlated with UCART19 exposure, although persistence started to decline by day 28 in most patients. The importance of lymphodepletion and immunosuppression was highlighted as when anti-CD52 monoclonal antibody (alemtuzumab) was omitted, UCART19 failed to expand and, consequently, no response was observed. These early data suggest that optimization of lymphodepleting regimen will be pivotal to facilitate donor cell activity while balancing the risk of infections during prolonged lymphopenia. Of importance, neither GvHD nor CAR-T specific severe toxicities (cytokine release syndrome, neurotoxicity) impeded the application of UCART19 cells. These early milestones showed

Table 1 Summary of first-in-human application of universal CAR-T cell therapy for B cell malignancies

Setting	Disease	Genome editing tool	Efficacy	Safety	Clinical trial
Pediatric (specials, off-trial) [19]	B-ALL	TALEN	Achieved complete remission (CR), successful HSCT, in both patients	No CRS, no neurotoxicity, mild GvHD	N/A
Pediatric (PALL trial) & adult (CALM trial) [15]	B-ALL	TALEN	Complete remission or CR with incomplete count recovery (CRi) obtained in 67%	CRS ≥ grade 3: 15% Neurotoxicity ≥grade 2: 5% GvHD grade 1: 10% Cytopenia: 32%	NCT02808442 NCT02746952
Adults	B-NHL FL LBCL	TALEN	Response rate 80%	No severe CRS/ neurotoxicity No GvHD	NCT03939026 NCT04416984
Adults	B-NHL	CRISPR/Cas9	Remission in 3/11 patients	No severe CRS/ neurotoxicity No GvHD	NCT04035434
Adults	B-NHL B-ALL	Meganuclease	Response in 2/3 patients	No severe CRS/ neurotoxicity	NCT03666000

ALL acute lymphoblastic leukemia, *FL* follicular lymphoma, *LBCL* large B cell lymphoma, *NHL* non-Hodgkin lymphoma, *CR* complete remission, *CRS* cytokine release syndrome, *GvHD* graft versus host disease

for the first time the feasibility of generating and delivering genome-edited allogeneic CAR T cells in the clinical arena, with minimal side effects, and promising response rates. Next generation CRISPR/Cas9 genome edited CAR-T cells, incorporating advances in editing techniques and automated cell manufacturing are underway in children at Great Ormond Street Hospital (London, UK) for R/R B-ALL (NCT04557436).

Following the promising experience of TALEN genome edited allogenic CAR-T cells in patients with ALL, clinical application has been directed towards other hematological malignancies that can be efficiently targeted using anti-CD19 CAR, such as non-Hodgkin lymphoma (NHL). Two phase 1, dose escalating clinical trials (ALPHA studies) are currently investigating safety and efficacy of UCART19 in adult patients with relapsed/refractory large B-cell or follicular lymphoma. Data on the first 9 patients treated were reported in early 2020 showing promising safety results: only mild CRS and neurotoxicity were observed, and one patient experienced multiple viral infections/reactivation (maximum grade III). Response rate was 80%, with complete response in 3/9 patients [16]. Updated results were lately communicated on 22 patients treated within this trial showing no dose-limiting toxicities, no GvHD and manageable CRS and neurotoxicity.

Emerging Experience with Next-Generation Genome Edited CAR19 T Cells in B-Cell Malignancies

The rapid evolution of genome editing tools has provided new and more efficient route to exploit the potential of allogeneic adoptive immunotherapies for cancer. New platforms for DNA editing, such as CRISPR/Cas9 have expanded the design of next generation allogenic CAR-T cell therapies. Simultaneous disruption of multiple targets and precision insertion of DNA sequences in specific sites can provide alternative strategies to overcome HLA-barriers and enhance anti-leukemic effect of CAR-T cells. New iterations of off-the-shelf CAR-T cells based on this technology have recently entered the clinic for treatment of B-cell malignancies. CRISPR Therapeutics has deployed CTX110, multiplexed genome edited T cells with a CAR19 cassette inserted into the TCR α-chain locus, generating a CD19-targeted T cell with CAR expression under the control of endogenous transcriptional machinery. This approach appeared attractive as pre-clinical data showed enhanced anti-tumor activity and reduced risk of early exhaustion. Insertion of the CAR gene into the TRAC locus simultaneously disrupted native TCR and cells were also knocked out for β2-microglobulin (B2M) leading to abrogation of MHC class I expression. Preliminary data from the first eleven patients with NHL were communicated in 2020, with remission in 3/11, and no GvHD or severe CRS/neurotoxicity were observed (NCT04035434). Precision Biosciences has developed another platform for genome editing (ARCUS®), using meganuclease to manufacture off-the-shelf CAR-T cells, again with a CAR gene in the TCR locus, albeit with an added internal promoter [17]. Interim analysis of the first three NHL patients treated at the lowest dose showed an encouraging safety profile and *in vivo* expansion (NCT03666000) [18].

Clinical applications of off-the-shelf CAR T cells for ALL and NHL have provided encouraging proof of principle for universal CAR-T cell therapy. While more robust data from patients treated using next-generation genome edited CAR-T cell are anxiously awaited, issues to be resolved include the most efficient lymphodepleting regimen, duration and persistence of T cell activity, and the need for stem cell transplant consolidation (Fig. 2).

Off-the-Shelf "Universal" Gene-Edited CAR-T Cells for Indications beyond B-Cell Malignancies

Allogeneic CAR-T for the Treatment of T Cell Malignancies

The inability to separate healthy T cells from malignant T cells due to the shared expression of T cell antigens, lends itself to the use of allogeneic CAR-T products for treating T cell cancers. The inadvertent generation of antigen negative, therapy resistant clones, has been observed in manufacture of autologous CART19 [20], in

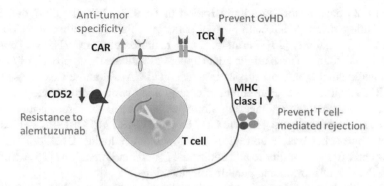

Fig. 2 Genome editing strategies to overcome HLA-barriers and generate universal CAR-T cells currently explored in clinical trials. Up-ward green arrow shows expression of CAR. Down-ward red arrows show disruption of T cell surface molecules: CD52 knock-out provide resistance to alemtuzumab; TCR genes knock-out prevent alloreactivity; Beta-2-Microglobulin knock-out blocks the formation and expression of MHC class I, providing resistance to immune-mediated rejection

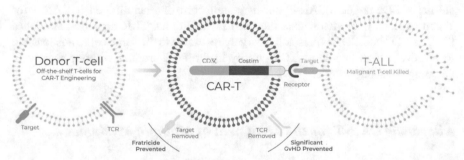

Fig. 3 Allogeneic CAR-T for the treatment of T cell cancers. The target is removed to prevent fratricide. The TCR is removed to mitigate the risk of GvHD

which removal of malignant B cells from the starting material is significantly less challenging. Additionally, the shared expression of target antigens between healthy T cells and malignant T cells has limited the development of CAR-T targeting T cell cancers because of unintended CAR-T fratricide in which the CAR-T recognize themselves as the target. Strategies to overcome fratricide include the use of gene-editing to delete the target from the CAR-T cell surface, preventing CAR-T from recognizing and killing each other [21]. Off-the-shelf fratricide-resistant CAR-T can be generated by suppressing expression of both the target and the TCR simultaneously (Fig. 3) [22]. UCART7, a multiplex gene-edited allogeneic CD7 targeted CAR-T demonstrated preclinical efficacy in vitro and against in vivo xenogeneic models of T-ALL [22]. This approach has since attracted the attention of companies seeking to deliver a commercially viable therapeutic product for the treatment of T cell cancers, including Wugen Inc., Gracell Bio, and Beam therapeutics. In an open-label single arm study (NCT04264078), 100% of patients (5/5) achieved a complete response 28 days following administration of GC027, Gracell's CD7 and TRAC deleted allogeneic CAR-T, with 80% of patients achieving a minimal residual disease (MRD) negativity [23]. Furthermore, no neurotoxicity or GVHD was observed in this initial cohort. These clinical data appear to validate the approach of targeting T cell malignancies with off-the-shelf gene edited CAR-T, and unlike the setting of UCART19, without the requirement of conditioning with alemtuzumab.

Alternative genome engineering strategies have been explored, both academically and commercially, to generate CD7 targeted CAR [24]. CRISPR guided base-editing approaches enable editing of genes without inducing DNA double strand breaks and offers the ability to add additional genetic modifications [25] while mitigating the risk of introducing genetic translocations.

Other T cell targets being explored in the setting of allogeneic CAR-T include CD2 [26] and CD3 [27], both of which are preferentially expressed on more mature T cell cancers such as T-NHL. CD3 targeted CAR, in which the TCR is also deleted, has the additional benefit of self-purification, harnessing fratricide as a mechanism for eliminating potentially GvHD inducing TCR+ CAR-T, and eradicating the requirement of additional mechanical depletion strategies [27]. Similarly, the co-culture of CD3 targeted CAR-T, during manufacture of other allogeneic CAR-T for T cell cancers, may also negate the need for additional TCR depletion strategies [24]. As CD3 and CD7 expression is largely restricted to the same cells, it is feasible to achieve a high degree of TCR- purity in the final product without negatively affecting the safety profile.

Allogeneic CAR-T for the Treatment of Multiple Myeloma

The autologous BCMA-targeted CAR-T, ide-cel (idecabtagene vicleucel, Abecma), is the lasted adoptive cellular therapy to gain FDA approval based on a response rate of 72% and a median duration of response of 11 Months [28]. With the recent approval of ide-cel, multiple myeloma is considered an optimal indication for translation of allogeneic CAR-T. Approaches for allogeneic CAR-T targeting BCMA include TALEN edited ALLO-715 [29] (Allogene NCT04093596), CRISPR/Cas9 edited CTX120 (CRISPR Therapeutics NCT04244656) [30], which utilizes an AAV vector to insert the CAR into the TRAC locus, and PBCAR269a manufactured using Precision Biosciences' proprietary ARCUS meganuclease platform (NCT04171843). A further alternative allogeneic BCMA targeted CAR-T, CYAD-211, utilizes a shRNA mediated approach to silence the TCR expression and mitigate GvHD (NCT04613557). All four platforms are currently in phase 1 clinical testing. In addition to BCMA, other targets include CS1 (SLAMF7). Cellectis has developed a TALEN edited, fratricide-resistant, allogeneic CAR-T targeting CS1 [31], which, in addition to high expression on malignant plasma cells, is expressed on CD8+ T cells. Phase 1 clinical testing of UCARTCS1 is currently ongoing (MELANI-01: NCT04142619).

Allogeneic CAR-T for the Treatment of AML

Identifying a selective target antigen for AML has proven challenging in the setting of both autologous and allogeneic CAR-T. Targeted AML antigens, such as CD33, FLT3 and CD123, which are expressed on hematopoietic stem cells or early myeloid progenitors, pose the risk of bone marrow failure. As such, targeting CAR-T therapy for AML is largely restricted to patient's pre-allogeneic transplantation. Targets such as CLL-1 (CD371), which are highly expressed on AML blasts but absent on normal HSC, may offer the ability to limit off-tumor toxicities in the setting of AML and are being pursued commercially in the allogeneic CAR-T setting (Caribou Biosciences).

Another potential strategy to mitigate off-tumor toxicities in the setting of AML includes transplantation of donor HSC in which the target epitope is genetically deleted or modified. In preclinical models, CD33 edited HSC maintain multilineage hematopoietic engraftment post-transplant while protecting HSC from CAR33 mediated cytotoxicity [32–34]. HLA compatible allogenic donor T cells, sourced from the HSC donor will not be subjected to the same degree of rejection as fully allogeneic CAR-T and will likely result in prolonged persistence but may still be subject to many of the current limitations of autologous CAR-T therapeutics. Phase 1 clinical trials assessing the safety of CD33 deleted HSC are expected to initiate later this year.

Allogene Therapeutics recently reported preclinical data supporting the role of a rituximab responsive suicide switch into their FLT3 targeted CAR-T construct (FLT3-CAR-R2, ALLO-819) as a mechanism to minimize bone marrow toxicity [35]. Following AML eradication, rituximab mediated CAR-T deletion enabled hematopoietic recovery in humanized mouse models suggesting a potential mechanism to clinically mitigate off-tumor targeting.

Considering the complexity of targeting AML, clinical data utilizing allogeneic CAR-T for AML is scarce. Cellectis developed UCART123, a TALEN edited, TRAC and CD52 disrupted, allogeneic CAR-T targeting CD123 [36] that is currently ongoing clinical testing. To enhance the safety profile, a suicide receptor (RQR8) [37] was incorporated into UCART123, enabling selective deletion of CAR expressing cells through rituximab administration. UCART123, has been tested clinically in two phase 1 clinical trials: AMELI-1 (NCT03190278) for AML and ABC123 (NCT03203369) for BPDCN (blastic plasmacytoid dendritic cell neoplasm). However, the first patient dosed in the ABC123 trial succumbed to severe cytokine release syndrome and vascular leak syndrome resulting in FDA clinical holds to both phase 1 trials. The BPDCN trial was discontinued, however, a revised clinical protocol, incorporating a lower UCART123 dose, was subsequently approved for the treatment of AML and results from AMELI-01 are eagerly awaited.

Summary

CAR-T cells have profoundly altered the therapeutic landscape for the treatment of hematologic malignancies. Increasingly sophisticated engineering strategies are being employed to build upon the success of autologous CAR-T to develop off-the-shelf allogeneic treatments. The initial clinical data from UCART19 is promising; however, off-the-shelf cellular therapies remain in their infancy and face several challenges if they are to expand to indications beyond B cell cancers. Key questions remain to be answered and how the field evolves will largely depend on the lessons learnt from the current clinical trials.

References

1. Schuster SJ, Svoboda J, Chong EA, et al. Chimeric antigen receptor T cells in refractory B-cell lymphomas. N Engl J Med. 2017;377(26):2545–54. (In eng). https://doi.org/10.1056/NEJMoa1708566.
2. Born WK, Kemal Aydintug M, O'Brien RL. Diversity of γδ T-cell antigens. Cell Mol Immunol. 2013;10(1):13–20. https://doi.org/10.1038/cmi.2012.45.
3. Lantz O, Bendelac A. An invariant T cell receptor alpha chain is used by a unique subset of major histocompatibility complex class I-specific CD4+ and CD4-8- T cells in mice and humans. J Exp Med. 1994;180(3):1097–106. (In eng). https://doi.org/10.1084/jem.180.3.1097.
4. Schmid H, Schneidawind C, Jahnke S, et al. Culture-expanded human invariant natural killer T cells suppress T-cell alloreactivity and eradicate leukemia. Front Immunol. 2018;9:1817. (In eng). https://doi.org/10.3389/fimmu.2018.01817.
5. Romee R, Rosario M, Berrien-Elliott MM, et al. Cytokine-induced memory-like natural killer cells exhibit enhanced responses against myeloid leukemia. Sci Transl Med. 2016;8(357):357ra123. (In eng). https://doi.org/10.1126/scitranslmed.aaf2341.
6. Osborn MJ, Webber BR, Knipping F, et al. Evaluation of TCR gene editing achieved by TALENs, CRISPR/Cas9, and megaTAL nucleases. Mol Ther. 2016;24(3):570–81. (In eng). https://doi.org/10.1038/mt.2015.197.
7. Berdien B, Mock U, Atanackovic D, Fehse B. TALEN-mediated editing of endogenous T-cell receptors facilitates efficient reprogramming of T lymphocytes by lentiviral gene transfer. Gene Ther. 2014;21(6):539–48. (In eng). https://doi.org/10.1038/gt.2014.26.
8. Torikai H, Reik A, Liu PQ, et al. A foundation for universal T-cell based immunotherapy: T cells engineered to express a CD19-specific chimeric-antigen-receptor and eliminate expression of endogenous TCR. Blood. 2012;119(24):5697–705. https://doi.org/10.1182/blood-2012-01-405365.
9. Qasim W, Zhan H, Samarasinghe S, et al. Molecular remission of infant B-ALL after infusion of universal TALEN gene-edited CAR T cells. Sci Transl Med. 2017;9:374. https://doi.org/10.1126/scitranslmed.aaj2013.
10. Cooper ML, DiPersio JF. Chimeric antigen receptor T cells (CAR-T) for the treatment of T-cell malignancies. Best Pract Res Clin Haematol. 2019;32(4):101097. (In eng). https://doi.org/10.1016/j.beha.2019.101097.
11. Kuhlen M, Willasch AM, Dalle J-H, et al. Outcome of relapse after allogeneic HSCT in children with ALL enrolled in the ALL-SCT 2003/2007 trial. Br J Haematol. 2018;180(1):82–9. (In en). https://doi.org/10.1111/bjh.14965.
12. Schrappe M, Hunger SP, Pui CH, et al. Outcomes after induction failure in childhood acute lymphoblastic leukemia. N Engl J Med. 2012;366(15):1371–81. (In eng). https://doi.org/10.1056/NEJMoa1110169.

13. Pasquini MC, Hu ZH, Curran K, et al. Real-world evidence of tisagenlecleucel for pediatric acute lymphoblastic leukemia and non-Hodgkin lymphoma. Blood Adv. 2020;4(21):5414–24. (In eng). https://doi.org/10.1182/bloodadvances.2020003092.

14. Maude SL, Laetsch TW, Buechner J, et al. Tisagenlecleucel in children and young adults with B-cell lymphoblastic leukemia. N Engl J Med. 2018;378(5):439–48. https://doi.org/10.1056/NEJMoa1709866.

15. Benjamin R, Graham C, Yallop D, et al. Genome-edited, donor-derived allogeneic anti-CD19 chimeric antigen receptor T cells in paediatric and adult B-cell acute lymphoblastic leukaemia: results of two phase 1 studies. Lancet (London, England). 2020;396(10266):1885–94. (In eng). https://doi.org/10.1016/s0140-6736(20)32334-5.

16. Neelapu SS, Munoz J, Locke FL, et al. First-in-human data of ALLO-501 and ALLO-647 in relapsed/refractory large B-cell or follicular lymphoma (R/R LBCL/FL): ALPHA study. J Clin Oncol. 2020;38(15_suppl):8002. https://doi.org/10.1200/JCO.2020.38.15_suppl.8002.

17. MacLeod DT, Antony J, Martin AJ, et al. Integration of a CD19 CAR into the TCR alpha chain locus streamlines production of allogeneic gene-edited CAR T cells. Mol Ther. 2017;25(4):949–61. https://doi.org/10.1016/j.ymthe.2017.02.005.

18. Jacobson CA, Herrera AF, Budde LE, et al. Initial findings of the phase 1 trial of PBCAR0191, a CD19 targeted allogeneic CAR-T cell therapy. Blood. 2019;134(Supplement_1):4107. https://doi.org/10.1182/blood-2019-128203.

19. Qasim W, Zhan H, Samarasinghe S, et al. Molecular remission of infant B-ALL after infusion of universal TALEN gene-edited CAR T cells. Sci Transl Med. 2017;9:374. (In eng). https://doi.org/10.1126/scitranslmed.aaj2013.

20. Ruella M, Xu J, Barrett DM, et al. Induction of resistance to chimeric antigen receptor T cell therapy by transduction of a single leukemic B cell. Nat Med. 2018;24(10):1499–503. (In eng). https://doi.org/10.1038/s41591-018-0201-9.

21. Gomes-Silva D, Srinivasan M, Sharma S, et al. CD7-edited T cells expressing a CD7-specific CAR for the therapy of T-cell malignancies. Blood. 2017;130(3):285–96. (In eng). https://doi.org/10.1182/blood-2017-01-761320.

22. Cooper ML, Choi J, Staser K, et al. An "off-the-shelf" fratricide-resistant CAR-T for the treatment of T cell hematologic malignancies. Leukemia. 2018. (In eng); https://doi.org/10.1038/s41375-018-0065-5.

23. Wang X, Li S, Gao L, et al. Safety and efficacy results of GC027: the first-in-human, universal CAR-T cell therapy for adult relapsed/refractory T-cell acute lymphoblastic leukemia (r/r T-ALL). J Clin Oncol. 2020;38(15_suppl):3013. https://doi.org/10.1200/JCO.2020.38.15_suppl.3013.

24. Georgiadis C, Rasaiyaah J, Gkazi SA, et al. Base-edited CAR T cells for combinational therapy against T cell malignancies. Leukemia. 2021; https://doi.org/10.1038/s41375-021-01282-6.

25. Gehrke J, Edwards A, Murray R, et al. 111 highly efficient multiplexed base editing enables development of universal CD7-targeting CAR-T cells to treat T-ALL. J Immunother Cancer. 2020;8(Suppl 3):A69. https://doi.org/10.1136/jitc-2020-SITC2020.0111.

26. Staser KW, Cooper ML, Choi J, et al. Modeling Sézary syndrome for immunophenotyping and anti-tumor effect of Ucart and long-acting Interleukin-7 combination therapy. Blood. 2018;132(Supplement 1):340. https://doi.org/10.1182/blood-2018-99-119375.

27. Rasaiyaah J, Georgiadis C, Preece R, Mock U, Qasim W. TCRαβ/CD3 disruption enables CD3-specific antileukemic T cell immunotherapy. JCI Insight. 2018;3:13. (In eng). https://doi.org/10.1172/jci.insight.99442.

28. Lin Y, Raje NS, Berdeja JG, et al. Idecabtagene Vicleucel (ide-cel, bb2121), a BCMA-directed CAR T cell therapy, in patients with relapsed and refractory multiple myeloma: updated results from phase 1 CRB-401 study. Blood. 2020;136(Supplement 1):26–7. https://doi.org/10.1182/blood-2020-134324.

29. Mailankody S, Matous JV, Liedtke M, et al. Universal: an allogeneic first-in-human study of the anti-Bcma ALLO-715 and the anti-CD52 ALLO-647 in relapsed/refractory multiple myeloma. Blood. 2020;136(Supplement 1):24–5. https://doi.org/10.1182/blood-2020-140641.

30. Dar H, Henderson D, Padalia Z, et al. Preclinical development of CTX120, an allogeneic CAR-T cell targeting Bcma. Blood. 2018;132(Supplement 1):1921. https://doi.org/10.1182/blood-2018-99-116443.
31. Mathur R, Zhang Z, He J, et al. Universal SLAMF7-specific CAR T-cells as treatment for multiple myeloma. Blood. 2017;130(Supplement 1):502. https://doi.org/10.1182/blood.V130.Suppl_1.502.502.
32. Borot F, Wang H, Ma Y, et al. Gene-edited stem cells enable CD33-directed immune therapy for myeloid malignancies. Proc Natl Acad Sci U S A. 2019;116(24):11978–87. (In eng). https://doi.org/10.1073/pnas.1819992116.
33. Humbert O, Laszlo GS, Sichel S, et al. Engineering resistance to CD33-targeted immunotherapy in normal hematopoiesis by CRISPR/Cas9-deletion of CD33 exon 2. Leukemia. 2019;33(3):762–808. (In eng). https://doi.org/10.1038/s41375-018-0277-8.
34. Kim MY, Yu KR, Kenderian SS, et al. Genetic inactivation of CD33 in hematopoietic stem cells to enable CAR T cell immunotherapy for acute myeloid Leukemia. Cell. 2018;173(6):1439–53. e19. (In eng). https://doi.org/10.1016/j.cell.2018.05.013.
35. Sommer C, Cheng H-Y, Nguyen D, et al. Allogeneic FLT3 CAR T cells with an off-switch exhibit potent activity against AML and can be depleted to expedite bone marrow recovery. Mol Ther. 2020;28(10):2237–51. https://doi.org/10.1016/j.ymthe.2020.06.022.
36. Guzman ML, Sugita M, Zong H, et al. Allogeneic Tcrα/β deficient CAR T-cells targeting CD123 prolong overall survival of AML patient-derived xenografts. Blood. 2016;128(22):765. https://doi.org/10.1182/blood.V128.22.765.765.
37. Philip B, Kokalaki E, Mekkaoui L, et al. A highly compact epitope-based marker/suicide gene for easier and safer T-cell therapy. Blood. 2014;124(8):1277–87. (In eng). https://doi.org/10.1182/blood-2014-01-545020.

Manufacturing of CAR-T Cells: The Assembly Line

Xiuyan Wang and Isabelle Rivière

Abstract The recent approval of five chimeric antigen receptor (CAR)-T cell products by the US food and drug administration (FDA) in the context of hematological malignancies has generated the impetus to broaden CAR-T cell therapy applications, resulting in growing production demand. Successful CAR-T cell manufacturing is not only the foundation of these promising therapies, but the choice of manufacturing platform and technology also contributes to defining the CAR-T cell product phenotype, therapeutic efficacy, potential toxicities, and affects the cost of goods. Although multiple methodologies and cell manufacturing platforms have become available, the core components of autologous CAR-T cell manufacturing such as source material collection, T cell isolation, activation, genetic modification, expansion, end of process formulation and cryopreservation remain constant. Current methodologies and cell manufacturing platforms are highlighted in the context of recent clinical trials. Quality requirement and quality control assays enabling the release of clinical CAR-T cell products for infusion are also underscored. The broadening of the scope of CAR-T cell applications beyond cancer therapies is also touched upon as this novel therapeutic paradigm is still evolving.

Keywords Manufacturing · CAR-T · Cell therapy · Collection · Selection · Activation · Gene transfer · Expansion · Large-scale · Product release · Vector · Platform · cGMP · Clinical trials

X. Wang · I. Rivière (✉)
Cell Therapy and Cell Engineering Facility, Memorial Sloan Kettering Cancer Center, New York, NY, USA
e-mail: rivierei@mskcc.org

© Springer Nature Switzerland AG 2022
A. Ghobadi, J. F. DiPersio (eds.), *Gene and Cellular Immunotherapy for Cancer*, Cancer Drug Discovery and Development,
https://doi.org/10.1007/978-3-030-87849-8_8

Introduction

The remarkable therapeutic efficacy of CD19 targeted CAR-T cells for hematological malignancies such as B cell acute lymphoblastic leukemia (ALL), non-hodgkin's lymphoma (NHL) and diffuse large B-cell lymphoma (DLBCL) [1] has led to the approval of five CAR-T cell products by the US food and drug administration (FDA): Tisagenlecleucel (Kymriah) for the treatment of pediatric ALL, DLBCL, high-grade B-cell lymphoma; Axicabtagene (Yescarta) for the treatment of relapsed or refractory large B-cell lymphoma; Brexucabtagene autoleucel (Tecartus) for relapsed and refractory mantle cell lymphoma; Lisocabtagene maraleucel (Breyanzi) for adults with relapsed or refractory large B-cell lymphoma, and idecabtagene vicleucel (Abecma) for relapsed/refractory multiple myeloma. Hundreds of early stage clinical trials using CAR-T cells targeting various tumor antigens, such as BCMA, CD33, CD123, GD2, mesothelin, PSMA, or using CAR-T cells in combination with immune checkpoint blockade such as anti-PD-1, anti-PD- L1 and CTLA-4, are registered at clinicaltrials.gov. [2].

The impetus for the establishment of new CAR-T cell therapies has resulted in growing production demands which are in turn fueling the rapid development of CAR-T cell manufacturing science and methodologies. Successful manufacturing is not only the foundation for every CAR-T cell clinical trial, but the choice of CAR-T cell manufacturing strategy and methodology also contributes to the phenotype and efficacy of the cells and drives the cost of goods. Despite the availability of multiple methodologies and cell manufacturing platforms, the core components of the CAR-T cell manufacturing procedure remain consistent between processes. They include source material collection, T cell isolation, activation, genetic modification, expansion, end of process formulation and cryopreservation. The quality of the CAR-T cell product is built within the manufacturing procedure and is demonstrated by the in-process and final product release testing. The stepwise CAR-T cell manufacturing procedure is described below and illustrated in Fig. 1.

CAR-T Cell Manufacturing

T Cell Collection: The Beginning

CAR-T cell therapy at present time is mostly an autologous therapy [2]. Emerging clinical studies aim at testing CAR-T cells in an allogeneic setting with additional genetic modification of T cells using gene-editing tools to mitigate the risk of graft versus host disease (GVHD) [3]. For both autologous and allogeneic CAR-T cell therapies, the manufacturing processes starts from the collection of patient or donor peripheral blood mononuclear cells (PBMCs), most commonly through a leukapheresis, whereby white blood cells are collected and all other components in the blood are returned to the circulation. Alternative T cell sources that have been reported so far include PBMCs enriched from Ficoll-Hypaque density gradient separation [4].

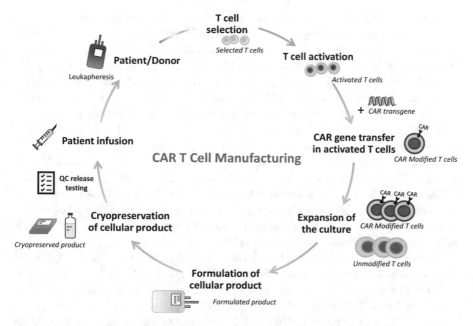

Fig. 1 Simplified CAR-T cell manufacturing scheme. T cells are first selected from patient or donor apheresis products and subsequently activated. After CAR transgene is introduced into activated T cells through various gene transfer methods, the culture is further expanded and formulated upon meeting the dose requirements. Formulated cells can be cryopreserved in either cryobags or vials. Cellular products are ready to be released for infusion upon meeting all release criteria

Collected PBMCs contain contaminants including anticoagulants that are included during PBMC collection, plasma, red blood cells (RBCs), and platelets. It is important to remove these contaminants to minimize their impact on downstream processing such as impairment of T cell activation and increased cell clumping [5]. Several cell-washing devices are suitable to remove the plasma, RBCs and platelets, such as COBE 2991, Haemonetics Cell Saver 5+, and Fresenius Kabi LOVO. Terumo Elutra [6, 7] and GE Sepax system [8] can further deplete monocytes and isolate lymphocytes with cell-size-based fractionation. Washed or fractionated cells can either be used directly for the next manufacturing step or cryopreserved until further processing.

T Cell Selection: Fine-Tuning the Starting Material

CD3+ T cell population is currently the most widely used starting cell population for CAR-T cell manufacturing [9]. Selection of CD3+ cells can be achieved by using the Dynabeads® magnetic separation technology. Washed apheresis product is first incubated with CD3/CD28 antibody-coated magnetic Dynabeads® to allow binding of beads to CD3+ T cells. T cells can subsequently be pulled out by a magnet, such as the ClinExVivo magnetic particle concentrator (MPC). CD3+ T cells selected using this method may contain high numbers of monocytes due to the engulfment of beads through phagocytosis, and high numbers of tumor cells if the patient has a large circulating tumor burden. High level of monocyte contamination poses a manufacturing challenge through inhibition of T cell expansion [10] and negatively impacts CAR-T cell function [11, 12]. The contaminating tumor cells can potentially be transduced and prevent the antitumor activity of CAR-T cells by tumor antigen epitope-masking [13]. To prevent these deleterious outcomes, T cells can be either positively selected by incubating the washed apheresis product with anti-CD4 and anti-CD8 microbeads and using CliniMACS [14] or by depleting CD19+, CD14+, and CD56+ cells using anti-CD19, anti-CD14, and anti-CD56 microbeads and CliniMACS (our unpublished data). In a phase I clinical trial of anti-CD22 CAR T-cells for children and young adults with relapsed/refractory CD22+ malignancies, it was shown that CD4/CD8 T-cell selection of the apheresis product improved CAR T-cell manufacturing feasibility as well as heightened inflammatory toxicities as compared to products that were derived from whole apheresis, leading to dose de-escalation [15].

Studies from several laboratories have further demonstrated that CAR-T cells derived from subpopulations such as naïve (T_N, CD45RA+CD62L+) [16], central memory (T_{CM}, CD45RA-CD62L+) [17, 18], or memory stem cell (T_{SCM}, CD45RA+ CD62L+CCR7+CD27+CD28+CD127+CD95+) [19] subsets, mediate stronger anti-tumor activities when compared to CAR-T cells derived from bulk T cell population in *in vivo* animal models. Despite challenging low numbers, investigators have used the T_{CM} subset as starting material in the clinical setting by combining CD14+, CD25+, and CD45RA+ depletion to CD62L+ positive selection, and subsequent manufacturing of CAR-T cells which led to glioblastoma regression in one patient [20]. CD8 T_{CM} subset was also successfully selected by depletion of CD4+, CD14+, and CD45RA+ cells followed by CD62L+ positive selection in pre-clinical models [17, 18, 21]. CAR-T cells with defined CD4+CAR+ and CD8+CAR+T_{CM} or CD4+CAR+ and CD8+CAR+ ratio have been infused in patients with B-ALL and NHL which potentially mitigated toxicity and improved disease-free survival [18]. Generation of CAR-T cells from a T cell population with defined properties is an attractive approach. A caveat related to the use of T cell subsets is the increased complexity of the manufacturing scheme and cost related to the selection procedure. The merit of using these refined T cell subsets still awaits long-term patient follow up and clinical outcome in larger patient cohorts to determine whether superior therapeutic benefit will emerge and outweigh simpler and yet robust manufacturing platforms.

T Cell Activation: Preparing T Cells for Gene Transfer and Expansion

Sustained and adequate T cell activation is needed for *in vitro* expansion of T cells and is required for transfer of the CAR transgene mediated by gamma-retroviral vectors. Activation of T cells *in vivo* requires the engagement of T cell receptor and its cognate antigen presented on the MHC molecule (signal 1) on antigen presenting cells (APCs) and activation of co-stimulatory molecules such as CD28, 41BB and OX40 by the APCs (signal 2). Various *in vitro* T cell activation methods have been established and they can be largely classified as T cell stimulation by either soluble antibodies, Expamer, antibody-coated beads, or artificial antigen presenting cells (AAPCs).

T Cell Activation by Soluble Antibodies: The engagement of CD3 monoclonal antibody OKT3 in the presence of high dose IL-2 has been used to activate and expand donor CD19-CAR T cells in numerous clinical trials [9]. Soluble tetrameric CD3, CD28, and CD2 antibodies have also been developed to cross-link CD3, CD28 and CD2 on T cell surface as T cell activator [22] . Guanylyl cyclase C-targeted CAR-T cells have been generated from T cells activated by this CD3/CD28 tetrameric antibody complexes and these CAR-T cells can significantly protect the syngeneic metastasis of colorectal cancer to the lung in an animal model [23].

T Cell Activation by Expamer: The core of the Expamer technology is the soluble multimer backbone of the mutated streptavidin molecule, Strep-Tactin. The strep-tags of Strep-Tactin bind to biotinalyted anti-CD3 and anti-CD28 Fab fragments, which facilitates the polyclonal stimulation of T cells. The interaction between biotinylated Fab to Strep-Tactin is reversible and Expamer can be removed by cell washing. It has been reported that Expamer can efficiently induce TCR signaling, activate T cells to enable transduction using retroviral vectors and support T cell expansion [24, 25]. Its soluble nature and ease of removal during cell washing makes Expamer an attractive T cell activation reagent.

T Cell Activation by Antibody-Coated Beads: the soluble anti-CD3 monoclonal antibody, OKT3, has been shown to be less effective for T cell activation when compared to its immobilized counterpart. In addition, the T cell activation function of OKT3 antibody can be enhanced by immobilized monoclonal antibodies against costimulatory molecules, such as CD28 [26–28]. A handful of companies have developed CD3- and CD28- antibody coated beads, such as Dynabeads™ human T-Activator CD3/CD28 (ThermoFisher Scientific), and the T cell TransAct™ CD3/CD28 (Miltenyi Biotech) [29, 30]. Dynabeads are paramagnetic beads that are used for both selection and activation of CD3+ T cells; they must be removed at the end of the culture before formulation. TransAct CD3/CD28 beads are polymeric nano-beads intended for the *in vitro* stimulation of pre-selected T cells. They are biodegradable and can be largely washed out during formulation, therefore they do not need to be removed at the end of the process. These off-the-shelf T cell activation cGMP reagents are currently the most widely used for the activation of T cells in the context of CAR-T cell manufacturing [9].

T Cell Activation by AAPC: Natural activators for T cells are autologous professional antigen presenting cells (APCs), including dendritic cells (DCs), B cells and macrophages. The preparation of DCs derived from apheresis products is not only tedious, the potency of primary DCs also significantly varies from patient to patient [31]. These limitations have hampered the application of DCs as a reliable source for T cell activation. Alternatively, artificial antigen presenting cells (AAPCs) have been developed from the chronic myelogenous leukemia (CML) cell line K562. K562 cells do not express MHC molecules or T cell costimulatory ligands, allowing investigators to customize the stimulatory and costimulatory molecules in these cells to activate, expand and amplify subsets of T cells. In comparison to antibody coated beads, K562 AAPCs are more efficient at activating and expanding CD8+ and antigen-specific T cells [17, 32, 33]. Irradiated K562-derived AAPCs have been successfully used to activate T cells and expand CD19-specific CAR-T cells [34]. Patient derived irradiated autologous PBMCs [35] as well as PBMCs together with EBV-specific lymphoblastoid B-cell lines (LCLs) [36] in combination with OKT3 anti-CD3 antibody and IL2 have also been reported for T cell activation as means to generate CD19- and CD20-specific CAR-T cells, respectively. Nonetheless, the usage of cell-based T cell activation is rather limited as compared to other T cell activation approaches due to the complexity of generating cGMP compliant AAPC lines [37].

Gene Transfer: Introduction of CARs into T Cells

CARs can be introduced into T cells either permanently or transiently by using viral or non-viral gene transfer methodologies. Current CAR-T cell therapies largely rely on the stable and robust expression of CARs. Gammaretroviral vectors, lentiviral vectors and transposon/transposases are the three major approaches for permanently incorporating CAR transgenes into the genome. Alternatively, AAV-CAR (Adeno-Associated Virus-CAR) expression cassettes flanked by homology arms are also used in conjunction with CRISPR/Cas gene editing tools for site-specific CAR integration [38, 39]. Transient CAR expression is advantageous for screening CAR specificity towards tumor antigens and for investigating the on-target off tumor effect, where short-term expression of CAR can mitigate the side effects of constitutive CAR expression. CAR mRNA electroporation is currently the method of choice to mediate transient expression of CARs. Each delivery system is described below and summarized in Table 1.

Gammaretroviral Vectors: Gammaretroviral vectors are widely used in cell and gene therapy applications as gene delivery vehicles. The first gammaretroviral vectors developed for gene delivery and still used up to this day are derived mostly from the Moloney murine leukemia virus (Mo-MLV) and the Myeloproliferative sarcoma virus (MPSV) [40, 41]. In addition to promoting high expression levels of the transgene(s), another instrumental advantage is the availability of multiple stable packaging cells lines that facilitate the generation of pseudotyped gammaretroviral vectors with a wide range of tropisms and are available for manufacturing according to cGMP [42, 43]. Despite the adverse events observed in SCID-X1 and WAS patients engrafted with gammaretroviral vector-transduced HPSCs, owing to the integration of the transgene near proto-oncogene sequences such as *LMO2, CCNDs, and MDS1-EVI 1* [44, 45], long-term patient follow up studies have shown the remarkable safety profile of gammaretroviral vectors in the context of adoptive T cell therapies [46–49]. Three of the five current FDA-approved CAR-T cell products, axicabtagene (Yescarta), brexucabtagene autoleucel (Tecartus) and

Table 1 Current major gene transfer platforms for CAR-T cells

Category	Platform	Theoretical Packaging capacity	CAR expression	Pros	Cons
Viral vectors [76, 77]	Gamma-retroviral vectors	7.5 kb	Permanent	Stable and high levels of transgene expression; availability of multiple packaging cell lines with wide tropism; feasibility to generate large vector lot	Unable to efficiently transduce non-dividing or slowly dividing cells; low probability of giving rise to replication competent retroviral virus; insertional genotoxicity in HSCs; expensive release testing; long-term monitoring of recipient
	Lentiviral vectors	7.8 kb	Permanent	Stable and high levels of transgene expression; transduce non-dividing cells; safer genome insertional profile	Lack of stable packaging cell lines; complex transient transfection manufacturing platform; larger lot to lot variability; possibility of giving rise to replication competent lentivirus; potential insertional genotoxicity; expensive release testing
	AAV	5 kb	Permanent	Facilitate site-specific incorporation of CAR transgene, persistent and stable transgene expression	Requires gene editing technology and special homologous sequences for site-specific incorporation.
Non-viral vectors [78–80]	Transposon/ transposase system	6 kb	Permanent	Plasmid based: Simpler to manufacture; simpler to test; lower cost comparing to viral vector; low immunogenicity	Low efficiency; potential insertional genotoxicity
	mRNA	10 kb	Transient	No genome toxicity; biodegradable; self limiting off-target toxicity of transgene	Transient expression of transgene; mRNA stability

lisocabtagene maraleucel (Breyanzi), utilize gammaretroviral vectors as the CAR delivery vehicle to transduce T cells [50]. cGMP gammaretroviral vectors can be manufactured in various scalable platforms [51–53] and are not at risk of promoting replication-competent retrovirus (RCR) during manufacturing [54].

Lentiviral Vectors: Lentiviral vectors present the advantage of being able to transduce non-dividing cells. The most common lentiviral vectors are derived from HIV-1 pseudotyped with VSV-G envelope (env). VSV-G env confers a high level of tropism to the viral particles and the ability to infect a wide variety of cell types [55]. Owing to the low level of expression of the receptor of VSV-G env, the low density lipoprotein receptor (LDLr), in unstimulated T cells, activation of T cells is also required to promote high levels of transduction with lentiviral vectors [56, 57]. Similar to retroviral vectors, lentiviral vectors mediate high levels of stable CAR expression. They also present a safer genome insertional profile [58]. The major drawback of lentiviral vectors is the lack of stable packaging cell lines due to the intrinsic fusogenic nature of the VSV-G env. Lentiviral vectors are typically produced via the multi-plasmid transient transfection process that requires large amount of plasmid DNA and downstream purification, which renders the process difficult to scale up and expensive [59]. Nonetheless, two FDA-approved CAR-T cell product, tisagenlecleucel (Kymriah) and idecabtagene vicleucel (Abecma), utilizes lentiviral vector produced by transient transfection as the vehicle for CAR delivery in T cells [60, 61]. Progress is being made in manufacturing these vectors using scalable platforms [62, 63]. Many researchers are also actively working on the development of stable producer cell lines for lentiviral vectors either by using elaborated inducible systems to control VSV-G env expression [59], or by employing alternative envelop glycoproteins such as the feline endogenous gamma retrovirus RD114 [64, 65] and the Baboon retroviral envelope glycoprotein [66].

Transposon and Transposase System: Transposon/transposase system is a relatively new plasmid-based CAR delivery method through electroporation of T cells. The CAR transgene is inserted into the genome via the transposase excision and insertion mechanism. This plasmid-based method is comparatively less expensive than retroviral and lentiviral vectors which are complex biologics requiring more intensive and expensive manufacturing and biosafety testing. It has been shown that sleeping beauty (SB) transposon/transposase has a theoretically higher safety profile [67]. Clinical trials have been conducted with CAR-T cells genetically modified via this SB platform with modest efficacy [68]. When compared to viral vector platforms, the drawbacks of the transposon/transposase system include the higher cell dose requirement due to less efficient gene transfer, hence longer *ex vivo* culture expansion period and the requirement for the selective propagation of CAR+ T cells via artificial antigen-presenting cells (AAPC) stimulation in addition to cytokines [37].

Adeno-Associated Viral Vectors: AAV vectors are used in a wide range of clinical applications [69]. In the context of CAR-T cell manufacturing, AAV vector has recently been used to facilitate the site-specific incorporation of CAR transgene in conjunction with gene editing tools. A site-specific double-stranded break at a targeted genomic location such as the *T-cell Receptor Alpha Chain (TRAC)* locus, enabled by gene editing tools such as CRISPR/cas9 and guide RNAs can subsequently be repaired by homology-directed repair (HDR). Transduction of gene edited T cells bearing a site-specific double-stranded break with an AAV-CAR expression cassette containing homology arms to the DNA break flanking sites facilitates the homologous recombination and enables the introduction of the CAR sequence at a specific location in the genome [38, 70].

mRNA: Unlike the gene transfer methods discussed above which enable permanent incorporation of CAR transgene into the genome and allow constitutive expression of CAR, transfer of *in vitro* transcribed CAR mRNA through electroporation mediates only transient expression. Since there is no genomic integration event associated with this platform, there are no concerns related to genotoxicity or formation of replication competent viruses. mRNA transfection has been successfully used to deliver mRNA encoding TCR [71], CAR [72], chemokine receptor and cytokines [73]. The self-limiting nature of CAR expression mediated by this platform is advantageous when serving as a safety check for on-target-off-tumor effect or off-tumor toxicities, and other unwanted side effects resulting from steady long term expression. mRNA-transfected mesothelin targeting CAR-T cells have been administered to patients with advanced solid tumors either through repeated systemic or intratumoral infusions [74, 75], indicating the feasibility of this gene transfer platform.

Large Scale CAR-T Cell Expansion: Growing Cells to Therapeutic Dose

For current CAR-T cell applications, cell expansion is typically needed to generate the amount of cells required for therapeutic clinical dose and release testing. Several platforms are available to enable this requirement. They are generally classified as static culture, wave-mixed bioreactor and expansion in continuous bioreactor.

Expansion in Static Culture: At the onset of CAR-T cell adoptive therapy, CAR-T cell expansion was mostly accomplished in static culture systems such as T flasks [81] or gas permeable cell bags [36]. As the cells expand, the large number of static vessels and volumes of culture become difficult to handle. The process is not only labor-intensive, but also requires highly trained operators working under the biosafety cabinet in a cGMP cleanroom environment. Although the handling of cell culture bags is simpler than that of tissue culture flasks, they are still not suitable for large-scale manufacturing. In recent years, a new type of cell culture flask with a gas permeable membrane at the base, the G-Rex bioreactor, was developed. This scalable cylindrical bioreactor allows initial low seeding density, one time upfront feeding regiment, growing of cells in an incubator, robust cell expansion, and ease of end of process volume reduction [82]. It mimics the format of the tissue culture flask but with features enabling a simple and cost-effective setting for early clinical application. Due to the static culture environment, G-Rex is especially suitable for co-culture of T cells with feeder cells, such as TILs [83] and expansion of T cell subset using AAPCs [84].

Expansion in Wave-Mixed Bioreactor: Wave-mixed bioreactors are more sophisticated bioreactors enabling efficient mixing and gas exchange using a low-shear rocking side-to-side wave motion. This type of scalable system comprises a single use cell bag bioreactor, a temperature enabling rocking base, a controller for gas and rocking speed, a pump enabling perfusion mode, and single use sensors monitoring pH and dissolved O2. Wave-mixed bioreactor is a functionally closed system with build-in automation features. It largely reduces the amount of labor required and allows cells to expand to higher cell density with the perfusion mode. This type of bioreactor has a working culture volume of 1–50 L with a minimal inoculation volume of approximately 300 mL, therefore requiring an initial seed train in either flasks or cell culture bags. This platform is wildly used by academic centers and biotech companies for CAR-T cell expansion to support early stage clinical trials [9, 85, 86].

Expansion in Continuous Culture Bioreactor: One of the newest technology for CAR-T cell expansion is the CliniMACS Prodigy System. It is a combination of a cell washer, a magnetic cell separation device, a shaker, a centrifuge, and a cell cultivation bioreactor. This system is fully enclosed and is designed to incorporate all steps of CAR-T cell manufacturing including T cell selection, activation, transduction, expansion and formulation. It enables a higher degree of automation, supports continuous cell culture, and largely decreases operator interpersonal variability. CAR-T cells generated in the CliniMACS Prodigy display significant anti-tumor activities in animal models and the transduction efficiency and T cell expansion were found comparable to those of CAR-T cells generated in Xuri/WAVE bioreactor [87]. Phase I clinical trials conducted with CD19 targeting CAR-T cells generated in CliniMACS Prodigy have generated encouraging results with 27 out of 31 pediatric patients with ALL (NCT03467256) [88] and 4 out of 5 adult patients with high risk NHL (NCT03434769) [89] achieving complete responses respectively. Additional trials using either CD19 specific CAR (NCT03434769) [90] and CD20.19 bi-specific CAR-T cells [91] were also successfully manufactured in academic cell processing facilities using this device. Another available integrated end-to-end cell manufacturing solution is the Cocoon platform, which also enables the activation, transduction, expansion and formulation steps of the manufacturing process. A clinical trial using CD19-targeted CAR-T cells manufactured with the Cocoon platform is currently being conducted (NCT02772198). These integrated and continuous culture bioreactors have the potential to enable the concept of point-of-care manufacturing.

Cryopreservation: Enabling Storage and Long Distance Shipment

Once the required cell dose is reached, expanded CAR-T cells are washed to remove the culture medium and contaminants such as cytokines, growth factors, magnetic beads, and resuspended in an infusion compatible formula, such as Plasmalyte with low percentage of human serum albumin [85]. The CAR-T cell product can be infused fresh within a short time frame (e.g. 24 h), upon passing all the release test criteria or be cryopreserved for infusion at a later time. Both practices are currently in use, but the time constraints relative to the rather complicated testing required to release CAR-T cell products for infusion (Table 2) and other logistics, such as real-time documentation review, real time issuance of certificate of analysis, and patient pre-treatment scheduling constitute major challenges for infusion of fresh products. The impact of cryopreservation on CAR-T cells has been evaluated in recent studies by comparing either the phenotypes and functions of fresh and cryopreserved CAR-T cells generated from healthy donor T cells or clinical outcomes of patients receiving either fresh or cryopreserved CAR-T cell products [92, 93]. Elevated expression of cell surface expression of apoptotic markers, activation of apoptosis and cell cycle pathways, as well as decreased *in vitro* secretion of IL-2, TNF and interferon-γ were observed in cryopreserved CAR-T cells when compared to fresh cells. However, no significant changes in transduction, T cell subsets composition, or antitumor activity in mouse models were found [92]. Moreover, retrospective studies in six clinical trials indicated that there was no difference in *in vivo* CAR-T persistence and clinical responses between fresh and cryopreserved CAR-T products in patients [93]. Further studies are warranted to evaluate the cell damage related to various cryoprotectant reagents [94], formulations and CAR-T cell freezing programs. However, cryopreservation of CAR-T cell product is currently a widely used strategy in many clinical applications and will be required for off-the-shelf applications and centralized manufacturing model.

Release of CAR-T Cell Products: Obtaining the Driver's License

Quality of the CAR-T products is built in the manufacturing procedure through current good manufacturing practices (cGMP) and current good documentation practices (cGDP). Because of the complexity of CAR-T cell manufacturing process, a cautiously designed set of in-process and release tests is needed to provide adequate evidence for product safety, identity, purity and potency. The release of the CAR-T cell product is governed by the certificate of analysis (CofA), that must include tests for the aforementioned critical quality attributes (CQA), the assay methods used, the identification of the testing facility, the release specification and the actual testing results. Examples of the general release testing and testing methods for CAR-T cell products are summarized in Table 2. Additional aspects of cell manufacturing quality checkpoints have been previously reviewed by Wang and Rivière [95].

Table 2 Example of quality control release assays for CAR-T cells [85, 96]

Critical quality attributes	Testing	Example assays	Example release criteria
Safety	Viability	Trypan blue, automatic cell count, or FACS	Typically ≥65–70%
	Sterility	USP	No growth for 14 days
		BACTEC/BACT ALERT	48 hr. or base on validation [97]
		Gram stain (for fresh product conditional release)	Negative
	Mycoplasma	PTC culture assay on indicator cell line	Negative
		PCR	Negative
		MycoAlert rapid test	Negative
	Endotoxin/Pyrogen	Kinetic chromogenic (LAL) assay	<5 EU/kg
	Average vector copy number	qPCR	≤4–5 copies/cells
	RCR or RCL	Marker rescue cell culture or qPCR	Negative
Identity	T cell marker	FACS	Application specific, such as >90%,
	CAR expression	FACS	Application specific, such as >4–10%
Purity	T cell markers and CAR expression	FACS	See above (purity and identity of CAR-T cell product could have some overlap)
	Contaminating cells (e.g. tumor, feeder cells)	FACS	Application specific
	Residual Dynabeads	Microscopy	<100 beads/3E6 cells
	Other residual reagents	Such as ELISA	Application specific
Potency	Cytotoxicity T cell assay	^{51}Cr release, or luciferase assay	Application specific
	Cytokine secretion, such as IFN-γ	ELISA or ELISpot	Application specific
	CD107a	FACS	Application specific

PTC point to consider, *PCR* polymerase chain reaction, *qPCR* quantitative real-time PCR, *ELISA* enzyme-linked immunosorbent assay, *ELISpot* Enzyme-linked immunospot

Future Perspectives

The last decade has witnessed a revolution in the development and application of autologous CAR-T cell therapy. The success of CAR-T cell engineering through the use of retroviral and lentiviral vectors has enabled this cell therapy to benefit thousands of patients and has led to the approval by the FDA of four CD19 targeted CAR-T cell products for hematological B-cell malignancies and one BCMA CAR for multiple myeloma [98, 99]. In the autologous setting, a seemingly minor change in the manufacturing process may have substantial impact on the quality of the final product, for example, usage of T cell subsets such as CD4/CD8 selected T cells [15], T_{SCM} [19] or T_N [16] in combination with better CAR design [38, 100] and could largely drive down the therapeutic dose requirements. The combination of gene editing and gene transfer technologies is currently being investigated. This rapidly evolving field is heading towards nucleases targeted CAR gene transfer at specific loci to alleviate random vector integration and towards off-the-shelf allogeneic CAR-T therapy to prevent inter-product variability in yield and phenotype and to overcome the impairment of anti-tumor functions of CAR-T cells derived from patients. New reagents, technologies and manufacturing platforms are being developed to meet the evolving needs [101]. In particular, minimally manipulated CAR-T cells kept in culture for less than 24 h. have demonstrated some level of anti-tumor activities in animal models. The optimization of this approach could simplify the CAR-T manufacturing process and has the potential to drastically decrease the overall cost [102, 103]]. Uniform batches of therapeutic T cells derived from induced pluripotent stem cells (iPSCs) [104, 105] could potentially mitigate the challenges posed by the poor quality of T cells derived from heavily pretreated cancer patients and generate a consistent product, although rejection by the host immune system remains to be solved [106].

Currently, CAR-T studies are largely geared toward the treatment of malignant diseases and have shown efficacy in hematological diseases. CAR-T cell inefficiencies in solid tumors are currently being tackled. In addition, this therapy could be applied to a much broader spectrum of diseases, including but not limited to (1) control of viral infection, such as hepatitis B [107], hepatitis C [108], CMV [109] and HIV [110]; (2) control of auto-reactive T cells [111]; and (3) control of graft-versus-host disease [112]. CAR-T cell therapy is becoming one of the pillars in modern immunotherapy and is poised to become incorporated into various types of applications. The future of CAR-T cell therapy relies on robust and reliable manufacturing processes, and the success in developing such processes is driven by our further understanding of the biology of the immune cells, the characterization of the products as well as the control of the processes.

References

1. Jain MD, Davila ML. Concise review: emerging principles from the clinical application of chimeric antigen receptor T cell therapies for B cell malignancies. Stem Cells. 2018;36:36–44.
2. Holzinger A, Barden M, Abken H. The growing world of CAR T cell trials: a systematic review. Cancer Immunol Immunother. 2016;65:1433–50.
3. Gao Q, Dong X, Xu Q, et al. Therapeutic potential of CRISPR/Cas9 gene editing in engineered T-cell therapy. Cancer Med. 2019;8:4254–64.
4. Enblad G, Karlsson H, Gammelgard G, et al. A phase I/IIa trial using CD19-targeted third-generation CAR T cells for lymphoma and Leukemia. Clin Cancer Res. 2018;24:6185–94.
5. Fesnak AD, June CH, Levine BL. Engineered T cells: the promise and challenges of cancer immunotherapy. Nat Rev Cancer. 2016;16:566–81.
6. Powell DJ Jr, Brennan AL, Zheng Z, Huynh H, Cotte J, Levine BL. Efficient clinical-scale enrichment of lymphocytes for use in adoptive immunotherapy using a modified counterflow centrifugal elutriation program. Cytotherapy. 2009;11:923–35.
7. Stroncek DF, Fellowes V, Pham C, et al. Counter-flow elutriation of clinical peripheral blood mononuclear cell concentrates for the production of dendritic and T cell therapies. J Transl Med. 2014;12:241.
8. Hamot G, Ammerlaan W, Mathay C, Kofanova O, Betsou F. Method validation for automated isolation of viable peripheral blood mononuclear cells. Biopreserv Biobank. 2015;13:152–63.
9. Vormittag P, Gunn R, Ghorashian S, Veraitch FS. A guide to manufacturing CAR T cell therapies. Curr Opin Biotechnol. 2018;53:164–81.
10. Stroncek DF, Ren J, Lee DW, et al. Myeloid cells in peripheral blood mononuclear cell concentrates inhibit the expansion of chimeric antigen receptor T cells. Cytotherapy. 2016;18:893–901.
11. Ino K, Ageitos AG, Singh RK, Talmadge JE. Activation-induced T cell apoptosis by monocytes from stem cell products. Int Immunopharmacol. 2001;1:1307–19.
12. Xiuyan Wang JQ, Stefanski J, Du F, Oriana, Borquez-Ojeda AH, Riviere I. Depletion of high-content CD14+ cells from apheresis products is critical for the successful transduction and expansion of CAR T cells during large-scale cGMP manufacturing. Mol Ther. 2015;23:S35.
13. Ruella M, Xu J, Barrett DM, et al. Induction of resistance to chimeric antigen receptor T cell therapy by transduction of a single leukemic B cell. Nat Med. 2018;24:1499–503.
14. Turtle CJ, Hanafi LA, Berger C, et al. CD19 CAR-T cells of defined CD4+:CD8+ composition in adult B cell ALL patients. J Clin Invest. 2016;126:2123–38.
15. Shah NN, Highfill SL, Shalabi H, et al. CD4/CD8 T-cell selection affects chimeric antigen receptor (CAR) T-cell potency and toxicity: updated results from a phase I anti-CD22 CAR T-cell trial. J Clin Oncol. 2020;38:1938–50.
16. Hinrichs CS, Borman ZA, Gattinoni L, et al. Human effector CD8+ T cells derived from naive rather than memory subsets possess superior traits for adoptive immunotherapy. Blood. 2011;117:808–14.
17. Berger C, Jensen MC, Lansdorp PM, Gough M, Elliott C, Riddell SR. Adoptive transfer of effector CD8+ T cells derived from central memory cells establishes persistent T cell memory in primates. J Clin Invest. 2008;118:294–305.
18. Sommermeyer D, Hudecek M, Kosasih PL, et al. Chimeric antigen receptor-modified T cells derived from defined CD8+ and CD4+ subsets confer superior antitumor reactivity in vivo. Leukemia. 2016;30:492–500.
19. Gattinoni L, Lugli E, Ji Y, et al. A human memory T cell subset with stem cell-like properties. Nat Med. 2011;17:1290–7.
20. Brown CE, Alizadeh D, Starr R, et al. Regression of glioblastoma after chimeric antigen receptor T-cell therapy. N Engl J Med. 2016;375:2561–9.
21. Wang X, Naranjo A, Brown CE, et al. Phenotypic and functional attributes of lentivirus-modified CD19-specific human CD8+ central memory T cells manufactured at clinical scale. J Immunother. 2012;35:689–701.

22. Devina Ramsaroop DS, Kee SL-Y, Hirsch C, Csaszar E, Aaron D-T. Moving towards a closed CAR-T cell manufacturing process. Mol Ther. 2019;27:288.
23. Magee MS, Abraham TS, Baybutt TR, et al. Human GUCY2C-targeted chimeric antigen receptor (CAR)-expressing T cells eliminate colorectal cancer metastases. Cancer Immunol Res. 2018;6:509–16.
24. Odendahl M, Grigoleit GU, Bonig H, et al. Clinical-scale isolation of 'minimally manipulated' cytomegalovirus-specific donor lymphocytes for the treatment of refractory cytomegalovirus disease. Cytotherapy. 2014;16:1245–56.
25. Bashour KT LR, Graef P, Stemberger C, Lothar G, Odegard V, and Ramsborg CG. Functional Characterization of a T Cell Stimulation Reagent for the Production of Therapeutic Chimeric Antigen Receptor T Cells. ASH 57th Annual Meeting & Exposition. Orlando, FL 2015.
26. Geppert TD, Lipsky PE. Activation of T lymphocytes by immobilized monoclonal antibodies to CD3. Regulatory influences of monoclonal antibodies to additional T cell surface determinants. J Clin Invest. 1988;81:1497–505.
27. Kalamasz D, Long SA, Taniguchi R, Buckner JH, Berenson RJ, Bonyhadi M. Optimization of human T-cell expansion ex vivo using magnetic beads conjugated with anti-CD3 and anti-CD28 antibodies. J Immunother. 2004;27:405–18.
28. Neurauter AA, Bonyhadi M, Lien E, et al. Cell isolation and expansion using Dynabeads. Adv Biochem Eng Biotechnol. 2007;106:41–73.
29. Casati A, Varghaei-Nahvi A, Feldman SA, et al. Clinical-scale selection and viral transduction of human naive and central memory CD8+ T cells for adoptive cell therapy of cancer patients. Cancer Immunol Immunother. 2013;62:1563–73.
30. Xiuyan Wang JQ, Stefanski J, Borquez-Ojeda O, Hack A, He Q, Wasielewska T, Du F, Sadelain M, Rivière I. Evaluation of Miltenyi ExpAct and TransAct CD3/28 beads for CAR-T cell manufacturing. Mol Ther. 2016;24:S182.
31. Sabado RL, Balan S, Bhardwaj N. Dendritic cell-based immunotherapy. Cell Res. 2017;27:74–95.
32. Maus MV, Thomas AK, Leonard DG, et al. Ex vivo expansion of polyclonal and antigen-specific cytotoxic T lymphocytes by artificial APCs expressing ligands for the T-cell receptor, CD28 and 4-1BB. Nat Biotechnol. 2002;20:143–8.
33. Suhoski MM, Golovina TN, Aqui NA, et al. Engineering artificial antigen-presenting cells to express a diverse array of co-stimulatory molecules. Mol Ther. 2007;15:981–8.
34. Singh H, Moyes JS, Huls MH, Cooper LJ. Manufacture of T cells using the sleeping beauty system to enforce expression of a CD19-specific chimeric antigen receptor. Cancer Gene Ther. 2015;22:95–100.
35. Kochenderfer JN, Dudley ME, Kassim SH, et al. Chemotherapy-refractory diffuse large B-cell lymphoma and indolent B-cell malignancies can be effectively treated with autologous T cells expressing an anti-CD19 chimeric antigen receptor. J Clin Oncol. 2015;33:540–9.
36. Till BG, Jensen MC, Wang J, et al. Adoptive immunotherapy for indolent non-Hodgkin lymphoma and mantle cell lymphoma using genetically modified autologous CD20-specific T cells. Blood. 2008;112:2261–71.
37. Singh H, Huls H, Kebriaei P, Cooper LJ. A new approach to gene therapy using sleeping beauty to genetically modify clinical-grade T cells to target CD19. Immunol Rev. 2014;257:181–90.
38. Eyquem J, Mansilla-Soto J, Giavridis T, et al. Targeting a CAR to the TRAC locus with CRISPR/Cas9 enhances tumour rejection. Nature. 2017;543:113–7.
39. Wang XZSE, Wu M, Zhu M, Del Casale C, Eyquem JE, Mansilla-Soto J, Sadelain M, Riviere I. Establishing cGMP manufacturing of CRISPR/Cas9-edited human CAR T cells. Mol Ther. 2020;28:66–7.
40. Mann R, Mulligan RC, Baltimore D. Construction of a retrovirus packaging mutant and its use to produce helper-free defective retrovirus. Cell. 1983;33:153–9.
41. Riviere I, Brose K, Mulligan RC. Effects of retroviral vector design on expression of human adenosine deaminase in murine bone marrow transplant recipients engrafted with genetically modified cells. Proc Natl Acad Sci U S A. 1995;92:6733–7.

42. Miller AD, Garcia JV, von Suhr N, Lynch CM, Wilson C, Eiden MV. Construction and properties of retrovirus packaging cells based on gibbon ape leukemia virus. J Virol. 1991;65:2220–4.
43. Ghani K, Wang X, de Campos-Lima PO, et al. Efficient human hematopoietic cell transduction using RD114- and GALV-pseudotyped retroviral vectors produced in suspension and serum-free media. Hum Gene Ther. 2009;20:966–74.
44. Hacein-Bey-Abina S, Garrigue A, Wang GP, et al. Insertional oncogenesis in 4 patients after retrovirus-mediated gene therapy of SCID-X1. J Clin Invest. 2008;118:3132–42.
45. Braun CJ, Boztug K, Paruzynski A, et al. Gene therapy for Wiskott-Aldrich syndrome—long-term efficacy and genotoxicity. Sci Transl Med. 2014;6:227ra33.
46. Bonini C, Grez M, Traversari C, et al. Safety of retroviral gene marking with a truncated NGF receptor. Nat Med. 2003;9:367–9.
47. Brenner MK, Heslop HE. Is retroviral gene marking too dangerous to use? Cytotherapy. 2003;5:190–3.
48. Muul LM, Tuschong LM, Soenen SL, et al. Persistence and expression of the adenosine deaminase gene for 12 years and immune reaction to gene transfer components: long-term results of the first clinical gene therapy trial. Blood. 2003;101:2563–9.
49. Scholler J, Brady TL, Binder-Scholl G, et al. Decade-long safety and function of retroviral-modified chimeric antigen receptor T cells. Sci Transl Med. 2012;4:132ra53.
50. Brudno JN, Kochenderfer JN. Chimeric antigen receptor T-cell therapies for lymphoma. Nat Rev Clin Oncol. 2018;15:31–46.
51. Wang X, Olszewska M, Qu J, et al. Large-scale clinical-grade retroviral vector production in a fixed-bed bioreactor. J Immunother. 2015;38:127–35.
52. Inwood S, Xu H, Black MA, Betenbaugh MJ, Feldman S, Shiloach J. Continuous production process of retroviral vector for adoptive T- cell therapy. Biochem Eng J. 2018;132:145–51.
53. Schambach A, Swaney WP, van der Loo JC. Design and production of retro- and lentiviral vectors for gene expression in hematopoietic cells. Methods Mol Biol. 2009;506:191–205.
54. Cornetta K, Duffy L, Feldman SA, et al. Screening clinical cell products for replication competent retrovirus: the National Gene Vector Biorepository Experience. Mol Ther Methods Clin Dev. 2018;10:371–8.
55. Wiznerowicz M, Trono D. Harnessing HIV for therapy, basic research and biotechnology. Trends Biotechnol. 2005;23:42–7.
56. Unutmaz D, KewalRamani VN, Marmon S, Littman DR. Cytokine signals are sufficient for HIV-1 infection of resting human T lymphocytes. J Exp Med. 1999;189:1735–46.
57. Amirache F, Levy C, Costa C, et al. Mystery solved: VSV-G-LVs do not allow efficient gene transfer into unstimulated T cells, B cells, and HSCs because they lack the LDL receptor. Blood. 2014;123:1422–4.
58. Mitchell RS, Beitzel BF, Schroder AR, et al. Retroviral DNA integration: ASLV, HIV, and MLV show distinct target site preferences. PLoS Biol. 2004;2:E234.
59. Merten OW, Hebben M, Bovolenta C. Production of lentiviral vectors. Mol Ther Methods Clin Dev. 2016;3:16017.
60. Levine BL, Miskin J, Wonnacott K, Keir C. Global manufacturing of CAR T cell therapy. Mol Ther Methods Clin Dev. 2017;4:92–101.
61. Raje N, Berdeja J, Lin Y, et al. Anti-BCMA CAR T-cell therapy bb2121 in relapsed or refractory multiple myeloma. N Engl J Med. 2019;380:1726–37.
62. Valkama AJ, Leinonen HM, Lipponen EM, et al. Optimization of lentiviral vector production for scale-up in fixed-bed bioreactor. Gene Ther. 2018;25:39–46.
63. Powers AD, Drury JE, Hoehamer CF, Lockey TD, Meagher MM. Lentiviral vector production from a stable packaging cell line using a packed bed bioreactor. Mol Ther Methods Clin Dev. 2020;19:1–13.
64. Sandrin V, Boson B, Salmon P, et al. Lentiviral vectors pseudotyped with a modified RD114 envelope glycoprotein show increased stability in sera and augmented transduction of primary lymphocytes and CD34+ cells derived from human and nonhuman primates. Blood. 2002;100:823–32.

65. Marin V, Stornaiuolo A, Piovan C, et al. RD-MolPack technology for the constitutive production of self-inactivating lentiviral vectors pseudotyped with the nontoxic RD114-TR envelope. Mol Ther Methods Clin Dev. 2016;3:16033.
66. Girard-Gagnepain A, Amirache F, Costa C, et al. Baboon envelope pseudotyped LVs outperform VSV-G-LVs for gene transfer into early-cytokine-stimulated and resting HSCs. Blood. 2014;124:1221–31.
67. Gogol-Doring A, Ammar I, Gupta S, et al. Genome-wide profiling reveals remarkable parallels between insertion site selection properties of the MLV retrovirus and the piggyBac transposon in primary human CD4(+) T cells. Mol Ther. 2016;24:592–606.
68. Kebriaei P, Singh H, Huls MH, et al. Phase I trials using sleeping beauty to generate CD19-specific CAR T cells. J Clin Invest. 2016;126:3363–76.
69. Naso MF, Tomkowicz B, Perry WL 3rd, Strohl WR. Adeno-associated virus (AAV) as a vector for gene therapy. BioDrugs. 2017;31:317–34.
70. MacLeod DT, Antony J, Martin AJ, et al. Integration of a CD19 CAR into the TCR Alpha chain locus streamlines production of allogeneic gene-edited CAR T cells. Mol Ther. 2017;25:949–61.
71. Zhao Y, Zheng Z, Cohen CJ, et al. High-efficiency transfection of primary human and mouse T lymphocytes using RNA electroporation. Mol Ther. 2006;13:151–9.
72. Yoon SH, Lee JM, Cho HI, et al. Adoptive immunotherapy using human peripheral blood lymphocytes transferred with RNA encoding Her-2/neu-specific chimeric immune receptor in ovarian cancer xenograft model. Cancer Gene Ther. 2009;16:489–97.
73. Rowley J, Monie A, Hung CF, Wu TC. Expression of IL-15RA or an IL-15/IL-15RA fusion on CD8+ T cells modifies adoptively transferred T-cell function in cis. Eur J Immunol. 2009;39:491–506.
74. Beatty GL, Haas AR, Maus MV, et al. Mesothelin-specific chimeric antigen receptor mRNA-engineered T cells induce anti-tumor activity in solid malignancies. Cancer Immunol Res. 2014;2:112–20.
75. Tchou J, Zhao Y, Levine BL, et al. Safety and efficacy of Intratumoral injections of chimeric antigen receptor (CAR) T cells in metastatic breast cancer. Cancer Immunol Res. 2017;5:1152–61.
76. Segura MM, Mangion M, Gaillet B, Garnier A. New developments in lentiviral vector design, production and purification. Expert Opin Biol Ther. 2013;13:987–1011.
77. Dong B, Nakai H, Xiao W. Characterization of genome integrity for oversized recombinant AAV vector. Mol Ther. 2010;18:87–92.
78. Vargas JE, Chicaybam L, Stein RT, Tanuri A, Delgado-Canedo A, Bonamino MH. Retroviral vectors and transposons for stable gene therapy: advances, current challenges and perspectives. J Transl Med. 2016;14:288.
79. Morgan RA, Kakarla S. Genetic modification of T cells. Cancer J. 2014;20:145–50.
80. Sahin U, Kariko K, Tureci O. mRNA-based therapeutics—developing a new class of drugs. Nat Rev Drug Discov. 2014;13:759–80.
81. Jensen MC, Popplewell L, Cooper LJ, et al. Antitransgene rejection responses contribute to attenuated persistence of adoptively transferred CD20/CD19-specific chimeric antigen receptor redirected T cells in humans. Biol Blood Marrow Transplant. 2010;16:1245–56.
82. Bajgain P, Mucharla R, Wilson J, et al. Optimizing the production of suspension cells using the G-Rex "M" series. Mol Ther Methods Clin Dev. 2014;1:14015.
83. Jin J, Sabatino M, Somerville R, et al. Simplified method of the growth of human tumor infiltrating lymphocytes in gas-permeable flasks to numbers needed for patient treatment. J Immunother. 2012;35:283–92.
84. Xiao L, Chen C, Li Z, et al. Large-scale expansion of Vgamma9Vdelta2 T cells with engineered K562 feeder cells in G-Rex vessels and their use as chimeric antigen receptor-modified effector cells. Cytotherapy. 2018;20:420–35.
85. Hollyman D, Stefanski J, Przybylowski M, et al. Manufacturing validation of biologically functional T cells targeted to CD19 antigen for autologous adoptive cell therapy. J Immunother. 2009;32:169–80.

86. Levine BL. Performance-enhancing drugs: design and production of redirected chimeric antigen receptor (CAR) T cells. Cancer Gene Ther. 2015;22:79–84.
87. Wang XSJ, Chaudhari J, Hall M, Thummar K, Zhao Z, Sadelain M, Riviere I. CAR-T cell manufacturing with CliniMACS Prodigy. Mol Ther. 2019;27:87.
88. Olga Molostova LS, Schneider D, Khismatullina R, Muzalevsky Y, Kazachenok A, Preussner L, Rauser G, Abugova J, Kurnikova E, Pershin D, Zubachenko V, Popov A, Illarionova O, Miakova N, Litvinov D, Novichkova G, Maschan AA, Orentas R, Dropulic B, Maschan M. Local manufacture of CD19 CAR-T cells using an automated closed-system: robust manufacturing and high clinical efficacy with low toxicities. Blood. 2019;134:2625.
89. Caimi PFRJ, Otegbeye F, Schneider D, Chamoun K, Boughan KM, Cooper BW, Galloway E, Gallogly M, Kruger W, Worden A, Kadan M, Malek E, Metheny LL, Tomlinson BK, Sekaly RP, Wald D, Orentas R, Dropulic B, De Lima MJG. Phase 1 trial of anti-CD19 chimeric antigen receptor T (CAR-T) cells with tumor necrosis alfa receptor superfamily 19 (TNFRSF19) transmembrane domain. J Clin Oncol. 2019;37:2539.
90. Kleinsorge-Block ÒS, Zamborsky JP-SK, Turney TL, Reese J, Wald D, Otegbeye F, de Lima M, Caimi PF. 258 Effective gmp-compliant point of care manufacturing of anticd19chimeric antigen receptor t cells for non hodgkin lymphomapatients using the clinimacs prodigy. Cytotherapy. 2020;22:S133.
91. Zhu FSN, Schneider D, Xu H, Chaney K, Luib L, Keever-Taylor CA, Dropulic B, Orentas R, Hari P, Johnson B. Point-of-care manufacturing of CD20.19 bi-specific chimeric antigen receptor T (CAR-T) cells in a standard academic cell processing facility for a Phase I Clinical Trial in Relapsed, Refractory NHL. Blood. 2018;132:4553.
92. Xu H, Cao W, Huang L, et al. Effects of cryopreservation on chimeric antigen receptor T cell functions. Cryobiology. 2018;83:40–7.
93. Panch SR, Srivastava SK, Elavia N, et al. Effect of cryopreservation on autologous chimeric antigen receptor T cell characteristics. Mol Ther. 2019;27:1275–85.
94. Li R, Johnson R, Yu G, McKenna DH, Hubel A. Preservation of cell-based immunotherapies for clinical trials. Cytotherapy. 2019;21:943–57.
95. Wang X, Riviere I. Clinical manufacturing of CAR T cells: foundation of a promising therapy. Mol Ther Oncolytics. 2016;3:16015.
96. Gee AP. GMP CAR-T cell production. Best Pract Res Clin Haematol. 2018;31:126–34.
97. Menchinelli G, Liotti FM, Fiori B, et al. In vitro evaluation of BACT/ALERT(R) VIRTUO(R), BACT/ALERT 3D(R), and BACTEC FX automated blood culture systems for detection of microbial pathogens using simulated human blood samples. Front Microbiol. 2019;10:221.
98. Deepu Madduri JGB, Saad Z. Usmani, Andrzej Jakubowiak, Mounzer Agha, Adam D. Cohen, A. Keith Stewart, Parameswaran Hari, Myo Htut, Elizabeth O'Donnell, Nikhil C. Munshi, David E. Avigan, Abhinav Deol, Alexander M. Lesokhin, Indrajeet Singh, Enrique Zudaire, Tzu-Min Yeh, Alicia J. Allred, Yunsi Olyslager, Arnob Banerjee, Jenna D. Goldberg, Jordan M. Schecter, Carolyn C. Jackson, William Deraedt, Sen Hong Zhuang, Jeffrey R. Infante, Dong Geng, Xiaoling Wu, Marlene J. Carrasco, Muhammad Akram, Farah Hossain, Syed Rizvi, Frank Fan, Sundar Jagannath, Yi Lin, and Thomas Martin III. Phase 1b/2 Study of Ciltacabtagene Autoleucel, a B-Cell maturation antigen–directed chimeric antigen receptor T cell therapy, in relapsed/refractory multiple myeloma. Blood. 2020;136:22–5.
99. Munshi NC, Anderson LD Jr, Shah N, et al. Idecabtagene Vicleucel in relapsed and refractory multiple myeloma. N Engl J Med. 2021;384:705–16.
100. Feucht J, Sun J, Eyquem J, et al. Calibration of CAR activation potential directs alternative T cell fates and therapeutic potency. Nat Med. 2019;25:82–8.
101. Xiuyan Wang IR. Gene editing platforms for T-cell immunotherapy. Cell Gene Ther Insights. 2019;5:705–18.
102. Cheng Zhang JH, Liu L, Wang J, Wang S, Liu L, Gao L, Gao L, Liu Y, Kong P, Liu J, Yu H, Zhang Y, Sun Z, Ye X, He Y, Shen L, Cao W, Zhang X. CD19-directed fast CART therapy for relapsed/refractory acute lymphoblastic leukemia: from bench to bedside. Blood. 2019;134:1340.

103. de Macedo Abdo L, Mariana LRCB, Saldanha Viegas LVCM, de Sousa Ferreira P, Bonamino LCMH. Development of CAR-T cell therapy for B-ALL using a point-of-care approach. OncoImmunology. 2020;9:e1752592.

104. Themeli M, Riviere I, Sadelain M. New cell sources for T cell engineering and adoptive immunotherapy. Cell Stem Cell. 2015;16:357–66.

105. Iriguchi S, Yasui Y, Kawai Y, et al. A clinically applicable and scalable method to regenerate T-cells from iPSCs for off-the-shelf T-cell immunotherapy. Nat Commun. 2021;12:430.

106. Depil S, Duchateau P, Grupp SA, Mufti G, Poirot L. 'Off-the-shelf' allogeneic CAR T cells: development and challenges. Nat Rev Drug Discov. 2020;19:185–99.

107. Kruse RL, Shum T, Tashiro H, et al. HBsAg-redirected T cells exhibit antiviral activity in HBV-infected human liver chimeric mice. Cytotherapy. 2018;20:697–705.

108. Sautto GA, Wisskirchen K, Clementi N, et al. Chimeric antigen receptor (CAR)-engineered T cells redirected against hepatitis C virus (HCV) E2 glycoprotein. Gut. 2016;65:512–23.

109. Proff J, Brey CU, Ensser A, Holter W, Lehner M. Turning the tables on cytomegalovirus: targeting viral fc receptors by CARs containing mutated CH2-CH3 IgG spacer domains. J Transl Med. 2018;16:26.

110. Wagner TA. Quarter century of anti-HIV CAR T cells. Curr HIV/AIDS Rep. 2018;15:147–54.

111. Blat D, Zigmond E, Alteber Z, Waks T, Eshhar Z. Suppression of murine colitis and its associated cancer by carcinoembryonic antigen-specific regulatory T cells. Mol Ther. 2014;22:1018–28.

112. Smith M, Zakrzewski J, James S, Sadelain M. Posttransplant chimeric antigen receptor therapy. Blood. 2018;131:1045–52.

Navigating Regulations in Gene and Cell Immunotherapy

Jaikumar Duraiswamy, Courtney Johnson, and Karin M. Knudson

Abstract By utilizing the inherent therapeutic properties of human cells, cellular immunotherapies and genetically-modified cellular immunotherapies are changing the treatment landscape of serious medical conditions such as autoimmune diseases, neuro-degenerative disorders, and cancer. These products, including autologous or allogeneic lymphocytes, chimeric antigen receptor (CAR)-T cells, antigen-presenting cells, or cancer cells manipulated or processed ex vivo, present unique manufacturing and validation challenges compared to other immunotherapeutics (e.g. monoclonal antibodies). In addition, cellular immunotherapies may produce long-acting changes in the human body, leaving patients at increased risk of unpredictable, delayed adverse events. As such, product development should produce a consistent, safe, pure, and potent product for a clinical trial that balances patient safety with a condition's severity and the unmet medical need. This chapter focuses on US Food and Drug Administration (FDA) regulatory considerations for human cellular immunotherapy products used for the treatment of cancer, including genetically-modified cellular immunotherapies.

Keywords Cellular immunotherapy · Regulatory considerations · CAR-T cells · Clinical trial · Gene therapy · Food and Drug Administration (FDA) · Cell and gene therapy (CGT) · Regulations · Chemistry, manufacturing, and control (CMC) · Manufacturing · Critical quality attributes (CQA) · Critical process parameters (CPP)

Introduction

Cellular immunotherapies and genetically-modified cellular immunotherapies, hereafter referred to as cell and gene therapy (CGT) to align with current Food and Drug Administration (FDA) guidance, are dramatically changing the treatment

All authors contributed equally to this book chapter

J. Duraiswamy · C. Johnson · K. M. Knudson (✉)
Office of Tissues and Advanced Therapies, Center for Biologics Evaluation and Research, Food and Drug Administration, Silver Spring, MD, USA
e-mail: Karin.knudson@fda.hhs.gov

© Springer Nature Switzerland AG 2022
A. Ghobadi, J. F. DiPersio (eds.), *Gene and Cellular Immunotherapy for Cancer*, Cancer Drug Discovery and Development,
https://doi.org/10.1007/978-3-030-87849-8_9

141

landscape of serious medical conditions by utilizing the inherent therapeutic properties of human cells (e.g.- hematopoietic stem cells, tissue-regenerating cells, cytotoxic lymphocytes) to treat disorders such as autoimmune diseases, neurodegenerative disorders, and cancer [1, 2]. In general, these products consist of autologous or allogeneic lymphocytes (e.g., T cells, natural killer (NK) cells, natural killer T (NKT) cells, B cells), antigen-presenting cells (e.g., dendritic cells (DCs), monocytes), or cancer cells manipulated or processed *ex vivo*. When human cells are genetically modified ex vivo, such products (e.g., chimeric antigen receptor (CAR)-T cells, T cell receptor (TCR)- engineered T cells, and CAR NK cells) are also considered gene therapies [3]. Most clinical investigations with CGT immunotherapy products focus on cancer indications [4]. See Table 1 for a list of FDA-approved CGT immunotherapy products for cancer indications.

In the United States, human CGT are reviewed by the FDA's Office of Tissues and Advanced Therapies (OTAT) in the Center for Biologics Evaluation and Research (CBER). CGT products are regulated as biologics under authority of the Public Health Service Act (PHS Act, 42 USC 262, section 351) and Federal Food, Drug, and Cosmetic Act (FD&C Act, Chapter 9 sections 321-399i). The implementing regulations are in Title 21 of the Code of Federal Regulations (21 CFR). CGT regulated under section 351 of the PHS Act[1] are evaluated in clinical studies under an Investigational New Drug (IND) application and licensed under a Biologics License Application (BLA) [5]. 21 CFR 312 contains procedures and requirements governing the use of investigational new biologics, including submission of IND applications and IND review by FDA [6]. Biologics must demonstrate both safety and efficacy in well-controlled clinical studies (21 CFR 314.126) for marketing approval under BLA (21 CFR 601.2) [6, 7].

This chapter focuses on FDA regulatory considerations for human cellular immunotherapy products used for the treatment of cancer, including genetically-modified cellular immunotherapies. Again, we refer to these products as CGT to align with current FDA guidance. This chapter pertains to US regulations only. FDA has published several useful documents applicable to these products, found at: https://www.fda.gov/vaccines-blood-biologics/biologics-guidances/cellular-gene-therapy-guidances and https://www.fda.gov/vaccines-blood-biologics/news-events-biologics/otat-learn.

---

[1] Some human cells, tissues, or cellular or tissue-based products (HCT/Ps), including CGT products, are regulated solely under section 361 of the PHS Act and 21 CFR part 1271 and do not require premarket review and approval. Briefly, these cellular products must be: (1) minimally manipulated; (2) intended for homologous use only; (3) not combined with other articles except for water, crystalloids, or the sterilizing, preserving or storage agent; and (4) either does not have a systemic effect or depend on the metabolic activity of living cells for its primary function or, if it has such an effect, be designated for autologous use, for allogeneic use in a first- or second- degree blood relative, or for reproductive use. See "Guidance for Industry and Food and Drug Administration Staff: Regulatory Considerations for Human Cells, Tissues, and Cellular and Tissue-Based Products: Minimal Manipulation and Homologous Use" (July 2020) and https://www.fda.gov/vaccines-blood-biologics/tissue-tissue-products/fda-regulation-human-cells-tissues-and-cellular-and-tissue-based-products-hctps-product-list for additional information and examples of cellular therapy products regulated under sections 361 or 351 of the PHS Act.

Table 1 Approved cellular immunotherapy products for cancer

Trade name	Manufacturer	Product	Indication	Approval date
Provenge (sipuleucel-T)	Dendreon Corporation	Autologous cellular immunotherapy	Asymptomatic or minimally symptomatic metastatic castrate resistant (hormone refractory) prostate cancer	April 2010
Kymriah (tisagenlecleucel)	Novartis Pharmaceuticals Corporation	CD19-directed genetically modified autologous T-cell immunotherapy	(1) 25 years of age with B-cell precursor acute lymphoblastic leukemia (ALL) that is refractory or in second or later relapse. (2) Adult patients with relapsed or refractory (r/r) large B-cell lymphoma after two or more lines of systemic therapy including diffuse large B-cell lymphoma (DLBCL) not otherwise specified, high grade B-cell lymphoma and DLBCL arising from follicular lymphoma	1. August 2017 2. May 2018
Yescarta (axicabtagene ciloleucel)	Kite Pharma, Incorporated	CD19-directed genetically modified autologous T-cell immunotherapy	Adult patients with relapsed or refractory large B-cell lymphoma after two or more lines of systemic therapy	October 2017
Tecartus (brexucabtagene autoleucel)	Kite Pharma, Incorporated	CD19-directed genetically modified autologous T-cell immunotherapy	Adult patients with relapsed/refractory mantle cell lymphoma (r/r MCL)	July 2020
Breyanzi (lisocabtagene maraleucel)	Juno Therapeutics, Inc., a Bristol-Myers Squibb Company	CD19-directed genetically modified autologous T-cell immunotherapy	Adult patients with relapsed or refractory large B-cell lymphoma after two or more lines of systemic therapy, including diffuse large B-cell lymphoma (DLBCL) not otherwise specified (including DLBCL arising from indolent lymphoma), high-grade B-cell lymphoma, primary mediastinal large B-cell lymphoma, and follicular lymphoma grade 3B	February 2021
Abcema (idecabtagene vicleucel)	Bristol-Myers Squibb	BCMA-directed genetically-modified autologous T-cell immunotherapy	Adult patients with relapsed or refractory multiple myeloma after four or more prior lines of therapy, including an immunomodulatory agent, a proteasome inhibitor, and an anti-CD38 monoclonal antibody	March 2021

Regulatory Chemistry, Manufacturing, and Control (CMC) Considerations for Cellular Immunotherapies

CGT products present unique manufacturing and validation challenges compared to other immunotherapeutics, such as monoclonal antibodies and recombinant cytokines. These challenges include lot-to-lot variability in the final product attributes due to patient-specific source material, inability to terminally sterilize the product due to presence of live cells, need for rigorous aseptic processing given lack of terminal sterilization, small lot/batch size due to planned administration to a single patient or small target population, stability issues as a result of short product shelf life, and manufacturing logistics due to patient conditioning prior to cell donation, short manufacturing time windows, and/or limited shelf life. Like all biologics, CGT product development should produce a consistent, safe, pure, and potent product through controlled and validated manufacturing processes. To help achieve these goals, critical quality attributes (CQA)[2] and critical process parameters (CPP)[3] should be employed based on the mechanism of action (MOA), active ingredient(s), and composition of the product [8].

All CGT INDs should include sufficient information to assure the identity, quality, purity, and potency of the investigational agent (21 CFR 312.23(a)(7)(i)). The information provided in the CMC section of the IND allows for evaluation of the manufacturing process, critical reagents, in-process intermediates and testing, and control of the final product safety and quality.

CGTP and CGMP Requirements for Manufacturing

CGT products are subject to applicable Current Good Tissue Practice (CGTP) requirements and Current Good Manufacturing Practices (CGMP). CGTP requirements under 21 CFR part 1271 (subparts C&D) govern the manufacturing methods, facilities, and controls to prevent introduction, transmission, or spread of communicable diseases [9, 10]. As CGT starting materials originate from human donors who can carry communicable diseases, CGTP requirements help ensure product safety. CGMP regulations assure proper design, monitoring, and control of manufacturing processes and facilities (21 CFR 210 and 21 CFR 211) [11–13]. CGMP and CGTP

---

[2] A critical quality attribute (CQA) is a physical, chemical, biological, or microbiological property or characteristic that should be within an appropriate limit, range or distribution to ensure the desired product quality. CQAs are generally associated with excipients, in-process materials, and the drug product. See "Guidance for Industry: Q8(R2) Pharmaceutical Development" (November 2009) for additional information.

[3] A critical process parameters is a process parameter whose variability has an impact on a CQA and therefore should be monitored or controlled to ensure the process produces the desired quality. See "Guidance for Industry: Q8(R2) Pharmaceutical Development" (November 2009) for additional information.

regulations also require established procedures for product tracking to prevent product contamination or mix up, which is especially important for patient-specific CGT. Certain requirements in 21 CFR part 211 may not be appropriate to the manufacture of most investigational drugs used for phase 1 clinical trials. Phase 1 studies should comply with appropriate manufacturing controls to ensure product quality and safety, as clarified in FDA guidance [13]. CGMP regulations under 21 CFR 211 and 21 CFR 600 s apply to Phase 2 and 3 studies, and full CGMP compliance is expected for licensure. CGMP compliance is verified through FDA inspection during BLA review.

Reagents and Raw Materials

Reagents are materials used for cell growth, differentiation, selection, purification, or other manufacturing steps [3, 14]. For many CGT products, reagents include serum, growth factors, cytokines, monoclonal antibodies, cell separation reagents such as antibody-conjugated magnetic selection beads, media, and media components. Qualification is required, especially if a reagent is not FDA-approved/cleared. Prior to introducing into the manufacturing process, a qualification program should be established for all critical materials, including appropriate safety tests (e.g., sterility, endotoxin, mycoplasma, adventitious agents (AA)), identity tests, functional analysis, and purity testing, as needed [3, 11, 14]. Additional requirements may be necessary for reagents derived from human or animal sources, including AA screening and/or testing [15, 16]. As these materials are not intended to be a part of the final product, the final product should be tested for residual manufacturing reagents, and lot release specifications may be required [3, 11, 14].

Cell Source Material and Donor Eligibility

Typical source materials for CGT products include peripheral blood mononuclear cells (PBMCs), hematopoietic stem/progenitor cells (HPCs), or tumor biopsy. The source material may come from either an autologous or allogeneic donor. Donor screening, donor testing, and making a donor eligibility determination are not required for donors of cells or tissue for autologous use (21 CFR 1271.90(a)(1)); however, if full donor eligibility is not determined for an autologous donor, then specific label regulations apply (21 CFR 1271.90). If autologous donors are screened/tested, compliance with 21 CFR 1271 is recommended. A donor eligibility determination based on donor screening and testing for relevant communicable diseases agents or diseases (RCDADs) (defined in 21 CFR 1271.3(r)) is required for allogeneic donors of cells or tissue as described in 21 CFR 1271 and FDA guidance [17, 18]. Donor screening is required for the following RCDADs: human immunodeficiency virus (HIV), hepatitis B virus (HBV), hepatitis C virus (HCV), human transmissible spongiform encephalopathy including Creutzfeldt-Jakob disease (CJD), Treponema pallidum (syphilis), sepsis, vaccinia, West Nile virus (WNV), and Zika virus (ZIKV) [17, 19–25]. Donors of viable, leukocyte-rich cells or tissue must be screened for risk factors for and clinical evidence of relevant cell-associated communicable disease agents and diseases, including human T-lymphotropic virus (HTLV) (21 CFR 1271.75) [26]. Donors must also be screened for communicable disease risks associated with xenotransplantation [17]. Donor testing must be performed by a laboratory that either is certified to perform such testing on human specimens under the Clinical Laboratory Improvement Amendments (CLIA) of 1998 and 42 CFR part 493 or has met equivalent requirements as determined by the Center for Medicare and Medicaid Services (CMS), using appropriate FDA-licensed, approved, or cleared donor screening tests (21 CFR 1271.80(c)) [27, 28]. A complete description of donor screening and testing should be included in the IND. Current required donor testing for RCDADs (21 CFR 1271.85) and a list of tests that adequately and appropriately reduce the risk of transmission of RCDADs (21 CFR 1271.80) are located in Table 2 [28, 29].

Cell Bank Systems

Cell banks may provide source material to produce a specific final product (e.g., *ex vivo* expansion, differentiation, activation) or could function itself as the final product. For example, undifferentiated induced pluripotent stem cells (iPSC) could serve as a master cell bank (MCB) for an allogeneic T cell product. Alternatively, a mesenchymal stem cell (MSC) bank could serve as an off-the-shelf allogeneic immunomodulatory cell product. Cell banks are typically scaled to treat a large number of patients, and therefore different patients will receive a more uniform product compared to patient-specific product lots manufactured from different donors. Due to the ability to be manufactured at a larger scale, more cells and volume are available for more comprehensive testing and extensive product characterization. Unlike immortalized cell lines, most cell bank-based CGT therapies are limited in passage number and scale. The cell bank history, source, derivation, and characterization should be included in the IND [3, 14]. Extensive cell bank safety testing (sterility, mycoplasma, in vitro and in vivo AA testing) is important as higher risk is associated with the larger number of doses to treat more patients [3, 14, 15, 30]. MCB will undergo more extensive characterization and safety testing than working cell banks (WCB), which are derived from one or more vials of the MCB [3, 14, 30–32]. However, WCB should still undergo AA, sterility, mycoplasma, and limited identity testing to ensure cell bank safety and identity [3, 14]. Please note that if the cell bank is the final drug product, additional release testing to ensure product safety, purity, identity, dose, and potency is required. Table 3 and Table 4 include non-exhaustive information on recommended characterization and safety testing for cell banks [3, 14, 15, 30–32].

Table 2 Donor Screening Tests for Allogeneic Cell or Tissue Donors

RCDAD[a]	Donor screening test(s)[b]	Additional information	References[c]
HIV, type-1	• Anti-HIV-1 • HIV-1 NAT	• Anti-HIV-1 or combination test for anti-HIV-1 and anti-HIV-2 is acceptable • NAT for HIV-1 or combination test including HIV-1 NAT is acceptable • Establishments not utilizing an FDA-licensed donor screening test that tests for group O antibodies must screen donors for risk associated with HIV group O infection	[24, 25]
HIV, type-2	• Anti-HIV-2	• Anti-HIV-2 or combination test for anti-HIV-1 and anti-HIV-2 is acceptable	[9, 24, 25, 32]
HBV	• HBsAg • anti-HBc (total IgG and IgM) • HBV NAT	• NAT for HBV or combination NAT including HBV is acceptable	[19, 23]
HCV	• Anti-HCV • HCV NAT	• NAT for HCV or combination NAT including HCV is acceptable	[18, 24, 25, 42]
Treponema pallidum (syphilis)	• Non-treponemal or Treponemal	• A donor whose specimen tests positive or reactive on a non-treponemal screening test for syphilis and negative or nonreactive on a specific treponemal confirmatory test may be determined eligible if all other required testing and screening are negative or nonreactive. A donor whose specimen tests positive or reactive on either a specific treponemal confirmatory test for syphilis or on a treponemal screening test is not eligible (21 CFR 1271.80(d)(1)).	[21]
WNV	• WNV NAT	• For living donors of cells or tissue during the timeframe described in the FDA WNV NAT guidance for donors of HCT/Ps	[20]
HTLV, Types I and II	• Anti-HTLV-I/II	• For donors of viable, leukocyte-rich cells or tissue only	[26]
CMV	• Anti-CMV (total IgG and IgM)	• For donors of viable, leukocyte-rich cells or tissue only • CMV is not an RCDAD, however, testing for CMV is required for donors of viable, leukocyte-rich cells or tissue. • A donor who tests positive or reactive for CMV (total antibody) is not necessarily ineligible. • Additional documentation is required for a CMV-positive donor.	[17]

CMV cytomegalovirus, *HBc* hepatitis B core antigen, *HBsAg* hepatitis B surface antigen, *HBV* hepatitis B virus, *HCV* hepatitis C virus, *HIV* human immunodeficiency virus, *HTLV* human T-lymphotropic virus, *IgG* immunoglobulin G, *IgM* immunoglobulin M, *NAT* nucleic acid test, *WNV* West Nile virus

[a]Relevant communicable disease agents or diseases (21 CFR 1271.3(r))
[b]FDA-licensed, approved or cleared donor screening tests (21 CFR 1271.80(c))
[c]For general references applicable to donor eligibility screening, see [17, 18, 27–29]

Table 3 Recommended cell bank characterization tests[a]

Test type[b]	Example
Identity[c]	• Cellular phenotype • Transgene expression • Genetic fingerprinting
Viability	• Doubling time
Purity	• Quantification of cell population of interest • Quantification of other cell populations that should be controlled (impurities)
Genetic stability	• Cytogenetic analysis • Stability of transgene
Biological assays	• Cellular activity • Cellular maturation
Cellular composition and heterogeneity	• Target cell phenotype

[a]If the cell bank is the final drug product, release testing to ensure product purity, identity, dose, and potency is required
[b]If using a two-tiered cell bank system (master cell bank (MCB) and working cell bank (WCB)), more extensive cell bank characterization is recommended for the MCB than the WCB
[c]Limited identity testing is recommended for the WCB

Vector Qualification and Testing

Genetic modification of cells is typically performed by delivering genetic material by physical, chemical, or viral methods to induce expression of a transgene. Recent advent of genome-editing technologies has enabled a new paradigm in which the sequence of the human genome can be precisely manipulated to achieve a therapeutic effect. This includes the correction of mutations that cause disease, the addition of therapeutic genes to specific sites in the genome, and the removal of deleterious genes or genome sequences [33, 34]. Retroviruses, most often gamma retroviruses and lentiviruses, are predominantly used to generate CGT such as TCR- and CAR-transduced T cells. The IND should contain information on the characterization and qualification of the vectors, including history and derivation of the source material, generation of recombinant vectors, description of all intermediate plasmids, complete annotated sequences of the plasmids, and sequencing of the vectors (for vectors smaller than 40 kb, complete sequencing is recommended at the IND stage) [3]. Vector preparations, including viruses, should be tested for safety (sterility, mycoplasma, endotoxin, AA), identity, purity, potency, and stability [3, 15]. If retroviruses are used, it is recommended that testing for replication-competent retrovirus/lentivirus be performed on the vector producer cell MCB, vector supernatant, end of production cells, and ex vivo transduced cells [3, 35].

Table 4 Recommended cell bank safety testing[a]

Test	Recommended method	Additional information		
Sterility	<USP 71>			
Mycoplasma	Culture-based assay PCR			
Endotoxin	<USP 85>			
Relevant human communicable disease agents	PCR	Recommended testing:		
		• CMV • HIV-1/2 • HTLV-1/2 • HHV-6/7/8 • JCV • BKV		• EBV • Parvovirus B19 • HBV • HPV • HCV
Retrovirus or other endogenous virus	In vitro infectivity assays	• Select sensitive cell cultures		
	Electron microscopy	• May also detect other infectious agents		
	Reverse transcriptase	• Not necessary if positive by retrovirus infectivity test		
	Other virus-specific tests	• As appropriate for cell lines known to be infected by such agents		
Species-specific nonendogenous or adventitious virus	In vitro assays	• Inoculation of test article into susceptible indicator cell cultures • Cell selection based on species of cell bank • Include human and/or nonhuman primate cell susceptible to human viruses		
	In vivo assays	• Inoculation of test article into suckling and adult mice and embryonated eggs		
	Antibody production tests	• Apply to cell banks exposed to animal-derived reagents • Usually applicable for detection of rodent viruses • e.g. MAP, RAP, HAP		
	Other virus-specific tests	• Tests for cell lines derived from other species – e.g. human, nonhuman primate • Tests for reagent-associated adventitious virus – e.g. bovine, porcine • Apply to cell banks exposed to animal-derived reagents		

BKV BK virus, *CMV* cytomegalovirus, *EBV* Epstein-Barr virus, *HAP* hamster antibody production, *HBV* hepatitis B virus, *HCV* hepatitis C virus, *HHV* human herpes virus, *HIV* human immunodeficiency virus, *HPV* human papillomavirus, *HTLV* human T-lymphotropic virus, *JCV* JC virus, *MAP* mouse antibody production, *PCR* polymerase chain reaction, *RAP* rat antibody production

[a]If the cell bank is the final drug product, additional release testing to ensure product safety and purity is required

Lot Release Testing and Product Specifications

Lot release specifications are defined as a group of tests, references to analytical procedures, and appropriate acceptance criteria used to assess product quality and safety [36]. Characterization of the CGT product (e.g., physicochemical properties, biological activity, immunochemical properties, purity, impurities) is necessary to establish relevant specifications [36]. Acceptance criteria should be based on defined CQA gained through prior scientific knowledge and/or data obtained from manufacturing experience [8]. However, setting acceptance criteria for CGT products can be challenging due to inherent lot-to-lot variability given the donor source material. Setting wide release acceptance criteria may allow for this variability but can present challenges for assuring manufacturing consistency, comparability after a manufacturing change, and quality of the final product. Thus, in-process and release specifications should be set with careful consideration. The final product must conform to the release specifications to be considered acceptable for use in clinical investigation. Typically, few specifications are validated or finalized in early stages of clinical development, but the IND should include proposed and justified acceptance criteria and test methods to assure product safety (e.g., sterility and purity), dose, potency, and identity in early studies [3, 14]. Evidence of product stability is also expected at all stages. It is anticipated that acceptance criteria be refined during product development, and optimized acceptance criteria should be based on safe and effective clinical lots. Release specifications to ensure product safety, purity, identity, dose, and potency should be fully validated for the BLA.

Safety Assays

Release safety testing is essential to ensure product safety during all phases of clinical development [3, 14]. Safety testing specifications should be established prior to the initiation of Phase 1 clinical investigation. Safety testing should be performed at the manufacturing stage most likely for detection of contaminants, and methods should be qualified for use with reagents, excipients, and other materials present in the test sample [3, 14]. Please note that release testing for potency, viability, and purity may also address product safety concerns (see relevant sections below).

Sterility: Product sterility is defined as the absence of viable microorganisms (bacterial and fungal) and is required for drug product testing under 21 CFR 610.12. Sterility testing should also be performed on all product intermediates, as applicable, and the final product formulation. The FDA recommends that a 14-day sterility test be performed according to USP<71> or an equivalent method, as appropriate [3, 14, 37, 38]. If the product is cryopreserved prior to use, it is recommended that USP<71> sterility testing be performed prior to freezing. This allows for sterility testing results to be available before product administration; however, if the product is manipulated after thawing, additional sterility testing should be performed. Some CGT products cannot be cryopreserved and require administration prior to obtaining the results of 14-day sterility testing. If complete sterility testing results are not available prior to product release, in process-sterility testing taken 48–72 h prior to the final harvest should be implemented, a qualified rapid microbial test (e.g., Gram stain) on the final product should be performed, and an action plan should be developed in the event of a positive sterility test results obtained after product administration [3, 14].

Mycoplasma Assay: Cultured CGT products should be tested for mycoplasma on the final harvest, prior to final product manipulations (e.g. washing). The cells and supernatant should be tested using a mycoplasma assay for release testing. Polymerase chain reaction (PCR)-based or other rapid detection assays may be qualified for products with a short shelf life, like many CGT [3, 14].

Endotoxin Assay: Endotoxin testing of final product is required to ensure product purity (12 CFR 610.13). The USP <85> Limulus Amebocyte Lysate (LAL) assay method is commonly used to detect endotoxin in cellular products [39, 40]. For any parenteral drug, except those administered intrathecally or intraocularly, the recommended upper limit of acceptance criterion for endotoxin is 5 Endotoxin Unit (EU)/kg body weight/hour [3, 14, 40, 41].

Adventitious Viral Agents: As appropriate, the final drug product should be tested for adventitious viral agents. A risk assessment can be used to determine the need for this release testing. Similar to mycoplasma testing, testing for adventitious viral agents should be performed on cell culture harvest material (cells and supernatant) prior to further processing [3].

Dose

Prior to initiating Phase 1 clinical studies, assays used to determine product dose (e.g., cell count) should be qualified [3, 14]. It can be a challenge to achieve a targeted dose for patient-specific products, so consideration should be given to the feasibility of a specified dose for these products. For many CGT products, the product dose may represent a population within the product, not the total number of viable cells (e.g., dose is based on number of $CD3^+$ T cells or transduced cells). As such, it should be documented in the IND whether a maximum number of cells per dose has been established and the justification for that level.

Identity

Identity assays are required to uniquely identify a product and distinguish it from other products manufactured in the same facility. Identity tests are performed on the final drug product to verify its contents (21 CFR 610 14), and the assay should adequately reflect the composition of product [3, 14]. Identity assays for CGT products typically use phenotypic cell surface markers or secreted molecules to identify target and residual populations (see purity section for more information on residual cells) [14, 42], while identity tests for genetically-modified CGT include a measure of the presence of the vector (i.e. transduced vs. non-transduced cells) and the cellular composition [3]. CGT are generally complex products containing more than one cell type, and the composition of these products may vary due to differences in donor-specific starting material. Thus, a single test may not distinguish the identity of the final product [3, 14]. It is recommended to qualify multiple test methods to confirm identity and continue characterizing the drug product throughout development.

Purity

Product purity is defined as the relative freedom from an extraneous matter in the finished product, whether or not it is harmful to the recipient or deleterious to the product (21 CFR 600.3(r)). Common impurities for CGT products include residual cell populations, proteins or peptides used for cell stimulation, or reagents used during the manufacturing process, such as cytokines, growth factors, antibodies, serum, or magnetic selection beads. These process- and product-related impurities should be measured throughout product development, and acceptance criteria should be set to ensure an appropriate level of product quality and safety [3, 14].

Viability

The function of many CGT products is dependent on the activity of live, viable cells. As such, a minimum release criteria for cell viability, usually set for at least 70%, should be established for CGT products [3, 14]. If 70% viability cannot be achieved, it is recommended that data are included in the IND to support a lower release criterion. It should also be demonstrated that non-viable cells will not affect the safety or efficacy of the product [3, 14, 42].

Potency

Potency assays measure the biological function of the drug product and are required to assure product quality, comparability following manufacturing changes, and stability [43]. Potency assays are typically unique for each product, and a product's potency assay should be supported by product characterization data collected through preclinical and clinical development. The selected potency assay should reflect a relevant biological property or the MOA of the product, a challenge when assessing complex CGT. For CGT immunotherapy products, the MOA typically involves multiple cellular attributes, such as cytokine secretion, expression of extracellular receptors, cytotoxicity, transgene expression, and/or function of the expressed transgene protein. The relevance of some of the attributes may not be firmly established during the early phases of development, so it is recommended that potency assays are developed to evaluate each biological function of the drug product. Thus, a potency assay may change significantly during product development due to increased understanding of the drug product. While it is recommended that the potency assay be quantitative, a matrix of both quantitative and qualitative measures of potency may be used to measure the product's strength/activity [3, 14,

43]. FDA regulations allow for considerable flexibility in determining an appropriate measure of potency; however, all potency assays used for release testing must comply with applicable biologics and CGMP regulations [43]. Potency assays should be qualified prior to initiating the clinical studies intended to provide the primary evidence of effectiveness for licensure. The potency assay should be fully validated for the BLA [3, 14, 43].

Stability

Many CGT products have a short shelf life and, if able to undergo cryopreservation, are administered within hours or days after manufacture. Stability studies are required to establish the dating period (shelf life) of the source material, intermediates, and the final drug product [44]. Stability testing must be performed during early stage development to demonstrate that the product remains within acceptable limits at the time of administration (21 CFR 312.23(a)(7)(ii)). Early stability analysis may be limited (e.g., viability, cell dose). For licensure, the stability analysis should include tests of product sterility, identity, purity, quality, and potency [3, 14, 44]. Transgene expression is a common additional test for genetically-modified CGT. Of note, changes in product formulation, manufacture, or storage conditions require additional stability testing [3, 14, 44].

Regulatory Preclinical Considerations for Cellular Immunotherapy Products

Adequate preclinical studies must be performed to conclude the product is reasonably safe to conduct proposed clinical trials (21 CFR 312.23(a)(8)). CGT are complex and diverse products, so conventional pharmacology and toxicity testing may not be appropriate to determine product safety and activity. Thus, the extent of preclinical studies for a product is determined on a data-driven, case-by-case basis [42, 45]. Please see the FDA's Guidance for Industry: Preclinical Assessment of Investigational Cellular and Gene Therapy Products [45] for additional information.

Regulatory Clinical Considerations for Cellular Immunotherapy Products

Early-Phase Trials

Early-phase trials should be designed to successfully identify a safe dose and regimen that can be used in later-phase trials [46]. The current FDA guidance "Considerations for the Design of Early-Phase Clinical Trials of Cellular and Gene

Therapy Products" provides OTAT's current recommendations regarding early-phase clinical trials, of which the primary objectives are assessment of safety, tolerability, and/or feasibility of administration of these agents [47]. Most of these trials are Phase 1 (including first in human studies); however, some are Phase 2.

The regulation of CGT is different from other pharmaceuticals as these products present unique challenges regarding dosing and administration and may pose substantial risks to human subjects, including unexpected off target organ toxicities and delayed clonal proliferation with risk of secondary malignancy [47]. When considering early-phase trial objectives, 21 CFR Part 312 IND regulations place importance on the assessment of trial risks/safeguards for subjects. Safety evaluations must include assessments of potential adverse events and the likelihood that these events are related to the investigational agent. The clinical components for an IND early-phase protocol should contain the rationale for the product's use in a specific patient population, information on previous human experience, anticipated risks, objectives, and inclusion/exclusion criteria. Other recommended objectives for early-phase trials include dose exploration, feasibility assessments, and activity assessments [46, 47]. The selection of the starting dose, dose-escalation scheme, and dosing schedule should be supported by data generated from preclinical and/or prior human experience [48]. Study protocols should clearly define a dose-limiting toxicity (DLT), off-treatment criteria, and the study stopping rules, irrespective of the dose-escalation scheme. It is recommended that the study should identify a maximum tolerated dose (MTD) in early development [47]. If the MTD or the optimal biological dose is not identified, this may lead to subsequent trials using subtherapeutic dose levels [47]. There should also be adequate safety and endpoint monitoring, information on adverse event reporting, and long term follow-up, where appropriate [46].

Patient Population

Patients with metastatic or relapsed/refractory disease have typically been the subjects for early-phase trials to demonstrate the safety and efficacy of investigational anti-tumor therapeutics [48]. When safety and efficacy were established in this population, the investigational agent would then typically be tested in patients with earlier-stage cancer. Selecting a patient population for a cellular immunotherapy trial can differ from this traditional model as patients with advanced disease may not have sufficient time to have an anti-tumor immune response or may have received multiple prior therapies which may mitigate the effectiveness of the CGT [48]. On the other hand, as CGT products may have uncertain benefits and significant risks, this argues for the enrollment of patients with advanced disease or those where there are no further treatment options [47]. Additionally, CGT trials may require the use of a companion diagnostic (e.g. for HLA or tumor neoantigen identification) to determine the subject population, making the knowledge of a product's mechanism of action in a specific disease essential. This may allow for an early assessment of the product's activity. [46]

It is equally important to consider the inclusion and exclusion criteria when designing a trial for CGT. Inclusion and exclusion criteria must be broad enough to achieve the proposed trial's objectives and endpoints while not restricting the enrollment of patients who may receive a potential benefit from the investigational agent [49]. This is particularly true in oncology, where patients are more likely to have a poor prognosis. This suggests the need for a standardized, evidence-based approach when developing inclusion/exclusion criteria.

There are CGT products developed for pediatric patients. Title 21 CFR Part 50 Subpart D (Subpart D) states specific safeguards for children in clinical trials. Subpart D requires that the Institutional Review Board (IRB) finds that the risk of the investigational agent holds out the prospect of direct benefit, the risk is justified by anticipated benefit, the relation of anticipated benefits to the risk is at least as favorable as that presented by alternative approaches, and adequate provisions are made for the assent of children and parental/guardian permission [47].

Trial Design and Endpoints

Trial design and endpoint selection are critical to support effectiveness claims in biologics license applications (BLAs), new drug applications (NDAs), or supplemental applications [50]. In oncology drug development, early phase clinical trials typically evaluate safety and identify evidence of biological drug activity. Later phase oncology studies typically evaluate whether a drug has a clinical benefit such as prolongation of survival. Additional endpoints based on tumor assessments typically used in oncology trials include disease-free survival, event-free survival, objective response rate, complete response rate, time to progression, progression-free survival, and time to treatment failure. Time to treatment failure is not encouraged as this endpoint may be subject to investigator bias. Additionally, it should be noted that time to event endpoints are difficult to interpret in single arm studies.

As early-phase trial objectives typically focus on feasibility, dose finding and tolerability, a control group (typically the current standard of care in oncology) may not be needed or appropriate [47, 51]. However, when feasible and appropriate, a control arm is recommended as it can facilitate interpretation of safety data and provide a comparator for the assessment of both activity and/or efficacy. This may prove useful in trials for subjects with a wide-range of disease severity. Control arms can also minimize the risk of bias in interpretation of study results. If a trial requires the use of a procedural device which may pose an unreasonable risk to the subjects in the control group, review by the FDA's Center for Devices and Radiological Health (CDRH) may be required. In addition, historical control groups present challenges in interpretation and are subject to multiple sources of bias—refer to ICH E10 Choice of Control Group and Related Issues in Clinical Trials at https://www.fda.gov/media/71349/download.

Dose Regimen

Finding an optimal dose and regimen should be one of the primary objectives of early clinical trials of investigational therapies for cancer therapies [46]. This process allows the investigator to define the acceptable range of the investigational agent's potential toxicities. In studies evaluating advanced cancer patients, a higher toxicity threshold is expected and may be acceptable, provided the benefit risk is acceptable and adequate justification is provided [46]. To determine the starting dose of an early-phase trial, proof-of-concept data from pre-clinical studies is typically needed and pharmacodynamic activity is preferred but not required [52]. The starting dose is typically based on the preclinical results from pharmacology, toxicology, and pharmacokinetic (pK) studies as well as data from prior human experience, recognizing that sometimes animal models are not feasible. Similarly, dose escalation decisions require balancing the individual subject's safety against the risk of failing to find the correct dose range that may be used in future studies or abandoning the development of a possibly beneficial agent.

Identifying the maximum-tolerated dose (MTD) and defining dose-limiting toxicity (DLT) is important in early-phase trials. The definition of a dose-limiting toxicity (DLT) is generally based on protocol and product-specific adverse events [49]. It usually is defined as a Grade 3 or higher toxicity according to the National Cancer Institute (NCI) Common Terminology Criteria (CTCAE) [49]. The primary objective is to generally identify the highest dose that can be administered and tolerated by an acceptable number of patients, which is defined as the maximum-tolerated dose (MTD). There are unique challenges to define DLTs and locating the MTD in CGT. CGT agents have the potential for both acute and long-term toxicity as they may expand in vivo [49] Consequently, the definition of a DLT and a MTD may not be the same. As CGT agents may cross react to off-target antigens, DLT definitions need to take this into consideration. This cross reactivity may be to vital tissues (brain, heart, liver, kidney, gut) and could potentially cause severe, life-threatening toxicity. In addition, significant toxicity which allows the identification of the MTD, may not occur in the expected therapeutic dose in some CGT agents, so the goal of dose exploration may need to shift to find the optimal feasible dose and regimen [46].

Staggering enrollment is also important when designing an early-phase trial as administering the investigational agent to subjects simultaneously may expose them to unreasonable risk [47]. There should be a specified follow-up interval between administration to subjects to allow evaluation of the agent's safety and to evaluate for acute and subacute adverse events. The cohort size and staggering interval within a dose escalation scheme are also important to consider when evaluating an agent's potential toxicity.

Adverse Event Monitoring and Reporting

Sponsors are legally required to report serious and unexpected adverse events (SAEs) to all stakeholders and the FDA (21 CFR 312.32) [53]. Investigators should report unanticipated events to the IRB under 21 CFR 56 (Institutional Review Boards), 21 CFR 312 (Investigational New Drug Application) and 21 CFR 812 (Investigational Device Exemption).

Evaluation and monitoring of expected and unexpected adverse events is imperative, as the major objective of an early-phase trial is to evaluate the safety of the investigational agent. Standard safety monitoring to include physical examinations, blood counts, blood chemistry, liver function tests, coagulation studies, etc., should be performed in a CGT early-phase trial. In addition to these studies, CGT has unique toxicities including cytokine release syndrome (CRS), hemophagocytic lymph histiocytosis/macrophage activation syndrome (HLH/MAS), and immune effector cell-associated neurotoxicity syndrome (ICANS). One of the most common toxicities in CD19 CAR-T cell therapy is CRS, which represents a common, expected and potentially delayed AE after infusion [54]. The use of standardized guidelines for the grading and treatment of CRS and HLH/MAS in the safety-monitoring is recommended. Guidelines for standardized grading (which guides treatment) of CRS have been developed by the American Society for Transplantation and Cellular Therapy (ASTCT) and may be used [55]. In addition, the National Comprehensive Cancer Network (NCCN) have provided guidance for the assessment and management of CRS and HLH/MAS. ICANS represents a range of neurological symptoms. Patients may initially develop a tremor, dysgraphia, mild expressive aphasia, apraxia and impaired attention [54]. The ASTCT have also developed a grading system for the severity of ICANS and NCCN guidelines for treatment exist.

There are other specific safety concerns for CGT including acute or delayed infusion reactions, autoimmunity, graft failure, GVHD, new malignancies, transmission of infectious agents from a donor and viral reactivation depending on the specific product. [47] Some CGT products can be locally administered (intratumorally or intraventricularly) and require safety assessments for both local and systemic toxicities [46]. The monitoring and assessment of the above listed toxicities are critical in the development and design of CGT trials.

Long-Term Follow-Up

Designing a long-term follow-up plan is essential to capture any delayed AE following the administration of CGT products [56]. Characteristics unique to human GT products that may be associated with delayed adverse events include the integration activity of the GT product, genome editing activity, prolonged expression and latency. The duration of follow-up can depend on pre-clinical study results, experience with related products, and knowledge of the disease process [47]. Some products may have an indefinite duration of activity and, in those cases, a longer follow-up may be required. Due to specific safety concerns and developmental outcomes of pediatric subjects, pediatric studies also may require a longer follow-up period [47]. In particular, novel gene therapy products such as transposon-based gene insertion and genome editing have unique genome modifying activities and can cause delayed adverse events [56]. It is important that long-term follow-up observations for novel CGT products are designed to consider product-specific characteristics, preclinical data and basic and translational knowledge developed in the field.

Treatment Discontinuation Criteria and Trial Stopping Criteria

Establishing treatment stopping rules is essential, especially when designing an early-phase trial. This protects patients from experiencing undue toxicity. The purpose of study stopping rules is to control the number of subjects put at risk if early experience with the investigational agent uncovers important safety problems [47]. These rules typically specify the number or frequency of events such as serious adverse events or deaths, that will result in the temporary suspension of enrollment until these events can be assessed. This can be challenging given the uncertainty regarding the severity of the adverse events with CGT products. Study stopping rules may not permanently stop the trial. Certain trials may resume after a dose reduction, change in product preparation/administration, or changes in the safety monitoring plan.

Sponsors should define acceptable toxicity and procedures for dealing with unacceptable toxicities when establishing treatment stopping rules [57]. Most criteria specify one of the following: (1) halting subject dosing or trial enrollment until toxicity data can be further studied; (2) evaluation of additional subjects in a particular dose cohort without exposing further subjects to a higher dose; (3) implementation of a smaller dose increase between dose cohorts and (4) exclusion of certain patients considered higher risk for a particular toxicity.

Later Phase Clinical Trials

Phase 2 trials are controlled clinical studies conducted to evaluate the effectiveness of the drug for a particular indication and to determine the drug's risks and short-term side effects and typically involve no more than several hundred subjects (21

CFR 312.21). Confirmatory studies are conducted after preliminary evidence suggesting effectiveness of the drug has been obtained and are intended to confirm effectiveness and safety of the investigational product and to assess the overall risk-benefit relationship of the drug (21 CFR 312.21).

Interaction with FDA

Due to the complexity of CGT products, there are significant challenges for product development. For sponsors of clinical trials, OTAT encourages early interaction through pre-scheduled meetings [58, 59]. Prior to submitting an IND, it is highly recommended that sponsors take advantage of the INTERACT and pre-IND meetings to obtain FDA's guidance on early stage product characterization, preclinical development, and clinical trial design [59–62]. After submitting an IND, sponsors may have formal meetings with the FDA, such as end of Phase 1, end of Phase 2, or pre-BLA. These meetings help support the clinical development program and provide specific guidance on clinical trials essential intended to provide evidence of both safety and effectiveness [58]. The following website contains information related to guidance, compliance and regulatory information: https://www.fda.gov/vaccines-blood-biologics/other-recommendations-biologics-manufacturers/references-regulatory-process-office-tissues-and-advanced-therapies.

Expedited Programs

The FDA implemented five programs to facilitate and expedite development and review of new drugs and biologics that address unmet medical need in the treatment of serious or life-threatening conditions: Fast Track (FT) Designation, Accelerated Approval Pathway, Priority Review Designation, Breakthrough Therapy (BT) Designation, and Regenerative Medicine Advanced Therapy (RMAT) Designation. Regenerative medicine products are defined in section 506(g)(8) of the FD&C Act as cell therapy, therapeutic tissue engineering products, human cell and tissue products, or any combination product using such therapies or products [63]. Additionally, FDA interpretation of Section 3033 of the 21st Century Cures Act considers RMAT to also include "gene therapies, including genetically modified cells, that lead to a durable modification of cells or tissues" [63]. Cellular immunotherapies, including CAR-T cells, qualify as regenerative medicine products. As of September 30, 2020, 55 of 145 RMAT designation requests were granted [64]. The majority of the RMAT requests were for cellular therapies [65]. Table 5 contains a summary of the expedited programs, including timing of application, qualifying criteria, and program features [63, 66].

Table 5 Expedited programs for serious conditions (adapted from [63, 66])

	Fast track (FT)	Accelerated approval (AA)	Priority review (PR)	Breakthrough therapy (BT)	Regenerative medicine advanced therapy (RMAT)
Type	Designation	Approval pathway	Designation	Designation	Designation
Date established	1988	1992	1992	2012	2016
Qualifying criteria	Intended to treat or treats a serious condition				
	• AND non-clinical or clinical data demonstrate potential to address unmet medical need	• AND provides a meaningful advantage over available therapies • AND demonstrates an effect on a surrogate endpoint likely to predict clinical benefit or measured earlier than IMM	• AND, if approved, would provide a significant safety or efficacy improvement over existing therapies	• AND early evidence shows substantial improvement over existing therapies on a clinically significant endpoint	• AND meets definition of a regenerative medicine therapy • AND clinical data demonstrate the potential to address unmet medical need
Key program features	• Frequent interaction with FDA • Eligible for PR or AA, if criteria met • Rolling BLA review	• Approval based on a surrogate endpoint or intermediate clinical endpoint that is likely to predict clinical benefit	• Shortened review process (6 months v.s. standard 10 months)	• All FT features • Intensive guidance on efficient drug development • Organization commitment	• All FT and BT designation features
Additional considerations	• Designation may be withdrawn if drug no longer meets qualifying criteria	• Confirmatory trials required to verify and describe the effect on IMM or other clinical benefit • Subject to expedited withdrawal	• Designation is assigned at the time of BLA or efficacy supplement filing	• Designation may be withdrawn if drug no longer meets qualifying criteria	• Designation may be withdrawn if drug no longer meets qualifying criteria
Application timeline	• With IND or after • Ideally prior to pre-BLA meeting	• No formal process • Discussion with FDA during drug development	• With BLA or efficacy supplement	• With IND or after • Ideally no later than end-of-phase II meeting	• With IND or after • Ideally no later than end-of-phase II meeting
FDA response	60 days	Not specified	60 days	60 days	60 days
Related regulations	• FD&C Act section 506(b)	• 21 CFR 314 subpart H • 21 CFR 601 subpart E • FD&C Act section 506(c)	• PDUFA	• FD&C Act section 506(a)	• FD&C Act section 506(g)
Reference	66	66	66	66	63

BLA biologics license application, *CFR* Code of Federal Regulations, *FD&C* Food, Drug, and Cosmetic, *IMM* irreversible morbidity or mortality, *IND* investigational new drug application, *PDUFA* Prescription Drug User Fee Act

Conclusions

Cellular immunotherapy and gene therapy products are diverse and prone to unique manufacturing challenges such as high lot-to-lot variability, complex composition, small batch size, patient-specific administration, and short shelf life. All CGT products are evaluated to ensure consistency, safety, purity, and potency.

CGT products may pose substantial risks to human subjects and produce permanent or long-acting changes in the human body. This may leave subjects at increased risk of unpredictable, delayed adverse events. When designing any clinical trial, important regulatory factors to consider include the patient population, trial design, objectives, endpoints, starting dose, treatment modifications, stopping rules, long term follow-up, and developing a safety monitoring plan. Clinical trials designed for cancer indications must balance safety with cancer's severe and life-threatening nature and the need to identify products to support unmet medical needs.

References

1. Aijaz A, Li M, Smith D, et al. Biomanufacturing for clinically advanced cell therapies. Nat Biomed Eng. 2018;2:362–76.
2. Weber EW, Maus MV, Mackall CL. The emerging landscape of immune cell therapies. Cell. 2020;181:46–62.
3. FDA. Guidance for Industry: Chemistry, Manufacturing, and Control (CMC) Information for Human Gene Therapy Investigational New Drug Applications (INDs). 2020.
4. Guedan S, Ruella M, June CH. Emerging cellular therapies for cancer. Annu Rev Immunol. 2018;37:145–71.
5. FDA. Guidance for industry and food and drug administration staff: regulatory considerations for human cells, tissues, and cellular and tissue-based products: minimal manipulation and homologous use. 2020.
6. Bross PF, Fan C, George B, Shannon K, Joshi BH, Puri RK. Regulation of biologic oncology products in the FDA's Center for Biologics Evaluation and Research. Urol Oncol. 2015;33:133–6.
7. FDA. Guidance for industry: providing clinical evidence of effectiveness for human drug and biological products. 1998.
8. FDA. Guidance for industry: Q8(R2) Pharmaeutical development. 2009.
9. FDA. Guidance for industry: current good tissue practice (CGTP) and additional requirements for manufacturers of human cells, tissues, and cellular and tissue-based products (HCT/Ps) 2011.
10. Good Tissue Practice (CGTP) Final rule questions and answers. 2018. at https://www.fda.gov/vaccines-blood-biologics/tissue-tissue-products/good-tissue-practice-cgtp-final-rule-questions-and-answers.)
11. FDA. Guidance for industry: Q11 development and manufacture of drug substances 2012.
12. FDA. Guidance for industry: Q7 good manufacturing practice guidance for active pharmaceutical ingredients. 2016.
13. FDA. Guidance for industry: CGMP for Phase 1 investigational drugs 2008.
14. FDA. Guidance for FDA reviewers and sponsors: content and review of chemistry, manufacturing, and control (CMC) information for human somatic cell therapy investigational new drug applications (INDs). 2008.

15. FDA. Guidance for industry: characterization and qualification of cell substrates and other biological materials used in the production of viral vaccines for infectious disease indications. 2010.
16. FDA. Points to consider in the manufacture and testing of monoclonal antibody products for human use. 1997.
17. FDA. Guidance for industry: eligibility determination for donors of human cells, tissues, and cellular and tissue-based products (HCT/Ps). 2007.
18. FDA. Guidance for industry: revised recommendations for determining eligibility of donors of human cells, tissues, and cellular and tissue-based products who have received human-derived clotting factor concentrates. 2016.
19. FDA. Guidance for industry: use of nucleic acid tests to reduce the risk of transmission of hepatitis B virus from donors of human cells, tissues, and cellular and tissue-based products. 2016.
20. FDA. Guidance for industry: use of nucleic acid tests to reduce the risk of transmission of west nile virus from living donors of human cells, tissues, and cellular and tissue-based products (HCT/Ps). 2017.
21. FDA. Guidance for industry: use of donor screening tests to test donors of human cells, tissues and cellular and tissue-based products for infection with Treponema pallidum (Syphilis). 2015.
22. FDA. Guidance for industry: donor screening recommendations to reduce the risk of transmission of zika virus by human cells, tissues, and cellular and tissue-based products. 2018.
23. FDA. Guidance for industry: adequate and appropriate donor screening tests for hepatitis B; hepatitis B surface antigen (HBsAg) assays used to test donors of whole blood and blood components, including source plasma and source leukocytes. 2007.
24. FDA. Guidance for industry: use of nucleic acid tests on pooled and individual samples from donors of whole blood and blood components (including source plasma and source leukocytes) to adequately and appropriately reduce the risk of transmission of HIV-1 and HCV. 2004.
25. FDA. Guidance for industry: nucleic acid testing (NAT) for human immunodeficiency virus type 1 (HIV-1) and hepatitis C virus (HCV): testing, product disposition, and donor deferral and reentry. 2017.
26. FDA. Guidance for industry: use of serological tests to reduce the risk of transfusion-transmitted human T-lymphotropic virus types I and II (HTLV-I/II). 2020.
27. Complete list of donor screening assays for infectious agents and HIV diagnostic assays. 2020. at https://www.fda.gov/vaccines-blood-biologics/complete-list-donor-screening-assays-infectious-agents-and-hiv-diagnostic-assays.)
28. Testing human cells, tissues, and cellular and tissue based product (HCT/P) Donors for relevant communicable disease agents and diseases. 2020. at https://www.fda.gov/vaccines-blood-biologics/safety-availability-biologics/testing-human-cells-tissues-and-cellular-and-tissue-based-product-hctp-donors-relevant-communicable.)
29. Testing donors of human cells, tissues, and cellular and tissue-based products (HCT/P): specific requirements. 2019. https://www.fda.gov/vaccines-blood-biologics/safety-availability-biologics/testing-donors-human-cells-tissues-and-cellular-and-tissue-based-products-hctp-specific-requirements.)
30. FDA. Q5D quality of biotechnological/biological products: derivation and characterization of cell substrates used for production of biotechnological/biological products; availability. 1998.
31. FDA. Points to consider in the characterization of cell lines used to produce biologicals. 1993.
32. FDA. Guidance for industry: Q5A viral safety evaluation of biotechnology products derived from cell lines of human or animal origin. 1998.
33. Bailey SR, Maus MV. Gene editing for immune cell therapies. Nat Biotechnol. 2019;37:1425–34.
34. Maeder ML, Gersbach CA. Genome-editing technologies for gene and cell therapy. Mol Ther. 2016;24:430–46.
35. FDA. Guidance for industry: testing of retroviral vector-based human gene therapy products for replication competent retrovirus during product manufacture and patient follow-up. 2020.

36. FDA. Guidance for industry: Q6B specifications: test procedures and acceptance criteria for biotechnological/biological products. 1999.
37. FDA. Amendments to sterility test requirements for biological products. Federal Register 2012:26162–75.
38. Pharmacopoeia US. Chapter <71> Sterility Tests. 23rd Edition ed1995.
39. Pharmacopoeia US. Chapter <85> Bacterial Endotoxins Test. 2001.
40. FDA. Guidance for industry: pyrogen and endotoxins testing: questions and answers. 2012.
41. FDA. Draft guidance for industry: setting endotoxin limits during development of investigational oncology drugs and biological products guidance for industry. 2020.
42. FDA. Guidance for industry: guidance for human somatic cell therapy and gene therapy. 1998.
43. FDA. Guidance for industry: potency tests for cellular and gene therapy products. 2011.
44. FDA. Guidance for industry: Q1A(R2) stability testing of new drug substances and products. 2003.
45. FDA. Guidance for industry: preclinical assessment of investigational cellular and gene therapy products 2013.
46. Husain SR, Han J, Au P, Shannon K, Puri RK. Gene therapy for cancer: regulatory considerations for approval. Cancer Gene Ther. 2015;22:554–63.
47. FDA. Guidance for industry: considerations for the design of early-phase clinical trials of cellular and gene therapy products. 2015.
48. Vatsan RS, Bross PF, Liu K, et al. Regulation of immunotherapeutic products for cancer and FDA's role in product development and clinical evaluation. J Immunother Cancer. 2013;1:5.
49. Jaggers JL, Giri S, Klepin HD, et al. Characterizing inclusion and exclusion criteria in clinical trials for chimeric antigen receptor (CAR) T-cell therapy among adults with hematologic malignancies. J Geriatr Oncol. 2020;12:235.
50. FDA. Guidance for industry: clinical trial endpoints for the approval of cancer drugs and biologics. 2018.
51. FDA. Guidance for industry: placebos and blinding in randomized controlled cancer clinical trials for drug and biological products. 2019.
52. Shen J, Swift B, Mamelok R, Pine S, Sinclair J, Attar M. Design and conduct considerations for first-in-human trials. Clin Transl Sci. 2019;12:6–19.
53. FDA. Guidance for clinical investigators, sponsors, and IRBs: adverse event reporting to IRBs-improving human subject protection 2009.
54. Kennedy LB, Salama AKS. A review of cancer immunotherapy toxicity. CA Cancer J Clin. 2020;70:86–104.
55. Lee DW, Santomasso BD, Locke FL, et al. ASTCT consensus grading for cytokine release syndrome and neurologic toxicity associated with immune effector cells. Biol Blood Marrow Transplant. 2019;25:625–38.
56. FDA. Guidance for industry: long term follow-up after administration of human gene therapy products. 2020.
57. FDA. Good review practice: clinical review of investigational new drug applications. 2013.
58. Takefman D, Bryan W. The state of gene therapies: the FDA perspective. Mol Ther. 2012;20:877–8.
59. FDA. Draft guidance for industry: formal meetings between the FDA and sponsors or applicants of PDUFA products. 2017.
60. INTERACT Meetings. 2020. https://www.fda.gov/vaccines-blood-biologics/industry-biologics/interact-meetings.)
61. FDA. Guidance for industry. IND meetings for human drugs and biologics: chemistry, manufacturing, and controls information. 2001.
62. Small business and industry assistance: frequently asked questions on the pre-investigational new drug (IND) meeting. 2020. https://www.fda.gov/drugs/cder-small-business-industry-assistance-sbia/small-business-and-industry-assistance-frequently-asked-questions-pre-investigational-new-drug-ind.)

63. FDA. Guidance for industry: expedited programs for regenerative medicine therapies for serious conditions. 2019.
64. Cumulative CBER Regenerative Medicine Advanced Therapy (RMAT) Designation Requests Received by Fiscal Year. 2020. https://www.fda.gov/vaccines-blood-biologics/cellular-gene-therapy-products/cumulative-cber-regenerative-medicine-advanced-therapy-rmat-designation-requests-received-fiscal.
65. Marks P. The FDA's regulatory framework for chimeric antigen receptor-T cell therapies. Clin Transl Sci. 2019;12:428–30.
66. FDA. Guidance for industry: expedited programs for serious conditions—drugs and biologics. 2014.

Bringing CAR-T to the Clinic

Michael D. Jain, Pselane Coney, and Frederick L. Locke

Abstract Chimeric antigen receptor (CAR)-T cell therapy is now a standard of care clinical therapy. The first United States Food and Drug Administration (US FDA) approval was in 2017 for CD19-directed CAR-T cell therapy using tisagenlecleucel (tisa-cel) for the treatment of pediatric patients (up to age 25) with relapsed or refractory (R/R) B-acute lymphoblastic leukemia (B-ALL). That same year, CD19 CAR-T cell therapy with axicabtagene ciloleucel (axi-cel) was approved for adults with R/R large B cell lymphoma (LBCL), which included histologies such as diffuse large B cell lymphoma, high grade B cell lymphoma, transformed follicular lymphoma, and primary mediastinal B cell lymphoma. In 2020, CD19 CAR-T cell therapy was approved for R/R mantle cell lymphoma (MCL) using brexucabtagene autoleucel (brexu-cel). Within the first few months of 2021, CD19 CAR-T cell therapy was approved for R/R follicular lymphoma (FL) using axi-cel and BCMA-targeted CAR-T cell therapy was approved for R/R multiple myeloma (MM) using idecabtagene vicleucel (ida-cel). In the case of R/R LBCL, three different CD19 CAR-T cell products are now approved, including axi-cel, tisa-cel, and lisocabtagene maraleucel (liso-cel), and in time multiple products are likely to be approved for most diseases. Altogether, over 8000 patients worldwide have been treated with approved CAR-T cell products as of 2020. The rapid growth in the number of patients receiving CAR-T cell therapies has created a need for physicians, nurses, and other health professionals to learn more about the clinical complexities of these patients and to develop the clinical management plans to optimize care. This chapter will review recent data about the clinical management of patients receiving CAR-T cell therapies in the standard of care setting.

M. D. Jain · P. Coney · F. L. Locke (✉)
Department of Blood and Marrow Transplant and Cellular Immunotherapy, Moffitt Cancer Center, USF Morsani College of Medicine, Tampa, FL, USA
e-mail: Frederick.Locke@moffitt.org

© Springer Nature Switzerland AG 2022
A. Ghobadi, J. F. DiPersio (eds.), *Gene and Cellular Immunotherapy for Cancer*, Cancer Drug Discovery and Development,
https://doi.org/10.1007/978-3-030-87849-8_10

165

Keywords Tisagenlecleucel (tisa-cel) · Axicabtagene ciloleucel (axi-cel) · Brexucabtagene autoleucel (brexu-cel) · Idecabtagene vicleucel (ida-cel) · Lisocabtagene maraleucel (liso-cel) · B-acute lymphoblastic leukemia (B-ALL) · Large B cell lymphoma (LBCL) · Diffuse large B cell lymphoma (DLBCL) · Mantle cell lymphoma (MCL) · Multiple myeloma (MM)

Overview of the CAR-T Patient Journey

The patient journey through CAR-T cell therapy begins with the recognition that disease has relapsed or is refractory to standard therapy. While the number of centers offering CAR-T cell therapy is growing, most patients require referral to a tertiary center with skills in cellular therapies and stem cell transplantation. The processes for patient selection and obtaining authorization to proceed to CAR-T cell therapy varies across regions and nations around the world . Upon identification of a potential patient for CAR-T cell therapy, testing of organ function such as heart and lung function is typically performed to identify and optimize any issues as well as to ensure overall fitness for therapy. Once approved, patients undergo leukapheresis to collect their T cells, which are then shipped to the manufacturer (Fig. 1). Manufacturing generally takes 3–6 weeks depending on product, and patients may require treatment during this time, termed "bridging therapy," to ensure disease stability. Upon confirmation of successful CAR-T cell product manufacturing meeting all defined release criteria and shipment of viably frozen CAR-T product, patients undergo lymphodepleting chemotherapy followed by CAR-T cell infusion. Early monitoring of patients involves management of well-known CAR-T cell toxicities such as cytokine release syndrome (CRS) and immune effector cell-associated neurologic syndrome (ICANS), as well as the effects of the lymphodepleting chemotherapy. After these early toxicities have resolved (generally within the first few weeks), patients need to be monitored for infection, disease relapse, and other issues, often involving the patient's local and specialist physicians. Finally, despite the success of CAR-T cells to generate durable remissions in some patients, many patients will relapse and will require additional management of their disease. With an increasing number of patients that are long term survivors without relapse, a clinical understanding of CAR-T survivorship is needed.

Patient Selection

Patient selection for CAR-T cell therapy depends on the disease being treated, alternative options, and willingness to undergo intensive therapy with close monitoring for weeks to months. Since clinical CAR-T cell therapy with autologous T cells requires a manufacturing period, patients with rapidly progressive disease or who

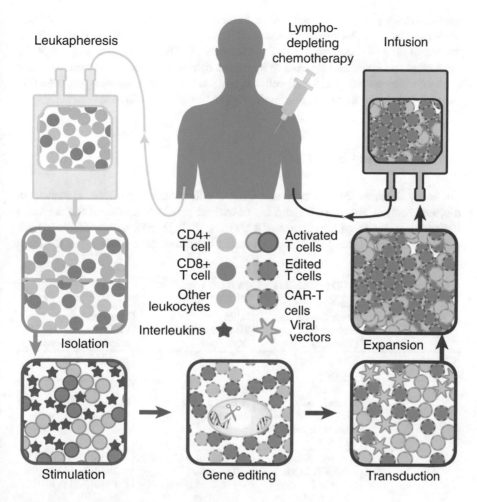

Fig. 1 CAR-T manufacturing and logistic schema

are symptomatic from their lymphoma may not survive long enough to obtain the benefits of treatment. On the other hand, chronic organ comorbidities or advanced age do not clearly affect CAR-T cell therapy outcomes. For example, patients over the age of 65 had equivalent outcomes to younger patients on the ZUMA-1 clinical trial [1]. Moreover, in the standard of care setting patients with comorbidities such as a prior solid organ transplant or chronic infections such as HIV or Hepatitis B and C, or CNS involvement of lymphoma have all been reported to have successful results with CAR-T cell therapies [2–4]. An emerging theme is that disease characteristics are the strongest determinant of outcome after CAR-T cell therapy, with high tumor burden associated with poorer outcomes. For example in B-ALL, patients with low marrow blast counts have the best outcomes [5, 6], and in DLBCL, patients with low metabolic tumor volume on PET/CT have higher efficacy and lower toxicity [7]. Indeed, high tumor burden is associated with higher LDH and higher levels of inflammatory markers such as ferritin and IL-6, markers that are known to be associated with inferior outcomes [8]. Therefore, it is important for physicians, patients, and systems to minimize delays that result in excessive tumor growth while awaiting CAR-T cell therapy, and to use caution when selecting patients with high tumor volume and/or rapidly progressive disease.

CAR-T Product Selection

For many diseases there is only one CAR-T cell product approved. However, in diseases such as R/R LBCL there are now three products approved for the same indication and in the future there are likely to be multiple products available in each disease category (Table 1). Currently, a center must undertake a new effort to obtain

Table 1 FDA approved CD19 CAR-Ts for large B cell lymphoma

	Zuma-1 Axicabtagene ciloleucel (Yescarta)	Juliet Tisagenlecleucel (Kymriah)	Transcend Lisocabtagene maraleucel (Breyanzi)
Company	Kite, a Gilead company	Novartis	Juno/Celgene/BMS
Source	Phase 1/2 **N Engl J Med** 2017;377:2531–44 **Lancet Oncol,** 2019; 20: 31–4	Phase2 **N Engl J Med** 2019; 380:45–56	Phase 2 **Lancet.** 2020 Sep 19:839–852
Population	• 76% DLBCL; 16% TFL; 8% PMBCL • 79% refractory • 21% relapsed post-ASCT	• 80% DLBCL; 18% TFL • 46% relapsed; 54% refractory • 49% post ASCT	• 51% DLBCL, 13% HGBCL, 6% PMBCL, 1% FL grade 3b • 67% chemorefractory • 35% post transplant
Enrollment	111 enrolled; 101 dosed and evaluable	165 enrolled; 111 dosed, 93 in efficacy analysis group	344 leukapheresed, 269 treated, 256 in efficacy analysis group
CAR	Second generation, CD28 Retroviral vector	Second generation, 41BB Lentiviral vector	Second generation, 41BB Lentiviral vector (CD4/ CD8: 1/1)
Dose	2.0×10^6 CAR-T cells/kg >100 kg 2.0×10^8 fixed	Median, 3×10^8 Range, $0.1–6.0 \times 10^8$ cells	DL1S 50×10^6 CAR-T cells ($N = 45$) DL1D 100×10^6 CAR-T cells ($N = 183$) DL2S 150×10^6 CAR-T cells ($N = 41$)

(continued)

Table 1 (continued)

	Zuma-1 Axicabtagene ciloleucel (Yescarta)	Juliet Tisagenlecleucel (Kymriah)	Transcend Lisocabtagene maraleucel (Breyanzi)
Lymphodepleting chemotherapy	Flu 30 mg/m² and cy 500 mg/m² on days −5, − 4, and −3	Flu 25 mg/m² and cy 250 mg/m² on days −5, − 4, and −3 or Bendamustine (90 mg/m²) daily for 2 days 1 week before infusion	Flu 30 mg/m² and cy 300 mg/m² × 3 days, 2–7 days before CAR infusion
Bridging chemotherapy	No	Yes (90%)	Yes (59%)
Efficacy	mITT = 108 • 24 month follow up • ORR: 82%; 58% CR • PFS: 12 m (44%), 24 m (39%) • Median DOR: 11.1 m	Minimum efficacy f/u: 3 m • 18 month follow up • ORR: 52%; CR: 40% • Median DOR: NR • DOR for responders: 12 m: 65%	mITT: 256 • ORR: 73%; CR: 53% • Median DOR: Not reached • PFS at 12 m: 44.1%
Safety	• Gr ≥ 3 CRS 11% (Lee) • Gr ≥ 3 NE 28% • Gr 5 AE 3% (2 due to CRS, one due to PE)	• Gr ≥ 3 CRS 22% (UPenn) • Gr ≥ 3 NE 12% • Gr 5 AE 3% (3 subject within 30d all due to disease progression)	• Gr ≥ 3 CRS 2% • Gr ≥ 3 NE 10% • Gr 5 AE: No death due to CRS or NE

Abbreviations: *DLBCL* diffuse large B cell lymphoma, *TFL* transformed follicular lymphoma, *HGBCL* high grade B cell lymphoma, *PBMCL* primary mediastinal B cell lymphoma, *ASCT* autologous stem cell transplant, *Flu* fludarabine, *Cy* cyclophosphamide, *mITT* modified intention to treat, *ORR* overall response rate, *CR* complete response, *DOR* duration of response, *NR* not reached, *PFS* progression free survival, *Gr* grade, *AE* adverse events, *CRS* cytokine release syndrome, *NE* neurologic events

and maintain approval to use each manufacturer's product, and depending on treatment volume, centers may limit the products they use. There are no randomized head-to-head studies nor well-conducted observational studies available to compare products. There is the temptation to compare the reported efficacy and toxicity rates across different clinical trials, but the enrolled patients may differ widely in key features such as tumor burden and inflammation, which strongly influence both efficacy and toxicity rates. In addition, the clinical management of CRS and neurotoxicity is evolving. In earlier clinical trials the use of anti-IL-6 and steroids were reserved for severe cases. However, clinical trials increasingly recommend treatment earlier in the treatment course and for patients with milder toxicity. The effect of earlier management of treatment is an overall reduction in CRS severity in newer trials, but with unclear effects on neurotoxicity and product efficacy [9]. Generally speaking, CAR-T products with 4-1BB endodomains appear to have lower toxicity rates than CD28-costimulated products [10], but whether this comes at the cost of efficacy is unknown, and early CRS management may mitigate this difference. A further consideration is the length of time needed for manufacturing and its reliability, since the failure to produce a CAR-T cell product after apheresis can be catastrophic to patients with rapidly progressive disease. Additional considerations include the ability to deliver CAR-T cell therapy in the inpatient versus outpatient settings, and an individual center's comfort with a particular product.

Approved CAR-T Cell Products in Clinical Use

Axicabtagene Ciloleucel

Axicabtagene ciloleucel (axi-cel) [Yescarta] is a CD19-directed CD3ζ/CD28-co-stimulated CAR-That utilizes a gamma-retrovirus vector without T cell selection during manufacturing. It is currently approved for patients with LBCL and FL that is relapsed or refractory (R/R) after 2 or more prior lines of systemic therapy.

For DLBCL, the pivotal ZUMA-1 clinical trial reported on 108 patients with R/R LBCL including DLBCL, TFL, and PMBCL who received axi-cel after flu/cy lymphodepletion [11, 12]. Best ORR was 82%, best CR 58%, and at a median follow up of 27 months, 39% of patients remained in durable remission. Severe CRS and neurotoxicity occurred in 13% and 28%, respectively. Different from the pivotal trials of the other CAR-T products, bridging therapy was not allowed on ZUMA-1. In patients treated as standard of care in the non-trial setting, results were similar. The 17-center US Lymphoma CAR-T cell Consortium reported on 298 patients with R/R DLBCL planned for standard of care axi-cel, of which 43% would not have met ZUMA-1 trial criteria for comorbidities, and over half received bridging therapies [13]. In that cohort, ORR was 82% and best CR was 64% at a median follow up of 12.9 months. On multivariate analysis, patients who had a poor ECOG performance status of 2 or lower and patients with an elevated LDH had shorter progression free survival (PFS) and shorter overall survival (OS). Non-relapse mortality was mainly due to infections and occurred in 4% of patients. Similarly, in a cohort of standard of care DLBCL patients described by Jacobson et al., patients who would not have met eligibility for the ZUMA-1 clinical trial had a shorter PFS and OS, but overall results were similar to clinical trials [14]. However, durable responders were still found among the higher risk patients in both studies and there is no comorbidity that has been identified that clearly excludes patients from CAR-T cell therapy eligibility.

As of March 2021, the FDA approved the use of axi-cel for follicular lymphoma (FL) that has relapsed after 2 or more lines of prior systemic therapy. This is based on data in the ZUMA-5 trial where among 81 evaluable patients the ORR was 91%, with 74% remaining in continued remission at 18 months [15]. Among 146 patients evaluable for safety, severe CRS and neurotoxicity occurred in 8% and 21%, respectively. The trial is ongoing and longer follow up is needed to determine the proportion of patients with FL who obtain long term remissions after CAR-T cell therapy.

Tisagenlecleucel

Tisagenlecleucel (tisa-cel) [Kymriah] is a CD19-directed, CD3ζ/4-1BB co-stimulated CAR-That is manufactured using a lentivirus vector after T cell selection. It is approved for clinical use in pediatric and young adult R/R B-ALL up to age 25 and adults with R/R LBCL. In pediatric and young adult B-ALL, the ELIANA phase 1/2 clinical trial demonstrated an EFS of 50% and OS of 76% at 12 months after infusion [16]. Overall, 77% of patients experienced CRS and 40% had neurological toxicities. For DLBCL, the JULIET clinical trial initially reported data from 93 infused patients with median age 56 (range 22–76). In this cohort the ORR was 52% with 40% of those in CR [17]. More recently, 115 patients from the study were reported at a median follow-up of 40 months [18]. The 24- and 36-month PFS in the infused patients are reported at 33% and 31%, respectively, highlighting the paucity of late relapses. Similar efficacy outcomes with tisagenlecleucel in the standard of care setting have been reported, with a CR rate and 12 month EFS rate of 86% and 52% in 255 ALL patients, and a CR rate and 6 PFS rate of 40% and 39% in 155 DLBCL patients [19]. The main toxicities seen in the trial included severe CRS in 22% and severe neurotoxicity in 12%. However, it should be noted that the toxicity grading system used in the JULIET trial differed from that used in other trials, and on re-grading to ASTCT criteria, the rate of severe CRS decreased to 13.5% while the rate of severe neurotoxicity remained similar [20, 21].

Lisocabtagene Maraleucel

Lisocabtagene maraleucel (liso-cel) [Breyanzi] is the third FDA-approved CAR-T cell therapy for the treatment of R/R LBCL after two prior lines of systemic therapy. One difference from the other two products is that it is also approved for FL grade 3B (although not FL grades 1–3A at the time of writing), due to the inclusion of FL 3B in the pivotal trial. It is a CD19-directed, CD3ζ/4-1BB costimulated CAR that is manufactured using a lentivirus. Uniquely, the manufacture of liso-cel results in the supply of a 1:1 ratio of CD4 and CD8-positive CAR T cells, with each component provided in separate vials. In preclinical studies the 1:1 ratio of CD4:CD8 improved CAR-T cell performance compared to unselected products [22], although it is unknown whether this is also true in the clinical setting. The TRANSCEND trial reported 344 patients who underwent leukapheresis, of which 269 received infusion, and among 256 evaluable patients the ORR was 73% with 53% remaining in CR at 18.8 months [23]. Grade 3 or higher adverse events included 2% CRS and 10% neurotoxicity. Interestingly, over half of patients had no CRS at all, and in a cohort of patients treated in the outpatient setting, 41% did not require any hospital admission [24].

Brexucabtagene Autoleucel

Brexucabtagene autoleucel (brexu-cel)[Tecartus] is a CD19 targeted, CD3ζ/CD28 co-stimulated CAR approved for the treatment of R/R MCL. The CAR construct is the same as axi-cel, but the manufacturing differs in that brexu-cel uses a T cell selection step. The reason for this difference is that MCL more often manifests with leukemic involvement than DLBCL, and selection reduces leukemia cell contamination during manufacturing. On the pivotal ZUMA-2 clinical trial, 94 patients underwent apheresis, 91 patients received CAR-T cells, and in the pre-specified primary analysis of 60 patients the ORR was 93% with 67% achieving CR. At 12.3 months, 57% remained in remission. Severe CRS occurred in 15% and severe neurotoxicity occurred in 31%. Key points include that bridging therapy with corticosteroids and/or BTK inhibitors was allowed and was given to 37% of patients. Moreover, although the US FDA label indicates use for R/R disease without specifying prior treatment, eligibility for ZUMA-2 required prior treatment with chemotherapy (anthracycline or bendamustine) and either intolerance or disease resistance to a BTK inhibitor.

Idecabtagene Vicleucel

Idecabtagene vicleucel (ide-cel) [Abecma] is the first approved B cell maturation antigen (BCMA)-targeted CAR-T cell therapy. It was approved by the US FDA in March 2021 for the treatment of R/R multiple myeloma (MM) after 4 or more prior lines of therapy including an immunomodulatory agent (i.e. lenalidomide), a proteasome inhibitor (i.e. carfilzomib), and an anti-CD38 (i.e. daratumumab). Ide-cel is a BCMA-targeted, CD3ζ/4-1BB costimulated CAR-That utilizes a lentiviral vector. BCMA is expressed on the surface of myeloma cells and normal late maturation B cells such as plasmablasts, plasma cells, and activated B cells. The pivotal phase 2 KarMMa study enrolled heavily pre-treated myeloma patients who had experienced a median of 6 prior lines of therapy (range 3–16), and 88% of patients received bridging therapy. Of 140 patients who underwent apheresis, 128 received ide-cel. Among treated patients, ORR was 73% and CR was 33%. At a median follow up of 13.3 months, the median PFS and OS were 8.8 and 19.4 months, respectively. Toxicities associated with treatment included CRS in 84% of participants, however, only 6% had severe CRS and 3% had severe neurotoxicity. Clinical trials are underway to determine if treating patients with fewer lines of prior therapy may increase the durability of myeloma remission after CAR-T cell therapy.

Clinical Management of Patients Receiving CAR-T Cell Therapy

Referral and Authorization

It is important to limit the length of time that elapses between relapse and CAR-T cell treatment, since tumor burden is a key determinant of outcome, and patients with aggressive disease may experience clinical decline in a short period of time. Therefore, it is useful to refer patients to a CAR-T cell therapy center early in their disease course, especially if the patient has high risk characteristics or is demonstrating signs of refractory disease. That way, once the patient meets the approved label indication they can be quickly moved through the authorization, vital organ testing, apheresis, and manufacturing periods and receive CAR-T cell infusion. The process for CAR-T cell therapy approval varies between systems or insurance carriers. Many centers utilize a multidisciplinary tumor board or expert committee to ensure appropriate allocation of this resource. However, these processes also may cause delays, and clinicians must advocate to quickly move patients to apheresis and infusion.

Patient Fitness Testing

There is no established consensus on the required tests or patient performance prior to CAR-T cell therapy. However, many centers have adopted testing in a manner analogous to that performed prior to autologous stem cell transplantation. The goal of the testing is to understand patient comorbidities early in the process, thereby allowing the opportunity for optimization while awaiting CAR-T cell manufacturing. Since CRS is commonly associated with cardiac dysfunction [25], reasonable workup includes a 2D echocardiogram, and ECG, and cardiology consultation in selected cases. CRS is also associated with hypoxia and pulmonary function testing may be helpful to assess pulmonary reserve. The NCCN guidelines recommend consideration of a baseline MRI brain, both to assess malignant involvement of the CNS and to provide a baseline to compare when a repeat MRI is performed as part of neurotoxicity workup. Neurology consultation and/or lumbar puncture may be indicated in specific patients. It is important to try to prevent the lymphoma from causing disability while awaiting CAR-T cell manufacturing, so restaging imaging is needed, allowing consideration of bridging therapy. In addition to routine blood-work, obtaining a baseline ferritin and C-reactive protein can help identify patients at higher risk for CAR-T toxicity [26]. Finally, patients are immunosuppressed in multiple ways after CAR-T cell therapy, including lymphopenia due to conditioning, B cell aplasia, cytopenias, and from the anti-cytokine or steroid treatment needed to manage CRS and neurotoxicity [27]. Therefore a thorough evaluation of infection including hepatitis B and C and HIV testing is needed.

Apheresis

Apheresis (alternatively called leukapheresis) is the process by which leukocytes are collected from a patient's peripheral blood. Among the apheresed leukocytes are the patient T cells that are used for autologous CAR-T cell manufacturing. The patient T cells are made up of a mixture of T cell subsets that varies between patients in terms of their relative quantity and quality. This influences the characteristics of the manufactured CAR-T cell product, which in turn affects the ability of the CAR-T cells to expand and eliminate the tumor. For example, in a biomarker study of the ZUMA-1 clinical trial, the percentage of CD8-positive T cells in the apheresis material strongly correlated with the percentage of CD8-positive T cells found in the manufactured CAR-T cell product [28]. Similarly, the study found that a higher proportion of stem and central memory-like T cells (CCR7 + CD45RA+) in the apheresis product was associated with a shorter CAR-T cell doubling time during manufacturing, which associated with greater CAR-T cell expansion after patient infusion. Therefore, patient T cell characteristics influence the quality of the manufactured CAR-T cell product, characteristics that are affected by prior or recent chemotherapy, tumor biology, or other factors. For this reason, manufacturers suggest guidelines for washout of prior therapies prior to apheresis, for patient blood lymphocyte counts at the time of apheresis, and for the blood volume that will be targeted for apheresis. Therapies that cause lymphocyte depletion (for example, bendamustine) may require a lengthy washout period to allow T cell recovery prior to apheresis. In addition, patients may require transfusion prior to apheresis. For example, hemoglobin >8 g/dl and platelets >50 k/µl allow patients to tolerate apheresis, while a total wbc count >1 k/µl allows efficient leukapheresis into a pellet that contains the desired CD3+ lymphocytes. Another consideration is the presence of circulating malignant cells and each manufacturer has a limit as to the number of leukemic cells recommended before apheresis. For products that utilize T cell selection to sort out the T cells from the malignant cells, some amount of circulating malignant cells may be tolerable, but in many cases therapeutic reduction of leukemic phase blasts or circulating malignant cells may be required prior to apheresis. The risk of including malignant cells in the apheresis product used for CAR-T cell manufacturing is that they may impair manufacturing, or worse, that the CAR transgene is inserted into a malignant cell leading to a CAR leukemia with downregulation of the CAR target on the malignant cells due to intracellular binding of CART and the target in the malignant cells [29]. Strategies to clear circulating malignant cells vary between diseases, including the use of monoclonal antibodies a few days before planned apheresis [30]. Finally, it may be possible to use treatments to improve patient T cell quality prior to apheresis. For example in chronic lymphocytic leukemia, use of the BTK/ITK inhibitor ibrutinib is associated with an improvement in T cell quality and improved outcomes when used prior to apheresis and continued concurrent to CAR-T cell therapy [31, 32].

Bridging Therapy

Bridging therapy includes chemotherapy, radiation, steroids, or targeted therapy given between apheresis and the completion of CAR-T cell manufacturing. Prior to apheresis clinicians must remain concerned about T cell quantity and quality, but once the cells are safely sent off for manufacturing, patients may be treated to prevent cancer progression and/or disability. The choice to use bridging therapy depends on balancing the expected anti-cancer effects of the therapy with the risk of toxicities or morbidity from the therapy itself. The initial clinical trials varied in terms of whether bridging therapy was allowed. For example in DLBCL, ZUMA-1 did not allow patients to receive bridging while JULIET (92% of patients) and TRANSCEND (59% of patients) did allow bridging. In diseases other than DLBCL, clinical trials typically allow bridging using therapies specific to the disease. For example, the BCMA CAR-T cell trials typically allow targeted anti-myeloma therapies while awaiting CAR-T manufacturing. Overall, the value of bridging therapy may depend on how effective it is at reducing tumor burden and morbidity. The US Lymphoma CAR-T Cell Consortium retrospectively reported the outcomes of standard of care patients receiving axi-cel for DLBCL and found that patients selected for bridging therapy had a higher proportion of high risk features compared to those who were not given bridging. When multivariate analysis or propensity matching was used to balance high risk features, bridging remained associated with a poorer outcome [13, 33]. In other cases radiation therapy has been used for bridging patients who are chemorefractory [34, 35]. Overall, the optimal bridging strategy has yet to be determined and may differ between diseases. Some patients may unexpectedly attain a complete remission (CR) from their bridging therapy but may still receive CAR-T cells. For example, 7 patients on the JULIET trial achieved CR from bridging, and after tisa-cel infusion there was observable CAR-T cell expansion and 5 of the 7 patients were progression-free at 12 months, with low rates of CRS and neurotoxicity [36].

Lymphodepleting Chemotherapy Prior to CAR-T Cell Infusion

Use of conditioning chemotherapy aimed at depleting lymphocytes (lymphodepletion) prior to CAR-T cell infusion has been shown to improve CAR-T cell expansion and tumor control, and is part of the FDA label for each product [37, 38]. The universally regimen consists of fludarabine and cyclophosphamide and may be given in the outpatient setting. Data is limited, but some patients with low baseline lymphocyte counts have been treated without using chemotherapy [17, 39]. The cytokine response to lymphodepletion allows for homeostatic repopulation of CAR-T cells and is associated with efficacy outcomes [8, 37, 40], but the optimal dosing and scheduling of lymphodepletion remains unknown. Clinicians must consider renal function as fludarabine is renally cleared, and dose reductions may be required in patients with low GFR.

Acute Monitoring after CAR-T Cell Infusion

Patients need to be monitored carefully after CAR-T cell infusion to identify and manage potential toxicities. On clinical trials, patients are typically monitored in the inpatient hospital setting for CRS, neurotoxicity, infection, and other complications that may occur after infusion (CAR-T complications are discussed in detail in the next chapter). However, due to considerations around resource utilization, efforts are underway to treat patients more commonly in the outpatient setting (discussed in detail in chapter "Roadmap for Starting an Outpatient Cellular Therapy Program") [41]. For example, 53 clinical trial patients with DLBCL were recently reported to be treated with liso-cel in the outpatient setting and 23 (43%) did not require hospitalization at any time [42]. A key requirement for patients who are outpatient after CAR-T cell therapy is a dedicated caregiver, which is generally a family member or friend. The caregiver needs to be educated on the acute toxicities of CAR-T cell therapy and to bring the patient to medical attention when toxicities occur (i.e. neurotoxicity) or when the patient cannot advocate for themselves. There is a strong desire to move the therapy into smaller community based practices, however it is important to note that CAR-T cell treatment in the outpatient setting requires significant infrastructure similar to, or in excess of, that needed for inpatient treatment. Another aspect of monitoring after CAR-T cell therapy is the Risk Evaluation and Mitigation Strategy (REMS) that is an FDA requirement that accompanies each product. For example, the REMS program for axi-cel and brexu-cel requires that each hospital has available at least 2 doses of tocilizumab for each CAR-T cell patient, that patients must remain within 2 h of the administering hospital for at least 4 weeks after CAR-T cell therapy, that patients must be issued a wallet card to indicate their CAR-T cell treatment, and specifies training requirements for adverse reaction management. In addition, there are processes in place for long-term, real-world data reporting that vary by region.

Disease Response Evaluation and Relapse Prevention

Outcomes of patients relapsing after CAR-T cell therapy are dismal [13, 43, 44]. There is no consensus on the optimal timing of disease response evaluation in the standard of care setting, and there is currently no relapse prevention strategy that is superior to observation in non-relapsed patients. Overall, outcomes of patients attaining CR are superior to those without CR and for aggressive diseases such as B-ALL or DLBCL most relapses occur within the first 6 months, with late relapses uncommon. In DLBCL, a partial response or stable disease identified on a day 30 PET/CT may deepen over time into a CR, so these patients are typically observed. Some patients with high risk B-ALL may benefit from consolidative allogeneic stem cell transplant to prevent relapse [45]. In pediatric B-ALL treated with 4-1BB-costimulated CAR-T cell therapy there is data that a loss of B cell aplasia coincides with shorter remissions [46]. In DLBCL this is not the case, and patients may recover B cells without lymphoma relapse [11]. Prospective trials are needed to identify high risk patients and determine if any early interventions can improve the outcomes of these patients.

CAR-T Cell Therapy Survivorship

Patients with durable remissions after CAR-T cell therapy remain in need of survivorship to address the physical, psychosocial, and immunologic issues that may remain. Apart from the known survivorship issues of patients with hematologic malignancies [47], CAR-T cell therapy poses some specific challenges to survivors. A major issue is the immune reconstitution that occurs after CAR-T cell therapy. Patients may have prolonged cytopenias, T cell quantitative and qualitative deficits, and/or B cell aplasia that create chronic infectious risks [27, 48]. Most centers provide prophylactic treatment against Pneumocystis jiroveci infection as well as against varicella zoster virus reactivation, although the duration and agents used vary [49]. There is also variation in the provision of intravenous immunoglobulin (IVIG) to patients with hypogammaglobulinemia due to B cell aplasia. Moreover, during the global pandemic caused by SARS-CoV2, vaccination has emerged as a key survivorship issue affecting return to normal life. The current data suggest that some antiviral antibodies persist after CAR-T cell therapies, presumably due to long-lived plasma cells, while others do not [50, 51]. It remains poorly described to what extent patients with B cell aplasia after CAR-T cell therapy can generate responses to new vaccines, such as those against SARS-CoV2, and whether patients need a different vaccine dose schedule than the general public. Finally, little data exists on the rate of secondary malignancies in CAR-T cell patients who have had high levels of prior chemotherapy and are left with immunologic deficits. More data is needed to understand the survivorship needs specific to the CAR-T cell patient population.

Conclusion

CAR-T cell therapy is now an established clinical standard of care for patients with R/R B-ALL, DLBCL, FL, MCL, and multiple myeloma. Best practices in clinical management continue to evolve as more patients receive these therapies for a broader range of indications. There are now also long term survivors after CAR-T cell therapy. Further research and dissemination of existing clinical knowledge are needed to meet the needs of this growing patient population.

References

1. Neelapu SS, Jacobson CA, Oluwole OO, et al. Outcomes of older patients in ZUMA-1, a pivotal study of axicabtagene ciloleucel in refractory large B-cell lymphoma. Blood. 2020;135:2106–9.
2. Abbasi A, Peeke S, Shah N, et al. Axicabtagene ciloleucel CD19 CAR-T cell therapy results in high rates of systemic and neurologic remissions in ten patients with refractory large B cell lymphoma including two with HIV and viral hepatitis. J Hematol Oncol. 2020;13:1.
3. Frigault MJ, Dietrich J, Martinez-Lage M, et al. Tisagenlecleucel CAR T-cell therapy in secondary CNS lymphoma. Blood. 2019;134:860–6.
4. Krishnamoorthy S, Ghobadi A, Santos RD, et al. CAR-T therapy in solid organ transplant recipients with treatment refractory posttransplant lymphoproliferative disorder. Am J Transplant. 2021;21:809–14.
5. Lu W, Wei Y, Cao Y, et al. CD19 CAR-T cell treatment conferred sustained remission in B-ALL patients with minimal residual disease. Cancer Immunol Immunother. 2021;
6. Park JH, Riviere I, Gonen M, et al. Long-term follow-up of CD19 CAR therapy in acute lymphoblastic leukemia. N Engl J Med. 2018;378:449–59.
7. Dean EA, Mhaskar RS, Lu H, et al. High metabolic tumor volume is associated with decreased efficacy of axicabtagene ciloleucel in large B-cell lymphoma. Blood Adv. 2020;4:3268–76.
8. Jain MD, Zhao H, Wang X, et al. Tumor interferon signaling and suppressive myeloid cells associate with CAR T cell failure in large B cell lymphoma. Blood. 2021;137(19):2621–33.
9. Strati P, Ahmed S, Furqan F, et al. Prognostic impact of corticosteroids on efficacy of chimeric antigen receptor T-cell therapy in large B-cell lymphoma. Blood. 2021;137(23):3272–6.
10. Johnson PC, Abramson JS. Patient selection for chimeric antigen receptor (CAR) T-cell therapy for aggressive B-cell non-Hodgkin lymphomas. Leuk Lymphoma. 2020;61:2561–7.
11. Locke FL, Ghobadi A, Jacobson CA, et al. Long-term safety and activity of axicabtagene ciloleucel in refractory large B-cell lymphoma (ZUMA-1): a single-arm, multicentre, phase 1-2 trial. Lancet Oncol. 2019;20:31–42.
12. Neelapu SS, Locke FL, Bartlett NL, et al. Axicabtagene Ciloleucel CAR T-cell therapy in refractory large B-cell lymphoma. N Engl J Med. 2017;377(26):2531–44.
13. Nastoupil LJ, Jain MD, Feng L, et al. Standard-of-care axicabtagene ciloleucel for relapsed or refractory large B-cell lymphoma: results from the US lymphoma CAR T consortium. J Clin Oncol. 2020:JCO1902104.
14. Jacobson CA, Hunter BD, Redd R, et al. Axicabtagene ciloleucel in the non-trial setting: outcomes and correlates of response, resistance, and toxicity. J Clin Oncol. 2020:JCO1902103.
15. Jacobson C, Chavez JC, Sehgal AR, et al. Primary analysis of Zuma-5: a phase 2 study of Axicabtagene ciloleucel (Axi-Cel) in patients with relapsed/refractory (R/R) indolent non-Hodgkin lymphoma (iNHL). Blood. 2020;136:40–1.
16. Maude SL, Laetsch TW, Buechner J, et al. Tisagenlecleucel in children and young adults with B-cell lymphoblastic leukemia. N Engl J Med. 2018;378:439–48.
17. Schuster SJ, Bishop MR, Tam CS, et al. Tisagenlecleucel in adult relapsed or refractory diffuse large B-cell lymphoma. N Engl J Med. 2018;
18. Jaeger U, Bishop MR, Salles G, et al. Myc expression and tumor-infiltrating T cells are associated with response in patients (Pts) with relapsed/refractory diffuse large B-cell lymphoma (r/r DLBCL) treated with Tisagenlecleucel in the Juliet trial. Blood. 2020;136:48–9.

19. Pasquini MC, Hu ZH, Curran K, et al. Real-world evidence of tisagenlecleucel for pediatric acute lymphoblastic leukemia and non-Hodgkin lymphoma. Blood Adv. 2020;4:5414–24.
20. Maziarz RT, Schuster SJ, Romanov VV, et al. Grading of neurological toxicity in patients treated with tisagenlecleucel in the JULIET trial. Blood Adv. 2020;4:1440–7.
21. Schuster SJ, Maziarz RT, Rusch ES, et al. Grading and management of cytokine release syndrome in patients treated with tisagenlecleucel in the JULIET trial. Blood Adv. 2020;4:1432–9.
22. Sommermeyer D, Hudecek M, Kosasih PL, et al. Chimeric antigen receptor-modified T cells derived from defined CD8+ and CD4+ subsets confer superior antitumor reactivity in vivo. Leukemia. 2016;30:492–500.
23. Abramson JS, Palomba ML, Gordon LI, et al. Lisocabtagene maraleucel for patients with relapsed or refractory large B-cell lymphomas (TRANSCEND NHL 001): a multicentre seamless design study. Lancet. 2020;396:839–52.
24. Bachier CR, Palomba ML, Abramson JS, et al. Outpatient treatment with lisocabtagene maraleucel (liso-cel) in three ongoing clinical studies in relapsed/refractory (R/R) B Cell Non-Hodgkin lymphoma (NHL), including second-line transplant ineligible patients: transcend NHL 001, outreach, and PILOT. Blood. 2019;134:2868.
25. Alvi RM, Frigault MJ, Fradley MG, et al. Cardiovascular events among adults treated with chimeric antigen receptor T-cells (CAR-T). J Am Coll Cardiol. 2019;74:3099–108.
26. Faramand RG, Jain MD, Staedtke V, et al. Tumor microenvironment composition and severe cytokine release syndrome (CRS) influence toxicity in patients with large B cell lymphoma treated with Axicabtagene ciloleucel. Clin Cancer Res. 2020;26(18):4823–31.
27. Logue JM, Zucchetti E, Bachmeier CA, et al. Immune reconstitution and associated infections following axicabtagene ciloleucel in relapsed or refractory large B-cell lymphoma. Haematologica. 2021;106(4):978–86.
28. Locke FL, Rossi JM, Neelapu SS, et al. Tumor burden, inflammation, and product attributes determine outcomes of axicabtagene ciloleucel in large B-cell lymphoma. Blood Adv. 2020;4:4898–911.
29. Ruella M, Xu J, Barrett DM, et al. Induction of resistance to chimeric antigen receptor T cell therapy by transduction of a single leukemic B cell. Nat Med. 2018;24:1499–503.
30. Kharfan-Dabaja MA, Jain MD, Aulakh S, et al. Obinutuzumab as bridging therapy for successful manufacturing of axicabtagene ciloleucel for transformed follicular lymphoma with circulating cells. Am J Hematol. 2019;94:E245–E7.
31. Fraietta JA, Beckwith KA, Patel PR, et al. Ibrutinib enhances chimeric antigen receptor T-cell engraftment and efficacy in leukemia. Blood. 2016;127:1117–27.
32. Gauthier J, Hirayama AV, Purushe J, et al. Feasibility and efficacy of CD19-targeted CAR T cells with concurrent ibrutinib for CLL after ibrutinib failure. Blood. 2020;135:1650–60.
33. Jain MD, Jacobs MT, Nastoupil LJ, et al. Characteristics and outcomes of patients receiving bridging therapy while awaiting manufacture of standard of care axicabtagene ciloleucel CD19 chimeric antigen receptor (CAR) T-cell therapy for relapsed/refractory large B-cell lymphoma: results from the US lymphoma CAR-T consortium. Blood. 2019;134:245.
34. Pinnix CC, Gunther JR, Dabaja BS, et al. Bridging therapy prior to axicabtagene ciloleucel for relapsed/refractory large B-cell lymphoma. Blood Adv. 2020;4:2871–83.
35. Sim AJ, Jain MD, Figura N, et al. Radiation therapy as a bridging strategy for CAR T cell therapy with axicabtagene ciloleucel in diffuse large B-cell lymphoma. Int J Radiat Oncol Biol Phys. 2019;
36. Bishop MR, Maziarz RT, Waller EK, et al. Tisagenlecleucel in relapsed/refractory diffuse large B cell lymphoma patients without measurable disease at infusion. Blood Adv. 2019;3:2230–6.
37. Hirayama AV, Gauthier J, Hay KA, et al. The response to lymphodepletion impacts PFS in patients with aggressive non-Hodgkin lymphoma treated with CD19 CAR T cells. Blood. 2019;133:1876–87.
38. Turtle CJ, Hanafi LA, Berger C, et al. Immunotherapy of non-Hodgkin's lymphoma with a defined ratio of CD8+ and CD4+ CD19-specific chimeric antigen receptor-modified T cells. Sci Transl Med. 2016;8:355ra116.

39. Brudno JN, Somerville RP, Shi V, et al. Allogeneic T cells that express an anti-CD19 chimeric antigen receptor induce remissions of B-cell malignancies that Progress after allogeneic hematopoietic stem-cell transplantation without causing graft-versus-host disease. J Clin Oncol. 2016;34:1112–21.
40. Kochenderfer JN, Somerville RPT, Lu T, et al. Lymphoma remissions caused by anti-CD19 chimeric antigen receptor T cells are associated with high serum Interleukin-15 levels. J Clin Oncol. 2017;35:1803–13.
41. Alexander M, Culos K, Roddy J, et al. Chimeric antigen receptor T cell therapy: a comprehensive review of clinical efficacy, toxicity, and best practices for outpatient administration. Transplant Cell Ther. 2021;27(7):558–70.
42. Bachier CR, Godwin JE, Andreadis C, et al. Outpatient treatment with lisocabtagene maraleucel (liso-cel) across a variety of clinical sites from three ongoing clinical studies in relapsed/refractory (R/R) large B-cell lymphoma (LBCL). J Clin Oncol. 2020;38:8037.
43. Spiegel JY, Dahiya S, Jain MD, et al. Outcomes of patients with large B-cell lymphoma progressing after axicabtagene ciloleucel. Blood 2020;137(13):1832-1835.
44. Wudhikarn K, Flynn JR, Riviere I, et al. Interventions and outcomes of adult patients with B-ALL progressing after CD19 chimeric antigen receptor T cell therapy. Blood. 2021;
45. Goldsmith SR, Ghobadi A, DiPersio JF. Hematopoeitic cell transplantation and CAR T-cell therapy: complements or competitors? Front Oncol. 2020;10:608916.
46. Summers C, Annesley C, Bleakley M, Dahlberg A, Jensen MC, Gardner R. Long term follow-up after SCRI-CAR19v1 reveals late recurrences as well as a survival advantage to consolidation with HCT after CAR T cell induced remission. Blood. 2018;132:967.
47. Damlaj M, El Fakih R, Hashmi SK. Evolution of survivorship in lymphoma, myeloma and leukemia: metamorphosis of the field into long term follow-up care. Blood Rev. 2019;33:63–73.
48. Baird JH, Epstein DJ, Tamaresis JS, et al. Immune reconstitution and infectious complications following axicabtagene ciloleucel therapy for large B-cell lymphoma. Blood Adv. 2021;5:143–55.
49. Hill JA, Seo SK. How I prevent infections in patients receiving CD19-targeted chimeric antigen receptor T cells for B-cell malignancies. Blood. 2020;136:925–35.
50. Walti CS, Krantz EM, Maalouf J, et al. Antibodies to vaccine-preventable infections after CAR-T-cell therapy for B-cell malignancies. JCI Insight 2021;6(11):e146743.
51. Hill JA, Krantz EM, Hay KA, et al. Durable preservation of antiviral antibodies after CD19-directed chimeric antigen receptor T-cell immunotherapy. Blood Adv. 2019;3:3590–601.

CAR-T Cell Complications

Emily C. Ayers, Dustin A. Cobb, and Daniel W. Lee

Abstract Autologous T-cells genetically modified to express a chimeric antigen receptor (CAR) have shifted the treatment paradigm for adults and children with relapsed and/or refractory B-cell malignancies. Multiple CD19-directed and now a B cell maturation antigen (BCMA) CAR T-cell therapies have been approved for use. Despite their differences, they all share the same toxicities and risks to patients. Cytokine release syndrome (CRS) and immune effector cell-associated neurotoxicity syndrome (ICANS), the two most common complications, appear to result from the exponential and uncontrolled expansion and supraphysiologic activation of CAR T-cells followed by the wider adaptive immune system. Though the exact mechanisms have yet to be elucidated, several animal models approximating the clinical effects have been developed. Until more mechanistic data is available, side effects in patients can be minimized via appropriate and timely interventions described herein such that the majority can be treated safely. Additional issues including prolonged cytopenias, on-target but off-tissue B-cell cytotoxicity and resulting aplasia and hypogammaglobulinemia, the theoretical development of replication-competent virus, and the risk of insertional mutagenesis resulting in secondary neoplasms will also be discussed.

E. C. Ayers
University of Virginia Cancer Center, Charlottesville, VA, USA

Division of Hematology/Oncology, Department of Medicine, University of Virginia, Charlottesville, VA, USA

D. A. Cobb
Division of Pediatric Hematology/Oncology, Department of Pediatrics, University of Virginia, Charlottesville, VA, USA

D. W. Lee (✉)
University of Virginia Cancer Center, Charlottesville, VA, USA

Division of Pediatric Hematology/Oncology, Department of Pediatrics, University of Virginia, Charlottesville, VA, USA
e-mail: DWL4Q@Virginia.edu; DWL4Q@hscmail.mcc.virginia.edu

© Springer Nature Switzerland AG 2022
A. Ghobadi, J. F. DiPersio (eds.), *Gene and Cellular Immunotherapy for Cancer*, Cancer Drug Discovery and Development,
https://doi.org/10.1007/978-3-030-87849-8_11

Keywords Complications · Cytokine release syndrome (CRS) · Immune effector cell-associated neurotoxicity syndrome (ICANS) · The immune effector cell-associated encephalopathy (ICE) · Cerebral edema · Prolonged cytopenias · On-target off-tissue cytotoxicity · B cell aplasia · Hypogammaglobulinemia · Replication-competent virus · Insertional mutagenesis · Secondary neoplasms

Introduction

Chimeric antigen receptor (CAR) modified T-cells are shifting the treatment paradigm for the management of relapsed or refractory B-cell malignancies, and many more indications are likely forthcoming in the next several years. Along with never-before-seen response rates in patient populations for which all viable therapies have been exhausted, CAR T-cells also bring never-before-seen toxicities, at least in terms of severity. Identifying and appropriately managing these toxicities is paramount to a successful outcome, and this chapter provides the basis for doing just that. Though we focus on the most common toxicities of CAR T-cell therapy, cytokine release syndrome (CRS) and immune effector cell-associated neurotoxicity syndrome (ICANS), additional complications including prolonged cytopenias and hypogammaglobulinemia and potential late effects of virally-modified, genetically engineered cells will be discussed.

Pre-Clinical Models of CRS and Neurotoxicity

It is essential that the development of strategies for pre-clinical modeling of CAR T cell-induced toxicities coincide with the advancing field of CAR T-cell therapeutics as it continues to grow and expand into the clinical setting. Thus far, the lack of animal models has impaired the ability of clinicians and researchers in predicting the development of CAR T-cell-induced toxicity, studying the underlying biology, and evaluating clinical intervention strategies. Recently, the establishment of two xenogeneic mouse models of CRS has facilitated the understanding of the biological factors involved. Modeling of CAR T-cell-induced neurotoxicity has also been lacking with the exception of a non-human primate model. However, one of the above-mentioned xenogeneic mouse models for CRS has also been shown to exhibit some features of neurotoxicity seen in patients.

In SCID-beige mice, severe CRS develops following CD19 CAR T-cell injection. In this model, CRS is characterized by a systemic inflammatory response that highly recapitulates human CRS, including IL-6 and IFN-γ production [1]. Several additional inflammatory cytokines, including human GM-CSF and IL-2 were also highly correlated with CRS severity and survival. Intervention with IL-6 receptor blockade or anakinra, an IL-1 receptor antagonist, abolished severe CRS in mice. Myeloid cells, particularly macrophages, were found to be key drivers of IL-6 production and exhibited increased inducible nitric oxide synthase (iNOS) expression, which leads to elevated nitric oxide and stimulation of vasodilation and hypotension, both features of severe CRS in patients.

In the second model, humanized mice (NSG mice expressing IL-3, stem cell factor, and GM-CSF human transgenes and engrafted with human hematopoietic stem cells) also develop CAR T-cell treatment-induced toxicity [2]. This model recapitulated important features of severe CRS, including fever and a systemic inflammatory cytokine response, with the addition of delayed neurotoxicity after CD19 CAR T-cell treatment. In this case, therapeutic blockade of either IL-6 (tocilizumab) or IL-1 (anakinra) prevented CRS, however, only inhibition of IL-1 was effective at preventing lethal neurotoxicity. Development of CRS in this model required human monocytes which were the primary producers of IL-6 and IL-1.

Lastly, a non-human primate model for CAR T-cell toxicities using rhesus macaques has also been developed. Upon injection of autologous CD20 CAR T-cells, animals exhibited clinical signs of CRS and neurotoxicity [3]. Systemic inflammatory cytokines, including IL-6, were increased. Further, high levels of pro-inflammatory cytokines were present in the cerebrospinal fluid (CSF) with accompanying T-cell infiltration. Similar to clinical observations in human patients experiencing neurotoxicity, significant accumulation of CAR and non-CAR T-cells were detectable in the CSF and brain parenchyma coinciding with neurologic symptoms.

Collectively, these animal models closely recapitulate key features of CAR T cell-induced toxicities and provide critical insights into the underlying mechanisms leading to CRS and neurotoxicity, which are summarized in Fig. 1. These and any future models in development will make it possible to further investigate the biology and provide improved pre-clinical tools for evaluating the efficacy of strategies to mitigate CRS and neurotoxicity.

CAR T-Cell Toxicity in Clinical Studies and Correlative Studies

The incidence and clinical phenotype of CRS and ICANS vary depending upon a number of different factors. Clinical studies report a range in the incidence and severity of toxicity between the different CAR T-cell products among the several hematologic malignancies for which patients are treated. Here we will review the incidence, clinical presentation, and kinetics of CRS and neurotoxicity in clinical studies (Table 1) as well as examine the correlative risk factors for severe toxicity identified by various analyses.

Cytokine Release Syndrome in Diffuse Large B-Cell Lymphoma

Three dominant clinical trials have informed our expectations regarding the incidence of CRS among patients with diffuse large B-cell lymphoma (DLBCL). The ZUMA-1 study, which first investigated the use of axicabtagene ciloleucel in 111

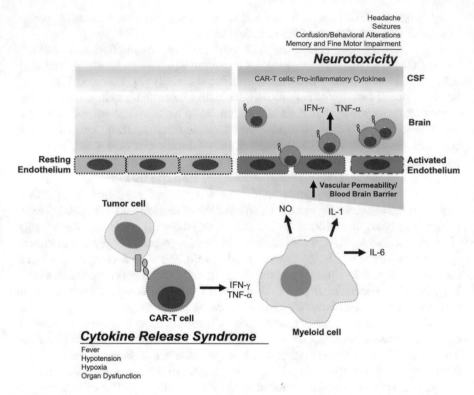

Fig. 1 Mechanisms of CRS and Neurotoxicity. Development of CAR T cell-induced CRS and neurotoxicity. Upon recognition of tumor cells and subsequent activation, CAR T-cells secrete IFN- γ and TNF- α, which stimulates myeloid cells including macrophages and monocytes, other non-immune cells, and endothelial cells. Activated myeloid cells secrete IL-6, IL-1, and other cytokines and chemokines. Macrophages also upregulate inducible nitric oxide synthase (iNOS) leading to abundant production of nitric oxide (NO) which promotes vasodilation and hypotension. Highly-activated CAR T-cells and recruited myeloid cells further exacerbate this systemic inflammatory response through elevated cytokine/chemokine release. The exacerbated inflammatory condition leads to endothelial cell activation and increased vascular permeability. This response can ultimately lead to a compromised blood brain barrier and capillary leak, allowing an influx of inflammatory cells including CAR T and non-CAR T-cells and other inflammatory mediators into the brain parenchyma and cerebrospinal fluid (CSF) that is concomitant with neurologic symptoms

patients with relapsed and/or refractory (R/R) DLBCL, identified any grade CRS in 93% of patients with a median time to onset of 2 days (range 1–12 days) [4]. Grade 3 or 4 CRS was seen in 13% of patients and median duration of toxicity lasted 8 days. In this trial, management of CRS included tocilizumab in 43%, corticosteroids in 27%, and vasopressors in 17% of patients.

The JULIET study describes the toxicity profile associated with tisagenlecleucel in the treatment of patients with R/R DLBCL [6]. In this study, median time to onset of CRS was similar to that seen with axicabtagene ciloleucel at 3 days with a range of 1–9 days from time of T-cell infusion. Median duration of CRS was 7 days with a range of 2–30 days in this study. The authors report any grade CRS in 58% with grade 3–4 CRS seen in 23% of patients. Tocilizumab, corticosteroids, and high-dose

Table 1 Incidence and severity of CRS and ICANS by CAR T-cell product

Study	Disease	CAR T-Cell product	Total patients (n)	CRS		ICANS		Grading system
				Any grade (%)	Grade ≥ 3 (%)	Any grade (%)	Grade ≥ 3 (%)	
ZUMA-1 [4]	R/R DLBCL	Axicabtagene ciloleucel	111	93	13	64	23	Lee [5]
JULIET [6]	R/R DLBCL	Tisagenlecleucel	111	58	23	20	11	Penn [7]
TRANSCEND [8]	R/R DLBCL	Lisocabtagene maraleucel	344	42	2	30	20	Lee [5]
ELIANA [9]	R/R B-ALL	Tisagenlecleucel	75	77	38	40	13	Penn [7]
ZUMA –2 [10]	R/R MCL	Brexucabtagene autoleucel	74	76	15	63	31	Lee [5]
ZUMA—5 [11]	R/R iNHL	Axicabtagene ciloleucel	146	NR	7	NR	19	Lee [5]
KarMMa [12]	R/R MM	Idecabtagene vicleucel	140	84	5	18	3	Lee [5]

Abbreviations: *CAR* chimeric antigen receptor, *CRS* cytokine release syndrome, *ICANS* immune effector cell-associated neurotoxicity syndrome, *R/R* relapsed or refractory, *DLBCL* diffuse large B-cell lymphoma, *B-ALL* B-cell acute lymphoblastic leukemia, *MCL* mantle cell lymphoma, *iNHL* indolent non-Hodgkin lymphoma, *MM* multiple myeloma, *NR* not reported

vasopressors were used for management in 16%, 11%, and 6% of patients with CRS, respectively, in addition to supportive care.

Most recently, the TRANSCEND study reports the experience with lisocabtagene maraleucel in this same patient population [8]. Of interest, this group reports lower incidence of CRS compared to the previously published clinical trials of CAR T-cell therapy in the R/R DLBCL patient group. The group reports any grade CRS in 42% of patients with only 2% classified as grade 3–4. In this study, tocilizumab was used in 21% and corticosteroids in 17% of patients. Use of vasopressors was not specified.

When comparing available CAR T-cell commercial products and their individual toxicity profiles, it is important to note the lack of a standardized grading system at the time of publication. Covered in more detail later in this chapter, the formalization of a cohesive grading system for both CRS and neurotoxicity did not exist at the time of these original clinical studies. As such, the cross comparison of the incidence of all grades and severity of CRS should be performed with extreme caution.

As the use of CAR T-cell therapy has been adopted into standard-of-care practice across the world, evidence in real-world settings has grown. In the last several years, a number of groups have published their experiences with available commercial products. In the real-world setting, axicabtagene ciloleucel has been associated with grade ≥ 3 CRS in 7–14% of patients with any grade CRS seen in up to 83% of patients [13–15]. CRS onset seems to mirror that seen on clinical trial with a median onset of 2–3 days and a median duration of 5–7 days. Tocilizumab was used in 62–70% of patients and steroids used in 26–57% of patients in these published series. Of note, the more frequent use of tocilizumab in these real-world studies suggests the earlier implementation of anti-IL-6 directed therapy in the standard-of-care setting compared to the initial clinical trials as we have a better understanding that cytokine-directed therapy does not alter antitumor efficacy.

In the real-world setting, tisagenlecleucel is associated with any-grade CRS in 45% of patients with grade 3–4 CRS seen in 1–4.5% of patients [15]. As expected, median onset is 3 days with a median duration of 5 days. Tocilizumab use has been reported in 13–43% of patients with corticosteroid use in 7–10%.

Cytokine Release Syndrome in B-Cell Acute Lymphoblastic Leukemia

The pivotal, multicenter, international ELIANA trial investigated the use of tisagenlecleucel across 11 different countries in children with B-cell acute lymphoblastic leukemia (ALL) [9]. Any grade CRS was reported in 77% with grade 3 or higher CRS seen in 38% of patients. With regards to management, 37% of patients received tocilizumab and 25% received high-dose vasopressors. Forty-seven percent of patients required admission to the ICU with a median duration of stay in the ICU of 7 days.

In the standard-of-care setting with commercially available CAR T-cell therapy, CRS was observed in 55% of patients with severe CRS seen in 16.1%, including 1 death [13]. Overall, tocilizumab was used in 25% of patients with 6% requiring corticosteroids as well.

Cytokine Release Syndrome in Mantle Cell Lymphoma

CAR T-cell therapy has also received approval based on results from the ZUMA-2 study in patients with relapsed or refractory mantle cell lymphoma treated with brexu-cabtagene autoleucel [10]. In patients on this study, 76% developed any grade CRS with 15% experiencing grade 3 or higher CRS. Onset of symptoms was similar to other disease subtypes with a median onset of 2 days, and all cases resolved at a median of 11 days. Patients were managed in a similar way as well, with 59% receiving tocili-zumab, 22% corticosteroids, and 16% of patients requiring vasopressors. As this product is newly approved, real-world studies have yet to be published in this setting.

Cytokine Release Syndrome in Indolent Non-Hodgkin Lymphoma

Compared to rates of CRS in aggressive non-Hodgkin lymphoma (NHL), patients with indolent NHL have experienced lower rates of toxicity. In the ZUMA–5 study, axicabtagene ciloleucel was associated with grade 3 or higher CRS in only 7% (6% in follicular lymphoma and 9% in marginal zone lymphoma) and 99% of CRS had resolved at time of data cut-off [11]. Again, experience in the standard-of-care setting is currently not available.

Cytokine Release Syndrome in Multiple Myeloma

The KarMMa study investigated the efficacy of anti BCMA-directed CAR T-cell therapy using idecabtagene vicleucel among multiple myeloma patients [12]. In this clinical trial, CRS occurred in 84% of patients with only 5% demonstrating grade 3 or higher CRS. Median time to onset was 1 day (range 1–12) and duration was 5 days (range 1–63) with tocilizumab used in 52% and glucocorticoids in 15%.

Neurotoxicity in Diffuse Large B Cell Lymphoma

Each of the aforementioned clinical trials of CAR T-cell therapy in relapsed or refractory DLBCL have also helped shape our understanding of expected neurotox-icities associated with available commercial products. ICANS had not been formally defined at the time the pivotal studies were performed, so neurologic side effects on these trials were largely described and graded as per the Common Terminology Criteria for Adverse Events (CTCAE) v4.0 [16], which is largely subjective. Therefore, comparisons across trials are not possible. In the ZUMA-1 study, neurotoxicity was seen in 64% of patients with 28% exhibiting grade 3 or greater neurotoxicity. Median onset among these patients was 5 days from T-cell infusion with a range of 1–17 days and a median duration of 17 days.

In the JULIET study, tisagenlecleucel demonstrated slightly lower rates of neurotoxicity with 20% of patients having any grade toxicity and 11% suffering from grade 3 or greater neurotoxicity. Similarly, lisocabtagene maraleucel showed slightly lower rates compared to axicabtagene ciloleucel in the TRANSCEND study with any grade reported in 30% of patients and 10% of patients experiencing grade 3 or higher. In this study, the median time to onset was 9 days (range 3–23) with a median duration of 11 days.

In a post-marketing safety analysis, axicabtagene ciloleucel has been associated with neurotoxicity in up to 61% of patients using data from the Center for International Blood and Marrow Transplant Research (CIBMTR) with a median onset of 6 days. Additional analyses performed in the real world setting have shown rates of neurotoxicity between 31 and 41% of patients with this product [14]. ICANS seems to be less commonly observed with tisagenlecleucel in the standard of care setting with rates ranging from 3–24% of patients receiving commercial product.

Neurotoxicity in B-Cell Acute Lymphoblastic Leukemia

Neurologic events were reported in 40% of patients in the ELIANA trial with 13% of patients experiencing grade 3 toxicity [9]. Symptoms began during the time of CRS or shortly after its resolution and 50% of grade 3 or higher neurologic episodes recovered within 10 days with an additional 25% recovering within 18 days. The authors report 2 deaths related to neurologic toxicity thought to be secondary to tisagenlecleucel in this study.

Neurotoxicity in Mantle Cell Lymphoma

Neurologic events among the mantle cell lymphoma patient group receiving brexucabtagene autoleucel were reported in 63% of patients [10]. Of patients with reported events, 50% were grade 1–2 and 50% were grade 3 or higher with a median onset of 7 days from T-cell infusion and a median duration of 12 days. Thirty-eight percent of patients received corticosteroids and 26% of patients received tocilizumab in the study. The group reports that neurotoxicity resolved completely in 86% of patients at the conclusion of follow-up.

Neurotoxicity in Indolent Non-Hodgkin Lymphoma

In the ZUMA-5 study of axicabtagene ciloleucel in patients with relapsed/refractory indolent NHL, grade 3 or higher neurologic events were reported in 19% of patients overall, with 15% in follicular lymphoma and 41% in marginal zone lymphoma [11]. The authors report 93% of neurologic events of any grade resolved at time of data cutoff.

Neurotoxicity in Multiple Myeloma

The KarMMa study reported neurotoxic effects in 18% of patients with 3% of grade 3. No grade 4 or 5 neurologic events were seen in the study. Median time to a neurotoxic event was 2 days with a duration of 3 days (range 1–26 days) [12].

Risk Factors and Predictors of Toxicity

Patient characteristics that predict severity of CRS include tumor burden, with the most robust data seen in the ALL population. Increased percentage of blasts in bone marrow as well as higher percentage of CD19+ cells in the marrow are predictive of CRS severity [17, 18]. Higher tumor burden has also been associated with both higher incidence and severity of CRS among DLBCL patients [8]. Elderly age and preexisting neurologic comorbidities have been associated with increased risk of neurotoxicity, although the data is not definitive [8, 19, 20]. Following T-cell infusion, earlier onset of fever (within 3 days) has also been associated with more severe CRS/ICANS [21].

With regards to treatment characteristics, some studies suggest higher CAR T-cell doses infused into the patient are potentially predictive of increased incidences of CRS and ICANS, although definitive data is lacking [19, 20]. In addition, lymphodepletion therapy with fludarabine and cyclophosphamide has been associated with increased risk of both neurotoxicity and CRS compared to other chemotherapeutic regimens used in this setting. Manufacturing CAR T-cells without selection of CD8+ central memory cells is predictive of CRS in one study [21]. There is also evidence that structural differences between the available commercial CAR products are responsible for the different kinetics of T-cell expansion and effector functions noted. For example, CARs with 4-1BB costimulatory domains, namely tisagenlecleucel, have been associated with more gradual T-cell expansion. In contrast, the CD28-based CARs, including axicabtagene ciloleucel and brexucabtagene autoleucel, induce more rapid expansion that is thought to explain the faster onset of symptoms reported using these commercial CAR products [22, 23].

With improved understanding into the pathogenesis of CRS and ICANS following CAR T-cell therapy, there has also been a significant effort to identify biomarkers which could predict severity of toxicity. In general, elevated inflammatory markers have been linked with higher-grade CRS and ICANS. In the ZUMA-1 trial, IL-15, IL-6, IL-1Ra, IL-2Rα, IFNγ, IL-10, IL-8, and granzyme B were all statistically significantly associated with grade ≥ 3 CRS compared to grade 1–2 CRS [4]. In the B-ALL population, higher peak levels of IL-6, soluble IL-2R, ferritin, IFNγ, and CRP predict more severe CRS [18, 24, 25].

Similarly, inflammatory markers including IL-15, IL-6, IL-2Rα, IFNγ, IL-10, and granzyme B also predict higher grade ICANS based on correlative studies on clinical trial [4]. Markers of diffuse intravascular coagulation have also been associated with severity of neurotoxicity [19, 26]. One study developed a model which predicted grade 4 or higher neurotoxicity with 100% sensitivity using fever ≥38.9

degrees Celsius, serum IL-6, and MCP-1 in the first 36 h after T-cell infusion [19]. Additionally, a more robust T-cell expansion *in vivo* portends more severe CRS and ICANS on several studies, although the data here is not consistent [4, 21].

Consensus CRS and Neurotoxicity Grading Systems

These early studies were hampered by a lack of agreed-upon definitions and grading systems for cytokine release syndrome and the unique neurotoxicity syndrome discovered with the advent of CAR T-cell therapy. While early CAR T-cell immunotherapists expected toxicities typically associated with immune system activation, such as with robust vaccination responses, the extent and severity of these toxicities as well as the narrow therapeutic window of CAR T-cell dosing was a surprise. The CRS term provided in the CTCAE in effect at the time was far from adequate to describe CAR T-cell-associated CRS. This prompted a small group of pediatric oncologists from the few institutions with CAR T-cell clinical trials in 2014 to redefine CRS and offer a more relevant grading system that was tied to a simplified management algorithm [5]. The Lee Criteria, as it came to be called, was widely adopted across most later trials though other grading systems were also published and utilized over the years [7, 27–29].

Concurrently, unique constellations of neurotoxicities appreciated for the first time with CAR T-cell therapy were subjected to definitions and grading in the CTCAE that were overlapping and highly subjective. Most grading was based on a patient's ability to perform activities of daily living, which does not typically apply to the already hospitalized patient. These challenges made comparing one CAR T-cell therapeutic to another across clinical trials impossible.

Finally, in 2018 a broader, international group of academicians, immunotherapists, industry and professional society partners assembled to develop consensus definitions and grading systems for CRS and CAR T-cell associated neurotoxicity, which they termed ICANS. Facilitated by the American Society for Transplantation and Cellular Therapy (ASTCT), the ASTCT criteria simplifies grading and can be applied by any care team member at the bedside in real time. Leaders in the field agree that the ASTCT grading system should be utilized for all future academic and industry sponsored clinical trials as well as for real-world reporting as encouraged by the CIBMTR [30].

Definition of CRS

The ASTCT consensus criteria defines CRS as, "a supraphysiologic response following any immune therapy that results in the activation or engagement of endogenous or infused T-cells and/or other immune effector cells. Symptoms can be progressive, must include fever at the onset, and may include hypotension, capillary leak (hypoxia) and end organ dysfunction."

In order to diagnose CRS, the patient must have developed a fever at the onset. After CRS has been diagnosed, fever is no longer required if the patient has been treated with antipyretics or anti-cytokine therapy. Similarly, absence of fever is required for CRS to be considered resolved but is not sufficient. If hypotension or hypoxia persist and are not attributable to another cause, then CRS is considered to persist even in the absence of fever. These must completely resolve in order to consider CRS resolved.

Many of the symptoms of CRS overlap with other disorders, such as sepsis, often seen in patients with refractory cancer. A prerequisite for CRS, therefore, must be an appropriate temporal relationship between the cell product infusion and the onset of symptoms accounting for known trends in toxicity kinetics between different cellular products, particularly when cells other than T-cells and/or engagement of tumor cells with methods other than CARs are used. Other causes that may result in overlapping symptoms, such as infections, must be excluded.

Severe CRS has many features that overlap with hemophagocytic lymphohistiocytosis or macrophage activation syndrome (HLH/MAS), though mild to moderate CRS is clearly distinct from HLH/MAS. Whether these represent a continuum of the same process or are due to distinct pathologies remains to be elucidated. For these reasons, the ASTCT consensus excludes HLH/MAS from the definition of CRS. Finally, while previously thought to be an extension of CRS, neurotoxicities are called out separately in the ASTCT criteria as its own, separate syndrome.

Grading of CRS

ASTCT consensus CRS grading allows any provider to assign CRS grade at the bedside if they know three basic facts: (1) presence or absence of fever (defined as temperature $\geq$ 38 °C), (2) presence or absence of hypotension and what management is being provided for it, and (3) type of oxygen delivery device, if any. Grading of CRS is shown in Table 2. The more severe symptom, hypotension or hypoxia if present, drives the grading of CRS. For example, if a patient requires one vasopressor for hypotension and is intubated and mechanically ventilated due to overwhelming pulmonary edema resulting in respiratory compromise, then he/she has Grade 4 CRS as the degree of hypoxia drives CRS grading in this circumstance.

Definition of Immune Effector Cell Associated Neurotoxicity Syndrome (ICANS)

Early CAR T-cell studies and the Lee Criteria initially considered the new and unusual constellation of neurotoxicities a manifestation of CRS. However, as the number of patients treated expanded it became clear that these neurotoxicities, termed ICANS by the ASTCT consensus group, represented a separate entity from CRS. Cytokines may be involved in its pathogenesis but its mechanism remains

Table 2 ASTCT CRS consensus grading [30]

CRS parameter	Grade 1	Grade 2	Grade 3	Grade 4
Fever[a]	Temperature ≥ 38 °C	Temperature ≥ 38 °C	Temperature ≥ 38 °C	Temperature ≥ 38 °C
With:				
Hypotension	None	Not requiring vasopressors	Requiring one vasopressor with or without vasopressin	Requiring multiple vasopressors (excluding vasopressin)
And/or[b]				
Hypoxia	None	Requiring low-flow nasal cannula or blow-by[c]	Requiring high-flow nasal cannula[c], facemask, non-rebreather mask, or Venturi mask	Requiring positive pressure (e.g.: CPAP, BiPAP, intubation and mechanical ventilation)

Organ toxicities associated with CRS may be graded according to CTCAE v5.0 but they do not influence CRS grading

CPAP continuous positive airway pressure, *BiPAP* bilevel positive airway pressure

[a]Fever is defined as temperature ≥ 38 °C not attributable to any other cause. In patients who have CRS then receive antipyretics or anti-cytokine therapy such as tocilizumab or steroids, fever is no longer required to grade subsequent CRS severity. In this case, CRS grading is driven by hypotension and/or hypoxia

[b]CRS grade is determined by the more severe event: hypotension or hypoxia not attributable to any other cause. For example, a patient with temperature of 39.5 °C, hypotension requiring one vasopressor and hypoxia requiring low-flow nasal cannula is classified as having Grade 3 CRS

[c]Low-flow nasal cannula is defined as oxygen delivered at ≤6 L/min. Low flow also includes blow-by oxygen delivery, sometimes used in pediatrics. High-flow nasal cannula is defined as oxygen delivered at >6 L/min

unclear. ICANS can present either concurrent with CRS or after CRS has completely resolved, further implicating a distinct process. The constellation of ICANS symptoms has not been previously described justifying its designation as a novel syndrome.

The ASTCT consensus group defines ICANS as, "a disorder characterized by a pathologic process involving the central nervous system following any immune therapy that results in the activation or engagement of endogenous or infused T-cells and/or other immune effector cells. Symptoms or signs can be progressive and may include aphasia, altered level of consciousness, impairment of cognitive skills, motor weakness, seizures, and cerebral edema." [30]

Typically, the initial symptoms of ICANS are tremor, dysgraphia, and impaired attention [30]. Expressive dysphasia, particularly with the ability to name objects, is common as the syndrome progresses, and patients ultimately may not be able to communicate. To help identify early ICANS, the ASTCT consensus group established the Immune Effector Cell-Associated Encephalopathy (ICE) score, which is a 10-point scale that focuses on the domains first affected by ICANS (Table 3). Modified from a similar score by the CARTOX group [28], this tool can be applied by any trained professional at the bedside several times a day, if needed, and takes just a few minutes to complete. The first identification of an ICE score < 10 or a

Table 3 ICE score [30]

Domain	Task	Points
Orientation	Orientation to year, month, city, hospital	4
Naming	Ability to name 3 objects (e.g., point to clock, pen, button)	3
Following commands	Ability to follow simple commands (e.g., "show me 2 fingers" or "close your eyes and stick out your tongue.")	1
Writing	Ability to write a standard sentence (e.g., "our national bird is the bald eagle.")	1
Attention	Ability to count backwards from 100 by 10	1

ICE immune effector cell-associated encephalopathy

significant drop in ICE score should be followed with prompt evaluation by the immunotherapy team. As ICANS progresses, patients may develop delirium, encephalopathy, aphasia, lethargy, difficulty concentrating, agitation, tremor, seizures, and rarely cerebral edema [30].

Grading of ICANS

The approach to grading ICANS is two-fold: 1) determine the encephalopathy score and 2) evaluate for other symptoms of particular concern. For most patients, the ICE score should be determined first and drives the grading assignment. Those who have a depressed level of consciousness, seizure, deep focal motor weakness, or evidence of increased intracranial pressure or cerebral edema are assigned a higher grade of ICANS regardless of their ICE score. In other words, the more severe symptom, including the ICE score, drives the grade of ICANS. The grading system is outlined in Table 4. Of note, an awake patient or one who awakens to voice or tactile stimulation may have an ICE score of 0 and would meet criteria for Grade 3 ICANS. However, a patient who is unarousable and therefore cannot perform any of the tasks involved in the ICE assessment will also have an ICE score of 0 but is considered to have grade 4 ICANS owing to his/her unarousable state.

ICANS grading for children is similar but utilizes the Cornell Assessment of Pediatric Delirium [31] (CAPD; Table 5) in place of the ICE score. Note that a higher CAPD score correlates to a lower ICE score and that the difference between grades 1 and 2 ICANS in children is determined by the level of consciousness [30].

Guidelines for Management

With the adoption of novel therapeutic strategies has come a unique set of toxicities described here that differs widely from previously seen adverse events associated with antineoplastic therapies. As such, the importance of newer, specific management strategies became palpably apparent with increased use of CAR T-cell therapy in both the clinical trial and standard-of-care settings. While a number of

Table 4 ICANS grading [30]

Neurotoxicity domain	Grade 1	Grade 2	Grade 3	Grade 4
ICE score for age $\geq$ 12 years[a]	7–9	3–6	0-2	0 (unarousable patient and unable to perform ICE)
CAPD score for age < 12 years	1–8	1–8	$\geq$ 9	Unable to perform CAPD
Depressed level of consciousness[b]	Awakens spontaneously	Awakens to voice	Awakens only to tactile stimulus	Patient is unarousable or requires vigorous or repetitive tactile stimuli to arouse. Stupor or coma
Seizure	None	None	Any clinical seizure focal or generalized that resolves rapidly or nonconvulsive seizures on EEG that resolve with intervention	Life-threatening prolonged seizure (>5 min); or repetitive clinical or electrical seizures without return to baseline in between
Motor findings[c]	None	None	None	Deep focal motor weakness such as hemiparesis or paraparesis
Elevated ICP/ cerebral edema	None	None	Focal/local edema on neuroimaging[d]	Diffuse cerebral edema on neuroimaging; decerebrate or decorticate posturing; or cranial nerve VI palsy; or papilledema; or Cushing's triad

ICANS grade is determined by the most severe event (ICE score, level of consciousness, seizure, motor findings, raised ICP/cerebral edema) not attributable to any other cause; for example, a patient with an ICE score of 3 who has a generalized seizure is classified as grade 3 ICANS

N/A indicates not applicable

[a]A patient with an ICE score of 0 may be classified as grade 3 ICANS if awake with global aphasia, but a patient with an ICE score of 0 may be classified as grade 4 ICANS if unarousable

[b]Depressed level of consciousness should be attributable to no other cause (eg, no sedating medication)

[c]Tremors and myoclonus associated with immune effector cell therapies may be graded according to CTCAE v5.0, but they do not influence ICANS grading

[d]Intracranial hemorrhage with or without associated edema is not considered a neurotoxicity feature and is excluded from ICANS grading. It may be graded according to CTCAE v5.0

publications have explored the optimal management of these syndromes, a better understanding into the pathophysiology and subsequently the appropriate treatment of CRS and ICANS has led to consensus guidelines which were published by the Society for Immunotherapy of Cancer (SITC) to help standardize treatment [26]. As always, these recommendations are not a substitute for carefully considered clinical decision making for each individual patient's circumstance.

Table 5 Encephalopathy assessment for children <12 years using the CAPD [30]

Answer the following based on interactions with the child over the course of the shift

	Never, 4	Rarely, 3	Sometimes, 2	Often, 1	Always, 0
1. Does the child make eye contact with the caregiver?					
2. Are the child's actions purposeful?					
3. Is the child aware of his/her surroundings?					
4. Does the child communicate needs and wants?					
	Never, 0	**Rarely, 1**	**Sometimes, 2**	**Often, 3**	**Always, 4**
5. Is the child restless?					
6. Is the child inconsolable?					
7. Is the child underactive; very little movement while awake?					
8. Does it take the child a long time to respond to interactions?					

Adapted from Traube et al [31]

For patients age 1–2 years, the following serve as guidelines to the corresponding questions:

1. Holds gaze, prefers primary parent, looks at speaker
2. Reaches and manipulates objects, tries to change position, if mobile may try to get up
3. Prefers primary parent, upset when separated from preferred caregivers. Comforted by familiar objects (i.e., blanket or stuffed animal)
4. Uses single words or signs
5. No sustained calm state
6. Not soothed by usual comforting actions, eg, singing, holding, talking, and reading
7. Little if any play, efforts to sit up, pull up, and if mobile crawl or walk around
8. Not following simple directions. If verbal, not engaging in simple dialog with words or jargon

Management of CRS

All patients with any-grade CRS require close monitoring with daily physical exam and laboratory tests including daily complete blood counts, comprehensive metabolic panel, magnesium, phosphorus, C-reactive protein, and ferritin. As cytokine levels have not been validated for use in clinical decision making, daily trending of these markers is not currently recommended. A thorough and appropriate infectious workup should be ordered for these patients and strong consideration should be given to the use of empiric antimicrobials if deemed appropriate by the treating physician.

Monitoring for disturbances in coagulation by measuring prothrombin and partial thromboplastin times and fibrinogen should be performed at the time of CRS onset and periodically (e.g., every 1 3 days) thereafter. Patients may develop profound hypofibrinogenemia later in the course of CRS or even after CRS has resolved despite an initial rise in fibrinogen, which is an acute phase reactant. Aggressive repletion of plasma and/ or cryoprecipitate should not be delayed when disturbances in coagulation are noted.

Treatment of CRS varies with severity of toxicity and ranges from supportive care including antipyretics and intravenous fluids (IVF) to anti-cytokine directed therapy, corticosteroids, and vasopressor support with close monitoring in the

Table 6 Foundations for CRS management

ASTCT CRS grade	Recommended management
1.	Daily physical exam, laboratory tests: CBC with differential, CMP, Mg, Phos, CRP, ferritin, PT/PTT, fibrinogen Infectious workup Anti-pyretics
2.	Manage symptoms as per grade 1 Intravenous fluids for hypotension Low-flow oxygen support if indicated Consideration of tocilizumab for elderly or patients with extensive comorbidities
3.	Management as per grade 2 Vasopressor support for hypotension Non-invasive oxygenation support as needed Tocilizumab recommended Consideration of steroids and second dose of tocilizumab if refractory
4.	Management as per grade 3 Invasive ventilator support as needed Consideration of siltuximab, anikinra, and/or high-dose methylprednisone

Note: See SITC guidelines [26] for comprehensive management recommendations
Abbreviations: *CBC* complete blood count, *CMP* comprehensive metabolic panel, *Mg* magnesium, *Phos* phosphorus, *CRP* C-reactive protein, *PT/PTT* prothrombin and partial thromboplastin time

intensive care unit when necessary. Suggested foundations for managing CRS are presented in Table 6. Vasodilatory hypotension, common in moderate to severe CRS, can be initially managed with 1–2 liters of IVF boluses but vasopressors should be initiated early and rapidly. Reliance on more than 2–3 liters of IVF boluses is counterproductive given the developing capillary leak.

While the earliest studies restricted the use of tocilizumab, an IL-6 receptor blocking antibody, for higher-grade CRS, current standards recommend earlier intervention to mitigate morbidity as there is no evidence to suggest that cytokine-directed therapy hinders treatment efficacy [32, 33].

Current SITC guidelines recommend consideration of tocilizumab for ASTCT grade 2 CRS and recommend its use in grade 3 or higher CRS. Elderly patients or patients with extensive comorbidities should be considered eligible for earlier administration in the course of CRS. If CRS does not improve following a single dose of tocilizumab, corticosteroids should be administered along with a second dose of tocilizumab. In patients with ongoing or progressive CRS following 2 doses of tocilizumab in conjunction with steroids, other agents such as siltuximab, anakinra, and high-dose methylprednisone can be considered but repeat broad infectious workup should also be performed. When steroids are employed in the management of CRS, it is recommended that the starting dose be no higher than 1 mg/kg prednisone equivalent with a rapid taper over 7–10 days [34, 35].

Management of ICANS

Management of ICANS is more varied in practice owing to its poorly understood pathophysiology and wider array of symptoms. We provide a foundation for managing ICANS in Table 7, though individual practitioners should heed additional issues detailed in the SITC guidelines [26].

Similar to the management of CRS, patients experiencing neurologic toxicity from CAR T-cell therapy should be monitored closely with daily physical exam and laboratory testing as described above. In addition to the standard infectious workup, a lumbar puncture should be considered when feasible and additional radiographic examination with a CT scan or MRI should be performed to rule out any other acute neurologic process. An electroencephalogram should be performed as well as subclinical, electroencephalographic seizures have been reported [26].

While cytokine directed therapy has marked success in the treatment of CRS, tocilizumab has not been effective in mitigating neurologic symptoms. Furthermore, there is a theoretical risk that transient increases in serum concentrations of IL-6 following tocilizumab administration may potentially worsen neurotoxicity of CAR T-cell therapy, as tocilizumab does not cross the blood-brain barrier [36, 37]. Corticosteroids, on the other hand, have demonstrated efficacy in the treatment of ICANS and remain the cornerstone of therapy [26].

In patients treated with 4-1BB CAR T-cell products, specifically tisagenlecleucel, SITC guidelines recommend corticosteroids for grade 3 or higher ICANS and state that steroids may be considered for grade 2 toxicity. For patients receiving CD28-based CAR products, steroids are recommended for grade 2 ICANS. Rapid

Table 7 Foundations for ICANS management

ASTCT ICANS grade	Recommended management
1.	Daily physical exam, laboratory tests: CBC with differential, CMP, MG, Phos, CRP, ferritin, PT/PTT, fibrinogen Infectious workup including lumbar puncture if able Imaging with head CT or MRI Electroencephalogram
2.	Manage symptoms as per grade 1 If CD28-based CAR construct, initiation of corticosteroids Consider prophylactic levetiracetam
3.	Management as per grade 2 If 4-1BB CAR construct, initiation of corticosteroids Levetiracetam for any seizure activity
4.	Management as per grade 3 Consider higher-dose corticosteroids Levetiracetam for any seizure activity

Note: See SITC guidelines [26] for comprehensive management recommendations

Abbreviations: *CBC* complete blood count, *CMP* comprehensive metabolic panel, *Mg* magnesium, *Phos* phosphorus, *CRP* C-reactive protein, *PT/PTT* prothrombin and partial thromboplastin time, *CT* computed tomography scan, *MRI* magnetic resonance imaging scan

taper is recommended following steroid initiation [26, 38]. While there is insufficient evidence to recommend prophylactic antiepileptics, levetiracetam is recommended for management of patients with seizures [26].

Prolonged Cytopenias and Their Management

In addition to CRS and ICANS, hematologic toxicity occurs frequently among patients receiving CAR T-cell therapy. As may be expected, the majority of patients will experience early cytopenias, predominantly neutropenia and thrombocytopenia, following lymphodepletion therapy with a median time to onset of 3 days from cell infusion and a median duration of 19.5 days [39]. The mechanism of these early cytopenias is thought to be directly related to expected myelosuppression as a result of cytotoxic chemotherapy and is not specific to CAR T-cell products. In addition, the cytokine milieu of CRS and ICANS have also been implicated in this process.

However, a substantial portion of patients will go on to experience a biphasic nature of post CAR hematologic toxicity with a second, separate nadir in neutrophil count and/or platelet count. Many patients will have a transient, intermediate count recovery, although this is also sometimes absent in patients with prolonged cytopenias. While the field is starting to understand more, the mechanism behind the second cell count nadir is still somewhat elusive. One group postulates that perturbations in SDF-1 levels, a chemokine responsible for neutrophil egress from the bone marrow, following rapid B-cell expansion in CAR T-cell patients is responsible for late-onset neutropenia [39].

The incidence of prolonged cytopenias varies in the literature with 20–50% of patients reported to experience cytopenias beyond 1 month following CAR T-cell infusion [39–41]. With median follow up of 5 years, median time to resolution of all cytopenias was 56 days from T-cell infusion in one study of tisagenlecleucel [41]. Similarly, 18 (17%) of 108 patients treated with axicabtagene ciloleucel for large-cell lymphoma experienced grade ≥ 3 cytopenia at 3 months or later with just 2 of these persisting long-term [42]. Patients with higher grade CRS and/or ICANS, as well as prior stem cell transplantation are at increased risk for prolonged cytopenias, and there is a correlation between late thrombocytopenia, anemia, and neutropenia. Additionally, the CAR construct has been implicated with higher rates of prolonged cytopenias reported with the use of axicabtagene ciloleucel compared to tisagenlecleucel or the BCMA CAR products [43].

Regarding management of cytopenias following CAR T-cell therapy, consensus guidelines recommend against the use of G-CSF within the first 14 days due to a theoretical aggravation of CRS and/or ICANS [26]. For persistent neutropenia after 28 days, growth factor support may be used, but a bone marrow biopsy should also be performed to evaluate for myelodysplasia. The use of colony stimulating factors for other cell lines, namely platelets and red blood cells, has not been formally investigated but may be indicated in some circumstances.

Antimicrobial Prophylaxis During CAR T Cell Therapy

Patients are at risk for opportunistic infections during the course of CAR T cell treatment beginning with the lymphodepletion regimen. No specific consensus or data-driven guidelines have been published, but most practitioners take a similar approach to prophylaxis as they do during allogeneic hematopoietic stem cell transplantation. Though differences in practice exist between institutions, in general most patients receive prophylaxis. A few expert opinion recommendations have been published and is the basis for the following [44, 45].

Those who are seropositive for herpes simplex viruses and/or varicella zoster virus should receive antiviral prophylaxis with acyclovir or valacyclovir beginning at the time of lymphodepletion and continuing throughout their therapy.

Patients with neutropenia from either their disease or lymphodepletion chemotherapy are at risk for bacterial infections. While many practitioners caring for adult patients will provide fluoroquinolone prophylaxis during the period of neutropenia (absolute neutrophil count <500/μL), this practice is not as widespread in the pediatric population.

Severely neutropenic patients are at risk for infections with fungus or mold. Hence, antimicrobials directed at *Candida* species, such as fluconazole or micafungin, are often employed while patients are neutropenic. For those who have more prolonged neutropenia, clinicians should consider voriconazole or posaconazole to minimize the risk of infections with mold.

Finally, prophylaxis for *Pneumocystis jiroveci* pneumonia using trimethoprim-sulfamethoxazole or an appropriate alternative is well accepted for most patients during all stages of their treatment irrespective of CAR T cell therapy. However, myelosuppression that is sometimes seen with trimethoprim-sulfamethoxazole use may prolong neutrophil recovery, so an alternative agent may need to be considered.

Hypogammaglobinemia and Management

A challenge for any CAR T-cell therapy is on-target but off-tumor cytotoxicity. For CD19, CD20, and CD22-targeted CAR T-cell therapies, normal B-cells and follicular dendritic cells are the only off-tumor casualty known. Fortunately, B-cell aplasia is well tolerated by most individuals. Antibodies may still be produced by plasma cells, which do not express these target antigens, but their priming will be compromised by the continuous elimination of B-cells by persistent CAR T-cells, particularly in children who have yet to develop full immunity to pathogens. Ultimately, this may result in profound hypogammaglobulinemia (as well as low IgA and IgM) potentially for years or even for a lifetime [26]. The implications of this is largely unknown, is the subject of much opinion and speculation, and may differ between adults and children.

Only a few groups have published primary data related to hypogammaglobulinemia in CAR T-cell treated patients. Cappell and colleagues reported on 43 adults with B-cell lymphomas or chronic lymphocytic leukemia (CLL) who received a CD19-directed, CD28 co-stimulated CAR T-cell product at a median follow up of

42 months [42]. Excluding infections in close proximity to CAR T-cell infusion, four patients required subsequent hospitalization for infections: one each with disseminated herpes zoster, pneumonia, and *Citrobacter* bacteremia and one patient hospitalized once with influenza and twice with pneumonia. These hospitalizations occurred over the course of 6 months to 3 years after CAR T-cell infusion and appear to have been in spite of intravenous gamma immunoglobulin (IVIG) administration for levels less than 400–500 mg/dL. Regardless, the incidence of serious infections well after CAR T-cell therapy in this patient population was high.

A subset of these patients had sufficient data to analyze immunoglobulin trends. The only patients who normalized all three immunoglobulins were those that lost CAR T-cell persistence. At last follow up, IgA, IgM, and IgG levels were below normal in 63%, 33%, and 21% of patients, respectively. 79% of patients with long-term IgG data available received at least one dose of IVIG with 17% still receiving regular IVIG at last follow up.

Corderio and colleagues described their experience with 86 adults with R/R ALL, NHL, or CLL who were treated with a 4-1BB containing CD19 CAR and survived at least 1 year [46]. 67% of patients had IgG <400 mg/dL or were administered IVIG at a median follow up of 28 months. Though the data is confounded by preexisting hypogammaglobulinemia prior to CAR T-cell infusion and a lack of control over indications for IVIG infusions, the infection density was 0.55 infections/100 days at risk or 2.08 infections per patient-year. While the vast majority were managed in an outpatient setting, 20% required admission with 5% necessitating admission to the intensive care unit.

The ZUMA-1 trial of 108 adults receiving axicabtagene ciloleucel recommended providing IVIG to maintain an IgG level > 400 mg/dL, especially during infections. As a result, 31% of all patients and 17 of 39 (44%) patients with an ongoing response received IVIG. Despite this, 28% of all patients developed a ≥ Grade 3 infection within the first 2 years [4, 47]. Similarly, 18% of the 111 adults with DLBCL treated on the JULIET study experienced a ≥ Grade 3 infection 8 weeks or later after CAR T-cell infusion, though the number of patients receiving IVIG was not reported and results are confounded by a high degree of prolonged, severe neutropenia seen in this population [6].

In the absence of data from randomized controlled trials, therefore, a panel of experts arrived at the consensus that adults deemed to be high risk for infections or those with recurrent infections should be considered for IgG replacement therapy when IgG levels are less than 400 mg/dL [26]. This is in contrast to current practice in adults after stem cell transplants where routine IVIG replacement is not recommended [48].

In children, where the only U.S. Food and Drug Administration (FDA) or European Medicines Agency (EMA) approved product is tisagenlecleucel, no long-term data exist regarding infections or IVIG use after the initial CAR T-cell treatment period. Since IVIG supplementation is standard of care at most pediatric centers for managing hypogammaglobulinemia after stem cell transplant, most pediatric CAR T-cell patients are likely receiving regular IVIG infusions. This is particularly important as children have not yet established mature immunity against common pathogens (via immunization or natural exposure) and so are thought to be at higher risk than most adults. Whether and when IVIG replacement in children can be discontinued is a matter of speculation, and well-designed clinical trials are needed to address this important issue. In the meantime, consideration should be given to transitioning patients to a weekly subcutaneous form of IgG replacement administered at home with lower cost as this has been demonstrated to produce adequate and stable serum IgG levels over time in children with agammaglobulinemia [49].

Monitoring for Replication Competent Retrovirus/Lentivirus, Mutagenesis, and Secondary Malignancies

Most CAR T-cells are manufactured using a viral-based system utilizing either gamma retroviruses or HIV-1-based lentiviruses. Replication-incompetent viral particles infect the target T-cell and incorporate its transgene permanently in the T-cell genome. This allows for *in vivo* expansion of CAR T-cell products and is a pivotal cornerstone of the success of the therapy. The FDA has identified the accidental gain of replication competence of these viral particles through mutagenesis or cross-over events as well as insertional mutagenesis as risks of interest following genetic engineering. As such, the FDA has established guidance and regulations to monitor for both events during the manufacturing process and after infusion in the patient.

Replication Competent Virus

Both academic and commercial producers of genetically engineered cellular products utilizing retro- or lentiviruses are subject to required testing for replication competent retrovirus (RCR) or replication competent lentivirus (RCL) at multiple points during manufacturing. Briefly, master cell banks or producer lines (retrovirus) as well as viral supernatant (retrovirus and lentivirus) prior to CAR T-cell manufacturing and aliquots of CAR T-cell products themselves after manufacturing (retrovirus and lentivirus) are subjected to RCR or RCL testing at each of these steps. Methods of RCR and RCL testing is summarized in Fig. 2 [50].

Patients infused with investigational CAR T-cell products are subject to additional scrutiny for RCR/RCL for up to 15 years after cell infusion, and the institution that infused them is often responsible for ensuring compliance. Current FDA Guidance documents require that blood samples from these patients be collected and tested for RCR or RCL at the following time points: pretreatment, 3, 6, and 12 months after infusion followed by an annual history and physical for a total of 15 years [51]. Additional testing beyond 12 months is required in the case of a positive test. While these requirements do not apply to patients infused with a commercially-available CAR T cell product, practitioners should be vigilant to the risk of replication competent virus and promptly investigate suspicious secondary malignancies with the aid of the manufacturer.

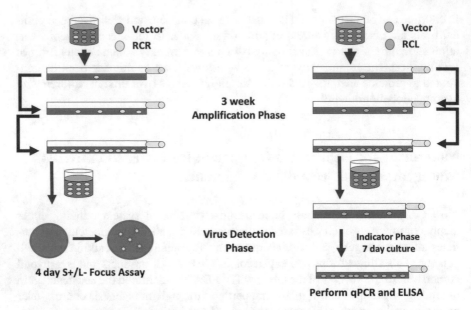

Fig. 2 Replication Competent Retrovirus (RCR) and Replication Competent Lentivirus (RCL) Testing. Current methods used in the National Gene Vector Biorepository at Indiana University are illustrated. The left figure depicts testing for RCR with RCL testing shown on the right. The 3 week amplification is mandated by the US FDA to allow slow growing recombinant viruses to expand to a detectable level. The PG4 Sarcoma+/Leukemia- (S+/L-) cell line is used to detect RCR. Gamma retroviruses transform S+/L- cell lines and foci of transformed cells indicate the presence of an RCR. For RCL detection, the combination of an ELISA method for detecting HIV capsid (p24), and a quantitative PCR (qPCR) based method for detecting reverse transcriptase (Product Enhanced Reverse Transcriptase, PERT), are used

Using the latest data published, no RCR has been detected in 282 samples across 14 clinical trials at the NIH-sponsored National Gene Vector Biorepository (NGVB) at Indiana University [52]. No RCR or RCL was detected in another study of 17 vector lots, 375 manufactured T-cell products, and 308 patients after cell infusion [53]. NGVB has tested a total of 1745 post-treatment patient samples for RCR, representing 64 different retroviruses, and 461 samples for RCL, representing 12 lentiviruses, which have all been negative (personal communication). By now, many more such products have been produced and infused in patients, particularly in the commercial setting, and there is no current indication that RCR or RCL events have occurred in a product administered to a patient. Nevertheless, it remains an unlikely possibility and required patient testing on clinical trials still applies.

Insertional Mutagenesis and Development of Secondary Malignancies

Previous experience with a retroviral vector transducing the *IL2RG* gene in hemato-poietic stem cells (HSCs) of 10 children with X-linked severe combined immuno-deficiency led to the development of T-cell leukemia in 4 of the 9 responding patients. Analysis revealed that the transgene was inserted within or near the proto-oncogenes *LMO2* or *CCND2,* which directly contributed to leukemogenesis [54]. Other trials utilizing retroviral modification of stem cells in children had similar experiences [55]. Vector copy number, or number of times the transgene is inserted in the host cell genome, is directly proportional to the risk of mutagenesis and is the subject of scrutiny at the regulatory level for every new investigational new drug application involving gene transfer.

Many clinical trials and even FDA-approved CAR and T-cell receptor (TCR) products still utilize retroviruses for gene transduction, and to date there has been no reported case of malignancy arising therefrom. This is likely due to both the improvements in viral vector design, resulting in fewer insertions per cell and tar-geting so-called "gene deserts," and the fact that mature T-cells are exceedingly less likely to redevelop stem-like properties that are active in undifferentiated HSCs [56]. Lentiviruses pose an even smaller risk of insertional mutagenesis and by extension secondary malignancy as the number of insertions per cell is limited to 1–3 on average when modern, fourth generation viruses are used [57].

Despite these data and advances in the field, disruptions of intact genes do occur on occasion and can lead to clonal expansion of an aberrant T-cell population. Such a discovery in a patient requires mandatory reporting via appropriate channels for the therapy being used and additional workup by experts in the field.

Conclusion

As promising as CAR T-cell therapies are, complications arising from uncontrolled, rapid and exponential expansion and activation of T-cells and the broader immune system creates a perfect storm of toxicities that if not managed promptly and appro-priately may have devastating outcomes for a patient. While we have provided a foundation for identifying and managing CAR T-cell-associated toxicities, includ-ing the ramifications of virally transducing and genetically engineering T-cells, optimal patient care requires more study and training as additional toxicities exist that are not addressed here. Understanding the pathophysiologies involved in CRS, ICANS, and prolonged cytopenias among others will require additional research, but is paramount to mitigating CAR T-cell complications.

The current cadre of FDA-approved CAR T-cell products are just the prototypes. Reestablishing control of T-cell and immune system activation to a more physio-logic state while maintaining anti-tumor efficacy should be the goal of investigators for the next generation of CAR T-cell therapies. In the meantime, prompt identification of toxicities and early intervention remains the best approach to delivering positive outcomes to patients.

References

1. Giavridis T, van der Stegen SJC, Eyquem J, et al. CAR T-cell–induced cytokine release syndrome is mediated by macrophages and abated by IL-1 blockade. Nat Med. 2018;24(6):731–8.
2. Norelli M, Camisa B, Barbiera G, et al. Monocyte-derived IL-1 and IL-6 are differentially required for cytokine-release syndrome and neurotoxicity due to CAR T-cells. Nat Med. 2018;24(6):739–48.
3. Taraseviciute A, Tkachev V, Ponce R, et al. Chimeric antigen receptor T cell-mediated neurotoxicity in nonhuman primates. Cancer Discov. 2018;8(6):750–63.
4. Neelapu SS, Locke FL, Bartlett NL, et al. Axicabtagene ciloleucel CAR T-cell therapy in refractory large B-cell lymphoma. N Engl J Med. 2017;377(26):2531–44.
5. Lee DW, Gardner R, Porter DL, et al. Current concepts in the diagnosis and management of cytokine release syndrome. Blood. 2014;124(2):188–95.
6. Schuster SJ, Bishop MR, Tam CS, et al. Tisagenlecleucel in adult relapsed or refractory diffuse large B-cell lymphoma. N Engl J Med. 2019;380(1):45–56.
7. Porter D, Frey N, Wood PA, Weng Y, Grupp SA. Grading of cytokine release syndrome associated with the CAR T cell therapy tisagenlecleucel. J Hematol Oncol. 2018;11:35.
8. Abramson JS, Palomba ML, Gordon LI, et al. Lisocabtagene maraleucel for patients with relapsed or refractory large B-cell lymphomas (TRANSCEND NHL 001): a multicentre seamless design study. Lancet. 2020;396(10254):839–52.
9. Maude SL, Laetsch TW, Buechner J, et al. Tisagenlecleucel in children and young adults with B-cell lymphoblastic leukemia. N Engl J Med. 2018;378(5):439–48.
10. Wang M, Munoz J, Goy A, et al. KTE-X19 CAR T-cell therapy in relapsed or refractory mantle-cell lymphoma. N Engl J Med. 2020;382(14):1331–42.
11. Jacobson C. Primary analysis of Zuma-5: a phase 2 study of axicabtagene ciloleucel (axi-cel) in patients with relapsed/refractory (R/R) indolent non-Hodgkin Lymphoma (iNHL). Blood. 2020;136(Suppl 1):40–1.
12. Munshi NC, Anderson LD, Shah N, et al. Idecabtagene Vicleucel in relapsed and refractory multiple myeloma. N Engl J Med. 2021;384(8):705–16.
13. Pasquini MC, Hu ZH, Curran K, et al. Real-world evidence of tisagenlecleucel for pediatric acute lymphoblastic leukemia and non-Hodgkin lymphoma. Blood Adv. 2020;4(21):5414–24.
14. Pasquini MC, Locke FL, Herrera AF, et al. Post-marketing use outcomes of an anti-CD19 chimeric antigen receptor (CAR) T cell therapy, axicabtagene ciloleucel (axi-cel), for the treatment of large b cell lymphoma (LBCL) in the United States (US). Blood. 2019;134(Suppl 1):764.
15. Riedell PA, Walling C, Nastoupil LJ, et al. A multicenter retrospective analysis of clinical outcomes, toxicities, and patterns of use in institutions utilizing commercial axicabtagene ciloleucel and tisagenlecleucel for relapsed/refractory aggressive B-cell lymphomas. Blood. 2019;134(Suppl 1):1599.
16. National Cancer Institute. Common terminology criteria for adverse events (CTCAE). Version 4.0. https://evs.nci.nih.gov/ftp1/CTCAE/CTCAE_4.03/CTCAE_4.03_2010-06-14_QuickReference_8.5x11.pdf. Accessed 15 March 2021.
17. Lee DW, Kochenderfer JN, Stetler-Stevenson M, et al. T cells expressing CD19 chimeric antigen receptors for acute lymphoblastic leukaemia in children and young adults: a phase 1 dose-escalation trial. Lancet. 2015;385(9967):517–28.
18. Maude SL, Frey N, Shaw PA, et al. Chimeric antigen receptor T cells for sustained remissions in leukemia. N Engl J Med. 2014;371(16):1507–17.

19. Gust J, Hay KA, Hanafi LA, et al. Endothelial activation and blood–brain barrier disruption in neurotoxicity after adoptive immunotherapy with CD19 CAR-T cells. Cancer Discov. 2017;7(12):1404–19.
20. Gajra A, Zettler ME, Phillips EG Jr, et al. Neurological adverse events following CAR-T cell therapy: a real-world analysis of adult patients treated with axicabtagene ciloleucel or tisagenlecleucel. Blood. 2019;134(Suppl 1):1952.
21. Hay KA, Hanafi LA, Li D, et al. Kinetics and biomarkers of severe cytokine release syndrome after CD19 chimeric antigen receptor–modified T-cell therapy. Blood. 2017;130(21):2295–306.
22. Van Der Stegen SJC, Hamieh M, Sadelain M. The pharmacology of second-generation chimeric antigen receptors. Nat Rev Drug Discov. 2015;14(7):499–509.
23. Salter AI, Ivey RG, Kennedy JJ, et al. Phosphoproteomic analysis of chimeric antigen receptor signaling reveals kinetic and quantitative differences that affect cell function. Sci Signal. 2018;11(544):eaat6753.
24. Teachey DT, Lacey SF, Shaw PA, et al. Identification of predictive biomarkers for cytokine release syndrome after chimeric antigen receptor T-cell therapy for acute lymphoblastic leukemia. Cancer Discov. 2016;6(6):664–79.
25. Porter DL, Hwang WT, Frey NV, et al. Chimeric antigen receptor T cells persist and induce sustained remissions in relapsed refractory chronic lymphocytic leukemia. Sci Transl Med. 2015;7(303):303ra139.
26. Maus MV, Alexander S, Bishop MR, et al. Society for Immunotherapy of cancer (SITC) clinical practice guideline on immune effector cell-related adverse events. J Immunother Cancer. 2020;8(2):1511.
27. Park JH, Rivi_ere I, Gonen M, et al. long-term follow-up of CD19 CAR therapy in acute lymphoblastic leukemia. N Engl J Med. 2018;378:449–59.
28. Neelapu SS, Tummala S, Kebriaei P, et al. Chimeric antigen receptor T-cell therapy - assessment and management of toxicities. Nat Rev Clin Oncol. 2018;15:47–62.
29. Brudno JN, Kochenderfer JN. Toxicities of chimeric antigen receptor T cells: recognition and management. Blood. 2016;127(26):3321–30.
30. Lee DW, Santomasso BD, Locke FL, et al. ASTCT consensus grading for cytokine release syndrome and neurologic toxicity associated with immune effector cells. Biol Blood Marrow Transplant. 2018;25(4):625–38.
31. Traube C, Silver G, Kearney J, et al. Cornell assessment of pediatric delirium: a valid, rapid, observational tool for screening delirium in the PICU. Crit Care Med. 2014;42:656–63.
32. Gardner R, Ceppi F, Rivers J, et al. Preemptive mitigation of CD19 CAR T-cell cytokine release syndrome without attenuation of antileukemic efficacy. Blood. 2019;134(24):2149–58.
33. Kadauke S, Myers RM, Li Y, et al. Risk-adapted preemptive tocilizumab to prevent severe cytokine release syndrome after CTL019 for pediatric B-cell acute lymphoblastic leukemia: a prospective clinical trial. J Clin Oncol. 2020;39(8):920–30.
34. Dholaria BR, Bachmeier CA, Locke F. Mechanisms and management of chimeric antigen receptor T-cell therapy-related toxicities. BioDrugs. 2019;33(1):45–60.
35. Teachey DT, Bishop MR, Maloney DG, Grupp SA. Toxicity management after chimeric antigen receptor T cell therapy: one size does not fit "ALL". Nat Rev Clin Oncol. 2018;15(4):218.
36. Chen F, Teachey DT, Pequignot E, et al. Measuring IL-6 and sIL-6R in serum from patients treated with tocilizumab and/or siltuximab following CAR T cell therapy. J Immunol Methods. 2016;434:1–8.
37. Nellan A, McCully CML, Garcia RC, et al. Improved CNS exposure to tocilizumab after cerebrospinal fluid compared to intravenous administration in rhesus macaques. Blood. 2018;132(6):662–6.
38. Strati P, Fateeha F, Westin J, et al. Prognostic impact of dose, duration, and timing of corticosteroid therapy in patients with large B-cell lymphoma treated with standard of care axicabtagene ciloleucel (Axi-cel). J Clin Oncol. 2020;38(15_suppl):8011.
39. Fried S, Avigdor A, Bielorai B, et al. Early and late hematologic toxicity following CD19 CAR-T cells. Bone Marrow Transplant. 2019;54(10):1643–50.

40. Hill JA, Li D, Hay KA, et al. Infectious complications of CD19-targeted chimeric antigen receptor-modified T-cell immunotherapy. Blood. 2018;131(1):121–30.
41. Chong EA, Ruella M, Schuster SJ. Five-year outcomes for refractory B-cell lymphomas with CAR T-cell therapy. N Engl J Med. 2021;384(7):673–4.
42. Cappell KM, Sherry RM, Yang JC, et al. Long-term follow-up of anti-CD19 chimeric antigen receptor T-cell therapy. J Clin Oncol. 2020;38(32):3805–15.
43. Jain T, Knezevic A, Pennisi M, et al. Hematopoietic recovery in patients receiving chimeric antigen receptor T-cell therapy for hematologic malignancies. Blood Adv. 2020;4(15):3776–87.
44. Hill JA, Seo SK. How I prevent infections in patients receiving CD19-targeted chimeric antigen receptor T cells for B-cell malignancies. Blood. 2020;136(8):925–35.
45. Jain T, Bar M, Kansagra AJ, et al. Use of chimeric antigen receptor T cell therapy in clinical practice for relapsed/refractory aggressive B cell non-Hodgkin lymphoma: an expert panel opinion from the American Society for Transplantation and Cellular Therapy. Biol Blood Marrow Transplant. 2019;25(12):2305–21.
46. Corderio Am Bezerra ED, Hirayama AV, et al. Late events after treatment with CD19-targeted chimeric antigen receptor modified T cells. Biol Blood Marrow Transplant. 2020;26(1):26–33.
47. Locke FL, Ghobadi A, Jacobson CA, et al. Long-term safety and activity of axicabtagene ciloleucel in refractory large B-cell lymphoma (ZUMA-1): a single-arm, multicentre, phase 1-2 trial. Lancet Oncol. 2019;20:31–42.
48. Bhella S, Majhail NS, Betcher J, Costa LJ, Daly A, Dandoy CE, et al. Choosing wisely BMT: American Society for Blood and Marrow Transplantation and Canadian blood and marrow transplant group's list of 5 tests and treatments to question in blood and marrow transplantation. Biol Blood Marrow Transplant. 2018;24:909–13.
49. Hill JA, Giralt S, Torgerson TR, et al. CAR-T - and a side order of IgG, to go? - immunoglobulin replacement in patients receiving CAR-T cell therapy. Blood Rev. 2019;38:100596.
50. Lee DW, Shah NN. Chimeric antigen receptor T-cell therapies for cancer: a practical guide. Cambridge, MA: Elsevier; 2020.
51. U.S. Food and Drug Administration, ed. Testing of retroviral vector-based human gene therapy products for replication competent retrovirus during product manufacture and patient follow-up: guidance for industry. Center for Biologics Evaluation and Research; 2020.
52. Cornetta K, Duffy L, Feldman SA, et al. Screening clinical cell products for replication competent retrovirus: the national gene vector biorepository experience. Mol Ther Methods Clin Dev. 2018;10:371e378.
53. Marcucci KT, Jadlowsky JK, Hwang WT, et al. Retroviral and lentiviral safety analysis of gene-modified T cell products and infused HIV and oncology patients. Mol Ther. 2018;26(1):269–79.
54. Hacein-Bey-Abina S, Garrigue A, Wang GP, et al. Insertional oncogenesis in 4 patients after retrovirus-mediated gene therapy of SCID-X1. J Clin Invest. 2008;118(9):3132–4.
55. Braun CJ, Boztug K, Paruzynski A, et al. Gene therapy for Wiskott-Aldrich syndrome—long-term efficacy and genotoxicity. Sci Transl Med. 2014;6:227ra33.
56. Cvazza A, Moiani A, Mavilio F. Mechanisms of retroviral integration and mutagenesis. Hum Gene Ther. 2013;24(2):119–31.
57. Cockrell AS, Kafri T. Gene delivery by lentivirus vectors. Mol Biotechnol. 2007;36:184–204.

Mechanisms of Resistance and Relapse After CAR-T Cell Therapy

Mehmet Emrah Selli, Prarthana Dalal, Sattva S. Neelapu, and Nathan Singh

Abstract Chimeric antigen receptor (CAR)-engineered T cells can mediate impressive responses in a subset of patients with B cell malignancies. Clinical trial and real-world data, however, reveal that most patients will not achieve durable remission. Therapeutic failure appears to segregate into two distinct models: inherent resistance, in which there is no meaningful disease response after treatment, or acquired resistance, in which disease recurrence follows a transient response. A host of studies have identified that both forms of failure can result from tumor-intrinsic evasion mechanisms which can be antigen-dependent or independent. Alternatively, resistance or relapse can occur due to T cell dysfunction, both intrinsic to the cells prior to infusion or that develops after delivery to patients. In this chapter, we review the mechanistic and correlative studies investigating resistance to CAR-T cells, and discuss strategies designed to overcome this significant hurdle to the broader success of this therapy.

Keywords Chimeric antigen receptor · Resistance · Antigen escape · Alternative splicing · Trogocytosis · T cell fitness · CD19 · BCMA · CD22 · Antigen masking · Exhaustion · T cell dysfunction

M. E. Selli · N. Singh (✉)
Division of Oncology, Washington University School of Medicine, St. Louis, MO, USA
e-mail: nathan.singh@wustl.edu

P. Dalal
Department of Medicine, Feinberg School of Medicine, Northwestern University, Chicago, IL, USA

S. S. Neelapu
Department of Lymphoma and Myeloma, The University of Texas MD Anderson Cancer Center, Houston, TX, USA

© Springer Nature Switzerland AG 2022
A. Ghobadi, J. F. DiPersio (eds.), *Gene and Cellular Immunotherapy for Cancer*, Cancer Drug Discovery and Development,
https://doi.org/10.1007/978-3-030-87849-8_12

Introduction

As outlined elsewhere in this volume, CAR-T cell therapy can enable durable remissions in select patients with B cell malignancies. In both adults and children with highly-refractory disease, CD19-directed CAR-T cells (CART19) therapy has been shown to eradicate chronic and acute B-cell leukemias (respectively) for >8 years—a milestone most would consider cure. Despite many instances of clinical success, mature clinical trial and commercial product data reveal that most patients will not experience long-term remission. The landmark clinical trials of CART19 in non-Hodgkin lymphoma (NHL) [1–4] and acute lymphoblastic leukemia (ALL) [5–10] highlight two distinct patterns of therapeutic failure. In NHL, failures primarily manifest as an up-front lack of disease regression, a phenomenon we have termed "inherent resistance" [11, 12]. Failure in ALL, however, is distinct. The majority (>85%) of patients will achieve minimal residual disease-negative remission 30 days after treatment [5, 6], but ~half of these patients will relapse within one year. Intriguingly, this pattern is also observed following therapy with CAR-T cells targeting B cell maturation antigen (BCMA) for multiple myeloma [13]. The mechanism of this "acquired resistance" has been heavily explored, with several distinct biological processes already identified as contributors. As with classical cancer immune surveillance and escape [14], a dynamic interplay between malignant cells and CAR-T cells determines disease control or progression. In this chapter, we will examine the cellular mechanisms that underlie both cancer cell-driven immunosuppression as well as T cell-intrinsic biological failure.

Tumor Evasion

The vast majority of clinical experience with CAR-T cells is in the treatment of hematologic malignancies. As such, we will focus this review on the mechanisms by which hematopoietic cancers evade CAR-T cell activity. Two fundamental paradigms have emerged that can lead to evasion: antigen-dependent and antigen-independent (Fig. 1). A great deal of research has focused on the biology that can lead to antigen modulation, while less has been reported about antigen-independent mechanisms.

Antigen Loss: Genomic and Transcriptional Modulation

Mechanisms that result in complete antigen loss have been heavily explored. In a study of 17 pediatric and young-adult patients who received tisagenlecleucel for B-cell ALL [15], specimens obtained at initial enrollment were compared to specimens obtained at the time of clinical relapse after CAR-T cell therapy. 12 of 17

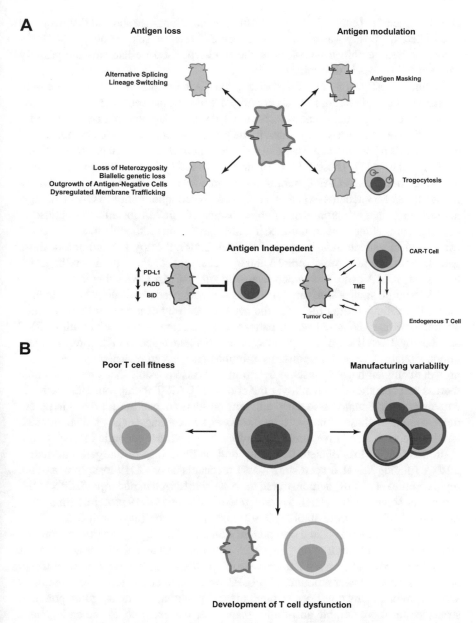

Fig. 1 Mechanisms of resistance and relapse. (a) Tumor-dependent and (b) T cell-dependent mechanisms that lead to CAR-T failure

patients had undetectable CD19 surface expression, highlighting the frequency of antigen loss as a mechanism of relapse. Deep sequencing of both DNA and RNA revealed several distinct mutations that were predicted to lead to truncated protein translation, resulting in nonfunctional or absent transmembrane domains. Analyzing allelic frequencies of the CD19 loss of function mutations also showed that acquired loss of heterozygosity was common at the time of relapse, suggesting that homozygous mutation combined with loss of the wild-type CD19 allele was the primary cause of CD19 loss in this cohort.

Parallel investigations in a BCMA-targeted CAR for multiple myeloma demonstrated similar biallelic loss of target antigen genes as the central cause of relapse [16]. Single cell genomic characterization showed a deletion of one allele and a mutation creating an early stop codon in the second. A second reported demonstrated complete loss of BCMA expression in a single patient at time of relapse after BCMA CAR-T therapy [17]. These authors found that loss of BCMA expression in patients relapsing after BCMA CART therapy was a rare event (~4–9% of patients) but more frequent; 28 of 33 patients in patients that were hyperhaploid prior to CART therapy manifested as loss or partial loss of chromosome 16 (*BCMA* locus) and duplication of the second allele with a mutated *BCMA* gene. Thus although loss of BCMA expression in patients relapsing after BCMA CART therapy is uncommon, those patients with loss of chromosome 16 and hyperhaploid appear to be at very high risk for loss of BCMA expression when relapsing after BCMA CART therapy.

While future studies with larger samples sizes are needed to validate this finding, these observations further highlight the need to carefully examine for target antigen alterations at the genomic level in patients being treated or re-treated with CAR-T cell therapy. Even if there is a very low level of biallelic deletion in the pre-treatment tumor, clonal selection in response to immune pressure can realistically lead to outgrowth of antigen-negative disease over time. It is also possible that a resistant clone merges and becomes dominant over the course of CAR-T therapy. In either setting, targeting multiple tumor-associated antigens presents an exciting approach to potentially overcome these genomic alterations, and upcoming trials of dual targeted CARs in leukemia and myeloma will demonstrate if similar genomic escape occurs.

In addition to loss of heterozygosity and biallelic loss of antigen, alternative mRNA splicing has also been shown as a mechanism for CD19 loss. In a seminal report, Sotillo et al. [18] demonstrated that CD19 mRNA can undergo distinct splicing events, some of which lead to production of truncated CD19 protein. Elimination of exon 2 leads to a more stable CD19 transcript than the full-length CD19; however, exon 2 contains a critical component of the CAR antigen recognition domain, leading to the production of an "invisible" antigen. Mechanistically, splicing factor SRSF3 was found to be a regulator of exon 2 inclusion. In two patients with CD19 negative relapses, lower amounts of SRSF3 were found compared to pre-treatment samples. While many questions remain, these findings can certainly guide potential strategies for more durable anti-tumor responses. For example, as the endogenous immune system is capable of epitope spreading and the generation of immune responses to epitopes distinct from the initial target, it may be useful to consider broad stimulation of the anti-tumor response with checkpoint blockade therapy combined with CAR-T cell therapy. Researchers are also developing CAR-T cells that are further modified to secrete immune stimulatory cytokines that can enhance the endogenous antitumor response in the tumor microenvironment to overcome loss of antigen in low-frequency clones [19].

Several reports have identified transitions in leukemic cell state from lymphoid to myeloid, a phenomenon known as lineage switching [20–22]. In two patients with rearrangements involving *KMT2A* (resulting in mixed-lineage leukemia, MLL), treatment with CD19 CAR-T cells was followed by transition from B-ALL to myeloid leukemia. In both cases the emergent disease was clonally related to the original lymphoid leukemia. Translocations leading to the MLL phenotype are known to induce a stem cell like-state that enables lineage conversion and the therapeutic pressure from CAR-T cell treatment may additionally facilitate or induce the lineage switch. These reports suggest that consideration of MLL status prior to treatment with a lineage-directed therapy may be needed if lineage switching emerges as a common cause of failure.

Mechanistic studies using murine models have explored the etiology of lineage switching after CAR therapy more closely [20]. Early relapses after CAR-T cell treatment retained a pre-B cell phenotype and demonstrated loss in CD19 exon 1 and exon 2 mRNA, consistent with previous reports of alternative splicing. However, late relapses showed complete loss of CD19 mRNA and protein expression with concurrent loss of *PAX5* and *EBF1* suggesting loss of the B-cell phenotype. RNA sequencing further confirmed the presence of myeloid, stem cell, or T-cell phenotypic markers, pointing to potential lineage switching. Furthermore, evidence of an intermediate phenotype with cells expressing both myeloid (Gr1, CD11b) and B cell markers (B220, CD22) was found suggesting divergent lineage identities as opposed to clonal selection.

Darwinian-like selection of preexisting antigen negative clones is also a mechanism for CAR-T cell treatment failure. Single cell RNA sequencing demonstrated the presence of CD19 negative leukemic cells before CAR-T cell therapy [23]. While relatively rare initially, the selective pressure caused these pre-existing subclones to expand, ultimately leading to targeted therapy failure. Other reports have also documented the presence of CD19 negative precursor cells in patients with ALL [24, 25]. This highlights the utility of pre-treatment screening in B-ALL patients potentially with single cell RNA sequencing to identify those at high risk of relapse after CAR-T cells therapy. Additionally, this is another mechanism of treatment resistance where dual antigen targeting would be an effective approach to decrease the likelihood of relapse.

Antigen Modulation: Structural

Trogocytosis is a cellular process in which membrane reorganization occurs at the immunological synapse between a T cell and an antigen-presenting cell. Hameih et al. identified that, in the context of CAR therapy, this reorganization can lead to transfer of the target antigen from malignant cells to the T cell surface, thus decreasing the density of the target antigen on the tumor cells [26]. This promotes tumor escape by reducing target detectability and T cell activity. It also leads to T cell fratricide as result of recognition of target antigen on other CAR+ cells. Beyond fratricide, the persistent activation of CARs by antigen expressed by other CAR-T cells led to exhaustion-like T cell dysfunction.

Antigen escape in CAR-T cell therapies targeting the B cell antigen CD22, however, appear to be mechanistically distinct. Fry and colleagues recently reported their findings of anti-CD22 CAR-T cell therapy in B-ALL. They observed that 12/21 patients achieved complete remission, and 9 of these 12 experienced an MRD-negative CR. Eight of 12 patients, however, relapsed 1.5–12 months post-infusion [27]. Intriguingly, all relapses were associated with reduced CD22 protein expression. Genomic analysis demonstrated that CD22 copy number profiles remained stable in the two patients studied, and none of the samples revealed the acquisition of mutations within the CD22 locus. RNA-sequencing analysis of samples prior to and following CAR-T cell infusion did not identify a reduced CD22 expression level after treatment. Furthermore, whereas Sotillo and colleagues identified alternative splicing as a contributing factor to anti-CD19 CAR-T cell escape [18], the investigators here observed no evidence of alternative CD22 isoforms underlying the reduced CD22 protein expression levels on tumor cells. These data therefore suggested that CD22 surface protein expression levels on tumor cells were regulated at the post-transcriptional level. A pre-clinical model consisting of a human ALL cell line reconstituted with low, intermediate, or high CD22 expression levels showed that mice infused with $CD22^{low}$ leukemia cells demonstrated negligible responses to CD22 CAR-T cell therapy. These findings suggest that the role of antigen density may vary depending on the target antigen, the CAR itself, or both.

While rare, unintentional transduction of the CAR into a single malignant cell resulting in antigen masking of CD19 has also been seen [28]. In this report, a patient who had relapsed with seemingly CD19-negative ALL was found to, instead, have a clonal leukemia which had undergone unintentional transduction with the CAR construct during manufacturing for the CAR-T product. The surface CAR on the ALL cell bound in *cis* to the CD19 epitope, thus masking it from recognition by the anti-CD19 CAR-T cells. As this clone grew under selective pressure, the patient experienced relapse nine months after initial infusion of tisagenlecleucel. These findings highlight the need for careful manufacturing technologies that can accurately delineate contaminating tumor cells from engineered T-cells.

Dysregulated antigen membrane trafficking can be another cause for treatment failure. Even if the CD19 protein is expressed and is structurally intact, defects in the membrane export process will result in failed CD19 surface expression. This has been previously identified following treatment with the CD19/CD-3 bispecific T-cell engager blinatumomab, in which the apparent CD19 negativity of the relapsed clone was attributed to a loss of expression of CD81 [29]. This protein is essential for CD19 membrane trafficking from the Golgi, and its absence led to lack of CD19 surface expression despite an intact CD19 transcription and translation.

Antigen-Independent Resistance

While the preponderance of data has focused on antigen modulation, a recent report from the University of Pennsylvania interrogated antigen-independent mechanisms of resistance [11]. Using a genome-wide loss-of-function screen in ALL, the investigators found that impairments in pro-apoptotic death receptor signaling proteins resulted in resistance to CAR-T cell cytotoxicity. Specifically, loss of Fas-associated protein with death domain (FADD) and BH3 interacting-domain death agonist (BID) enabled ALL to progress nearly unabated in mice. This inherent resistance in turn led to the persistent presence of CD19 antigen that led to T cell dysfunction, further impairing anti-tumor activity and permitting disease progression. Impressively, evaluation of pre-infusion bone marrow from patients receiving CD19 CAR-T cells suggested that baseline expression of death receptor genes was predictive of response.

Crosstalk between the tumor microenvironment (TME) and CAR-T cells also affects the development of antigen-independent resistance. The TME can affect both the infiltration and function of CAR-T cells. As an example, tumor cells can upregulate PD-L1 to induce apoptosis of local immune effector cells and can also release PD-L1 into the circulation to affect the global response to immunotherapy and cellular therapy. Local hypoxia, glucose depletion, and lactic acid accumulation leading to low pH can also suppress T-cell effector function [30]. On the other hand, CAR-T cells can substantially modify the TME and enhance endogenous T cell activation. Multiplex immunostaining of lymphoma biopsies after CAR-T cell therapy showed that CAR-T cells surprisingly constitute only a small fraction of all T cells in the TME after 5 days. However, not only did the CAR-T cells show evidence of an activated phenotype, but endogenous T cells were also activated in large numbers [31]. A recent study showed that CART-cells specifically produce interferon-γ which enhances endogenous T cell and natural killer cell activity and helps sustain cytotoxic function [32]. These studies together suggest a model where CART cell therapy supports the activation of larger numbers of endogenous immune cells. However, tumor cells also employ mechanisms to confer resistance and more studies to better understand this complex interplay in the TME are required.

While CAR-T cell therapy has been a sea change in the care for patients with B cell malignancies, the multiplicity of mechanisms by which cancer cells evade and resist infused cells highlights the need for continued improvements. While each of these mechanisms have been described individually, there is likely a dynamic and multifactorial interplay between each. Emerging combination therapies that can target multiple resistance mechanisms represent some of the most promising strategies to overcome CAR-T cell treatment resistance.

T Cell Failure

In contrast to malignant cell evasion, T cell failure has also recently been identified as an etiology of therapeutic failure. This can occur either as a result of defects in the product itself, or as a result of the development of dysfunction after infusion.

T Cell Fitness

Health of the T cells collected for CAR-T cell manufacturing can vary dramatically between patients, and this health has a direct impact on the quality and quantity of CAR-T cells that compose the final product. Many factors can influence T cell health. Data suggest that different cancers differentially impair circulating T cell biology, wherein chronic malignancies appear to cause more T cell dysfunction than acute diseases [33, 34]. Additionally, previous chemotherapy also can differentially impair T cell effector potential [34, 35]. A study conducted in pediatric patients with ALL and non-Hodgkin lymphoma found that the fraction of less-differentiated T cells, defined as having either naïve or stem central memory phenotypes, directly correlated with the ability of harvested T cells to produce an effective CAR-T cell product. This study further demonstrated that chemotherapy given early in therapy for ALL, such as cyclophosphamide and cytosine arabinoside specifically depleted less-differentiated cells [34]. The addition of cytokines that support early-lineage cells, such as interleukin-7 (IL-7) and interleukin-15 (IL-15), into manufacturing culture media can help T cells to recover from the detrimental effects of chemotherapy. Notably, inclusion of IL-7 and IL-15, but not IL-2, in culture media may specifically help by enriching naïve and central memory-like T cells without also enriching more terminally-differentiated cells [36]. Finally, it has long been observed that age has a direct impact on T cell function, wherein T cells from older adults have less expansion potential than those from younger adults or children. Interestingly, T cells from older adults have also been shown to secrete cytokines that can support cancer growth, adding further complexity to the dynamics of immune surveillance [37, 38]. Intriguingly, a recently published post-hoc subgroup analysis from the ZUMA-1 trial studying axicabtagene ciloleucel showed better investigator-assessed objective response rates and higher complete response rates at two years among patients aged ≥65 years than those patients aged <65 years [39].

Product Manufacturing

The process of CAR-T cell manufacturing is discussed in detail elsewhere in this volume. The process of manufacturing occurs at either an academic or private laboratory, and while there is not significant variability in procedure, this process remains to be standardized. As such, distinctions in product quantity and quality exist as a direct result of distinctions in process.

Collected T cells can enter the manufacturing process either as a bulk pool, or manipulations can be made to alter the "pre-production" composition. It has been speculated that using standardized ratios of CD4:CD8 cells can improve the predictivity of the clinical outcome [40, 41]. In a variation on this strategy, a recent phase I anti-CD22 CAR-T cell trial applied a CD4/CD8 T cell selection approach to purify T cells prior to manufacturing. They found that this approach improved successful product manufacturing rates, and was associated with more inflammatory toxicities; it is not clear if this enhanced responses, but did increase the number of patients who were able to receive therapy. Another study showed that using elutriation, a method to separate monocyte/granulocyte contaminants from lymphocytes, during manufacturing increased CAR-T cell yield, suggesting an inhibitory effect of monocytes/granulocytes on CAR-T cell expansion [42].

In an intriguing case report Fraietta et al. found that, in a patient who achieved remission following CD19 CAR-T cell infusion, there was outgrowth of a single T cell clone [43]. Deep sequencing found that this clone had undergone CAR lentiviral integration within in the *TET2* locus, disrupting the activity of this regulator of DNA methylation and promoting a beneficial central memory phenotype. This finding, while isolated, further highlights the need to infuse the "right" cell lineage.

Analysis of axicabtagene ciloleucel infusion products from adult large B-cell lymphoma patients by single-cell RNA sequencing revealed that products with a higher proportion of central memory CD8+ T cells associated with durable clinical benefit whereas an exhausted phenotype characterized by dual expression of LAG3 and Tim3 was associated early progression [44].

CAR-T Cell Dysfunction

T cell exhaustion is defined as a dysfunctional state triggered by prolonged antigen exposure due to chronic infection or cancer [45]. Several recent studies have identified that CAR-T cell dysfunction also limits anti-tumor activity. In a model of persistent exposure to CD19+ ALL cells, CD19-targeted CAR-T cells rapidly become dysfunctional as a direct result of prolonged antigen engagement [11]. These cells, while appearing functionally exhausted, do not bear the classical phenotypic features of exhausted T cells, such as high PD-1, Tim3 or LAG3 surface expression, or the epigenetic changes that define exhaustion [46, 47], suggesting that CARs may drive the development of dysfunction via distinct pathways. Studies in murine models of solid tumors have found that tumor-infiltrating dysfunctional CD8+ CAR-T cells have upregulated expression of nuclear receptor transcription factors, NR4A1, NR4A2 and NR4A3, which are regulators of the inhibitory surface proteins PD-1 and Tim3. Loss of all three NR4A transcription factors in CAR-T cells improved tumor regression and survival in mice, drawing a direct link between expression of these transcription factors and CAR-driven T cell dysfunction [48]. In parallel to this study, Liu et al. independently identified NR4A1 as a key regulator of T cell exhaustion in a genome wide screen [49]. The investigators found that NR4A1 mediates T cell dysfunction via its preferential recruitment to AP-1 binding sites, where it blocks the expression of AP-1 associated activator genes. Consistent with this finding, Lynn et al. [50] used a tonically signaling CAR model system to demonstrate that the overexpression of canonical AP-1 factor c-Jun alleviates T cell dysfunction. Collectively, these data identify several key transcription factors that may regulate the development of CAR-driven T cell dysfunction in an antigen-dependent manner.

Single cell profiling of CAR-T cells from infusion products and patient blood also provided interesting insights on CAR-T cell behavior [51]. For example, clonal diversity of CAR-T cells is highest before infusion and the most dominant clones that expand after infusion originate from cells that highly express cytotoxicity and proliferation genes. Soon after infusion CAR-T cells display a gene expression phenotype similar to activated CD8+ effector T-cells; however, over time the transcriptional signatures marking activation and proliferation progressively decline. No enrichment of an exhaustion gene signature or increase in inhibitory receptor expression was detected at later times after infusion but further studies are required to detail the exhaustion state of CAR-T cells after infusion both in the blood and at the site of the tumor.

CAR structural design itself can also contribute to dysfunction in an antigen-independent manner. Several reports have identified that tonic signaling of CARs with CD28 co-stimulatory domains leads to the development of dysfunction [52, 53]. Intriguingly, replacement of CD28 with 41BB in the setting of tonic signaling alleviates the development of dysfunction, and may in fact improve CAR-T cell function.

Next Steps

Improving outcomes after CAR-T cell therapy in hematologic cancers will require several approaches that are directed specifically at the mechanism of failure. A central feature during the next decade of cellular immunotherapy will be appropriate patient selection, matching the right patients with the right cell products. Patients with disease that has evidence of an underlying antigen-low or negative population may mandate therapy that is multi-antigen targeted, using novel products such as dual CARTs, T cells that contain to full-length CARs targeting different antigens [54], or tandem CARTs, T cells that contain one CAR with two scFvs each targeting a distinct antigen [55]. Targeting antigen-independent mechanisms of resistance will rely on deep understanding of the underlying biology. For example, pairing CAR-T cells with small molecule regulators that can inhibit anti-apoptotic signaling to enhance effective T cell cytotoxicity [56].

Addressing T cell failure will require distinct strategies. A great deal of work is ongoing to identify the ideal pre-manufacture T cell populations to include in the production process. While this is certain to lead to innovation in product manufacturing, without standardized practice across institutions to rigorously compare CAR-T products to each other we are likely to remain clouded in our ability to declare winners. Several groups have worked to design T cells that bear CARs as well as additional therapeutic or support proteins, such as cytokines [57, 58] or secreted bi-specific antibodies [59]. Deletion of suppressive proteins such as PD-1 has also demonstrated success in improving CAR-driven T cell function [60]. A provocative recent report by Weber et al. demonstrated that transient rest of CART in vitro or in vivo using multiple approaches can dramatically restore functionality and reverse exhausted phenotype of these CART resulting in enhanced survival and anti-tumor efficacy [61].

Conclusions

CD19-directed CAR-T cell therapy represents a watershed in the management of B cell cancers. Its promise, however, remains to be achieved. Careful and detailed understanding of the biology leading to therapeutic failure that is driven both by tumors and T cells has begun to identify strategies to improve the efficacy of this platform. The combination of product innovation as well as basic discovery will no doubt lead to a new cadre of CAR-based therapies in the coming years that are more successful than their first-generation predecessors, moving us closer to the widespread use of this therapy for both hematologic and solid tumors.

References

1. Neelapu SS, Locke FL, Bartlett NL, et al. Axicabtagene ciloleucel CAR T-cell therapy in refractory large B-cell lymphoma. N Engl J Med. 2017;377:2531–44.
2. Schuster SJ, Bishop MR, Tam CS, et al. Tisagenlecleucel in adult relapsed or refractory diffuse large B-Cell lymphoma. N Engl J Med. 2019;380:45–56.
3. Chong EA, Ruella M, Schuster SJ, Lymphoma Program Investigators at the University of P. Five-year outcomes for refractory B-cell lymphomas with CAR T-Cell therapy. N Engl J Med. 2021;384:673–4.
4. Abramson JS, Palomba ML, Gordon LI, et al. Lisocabtagene maraleucel for patients with relapsed or refractory large B-cell lymphomas (TRANSCEND NHL 001): a multicentre seamless design study. Lancet. 2020;396:839–52.
5. Frey NV, Shaw PA, Hexner EO, et al. Optimizing chimeric antigen receptor T-cell therapy for adults with acute lymphoblastic leukemia. J Clin Oncol. 2020;38:415–22.
6. Maude SL, Laetsch TW, Buechner J, et al. Tisagenlecleucel in children and young adults with B-cell lymphoblastic leukemia. N Engl J Med. 2018;378:439–48.
7. Gardner RA, Finney O, Annesley C, et al. Intent-to-treat leukemia remission by CD19 CAR T cells of defined formulation and dose in children and young adults. Blood. 2017;129:3322–31.
8. Lee DW, Kochenderfer JN, Stetler-Stevenson M, et al. T cells expressing CD19 chimeric antigen receptors for acute lymphoblastic leukaemia in children and young adults: a phase 1 dose-escalation trial. Lancet. 2015;385:517–28.
9. Davila ML, Riviere I, Wang X, et al. Efficacy and toxicity management of 19-28z CAR T cell therapy in B cell acute lymphoblastic leukemia. Sci Transl Med. 2014;6:224ra25.
10. Park JH, Riviere I, Gonen M, et al. Long-term follow-up of CD19 CAR therapy in acute lymphoblastic leukemia. N Engl J Med. 2018;378:449–59.
11. Singh N, Lee YG, Shestova O, et al. Impaired death receptor signaling in leukemia causes antigen-independent resistance by inducing CAR T-cell dysfunction. Cancer Discov. 2020;10:552–67.
12. Singh N, Orlando E, Xu J, et al. Mechanisms of resistance to CAR T cell therapies. Semin Cancer Biol. 2020;65:91–8.
13. Raje N, Berdeja J, Lin Y, et al. Anti-BCMA CAR T-cell therapy bb2121 in relapsed or refractory multiple myeloma. N Engl J Med. 2019;380:1726–37.
14. Dunn GP, Bruce AT, Ikeda H, Old LJ, Schreiber RD. Cancer immunoediting: from immunosurveillance to tumor escape. Nat Immunol. 2002;3:991–8.
15. Orlando EJ, Han X, Tribouley C, et al. Genetic mechanisms of target antigen loss in CAR19 therapy of acute lymphoblastic leukemia. Nat Med. 2018;24:1504–6.

16. Samur MK, Fulciniti M, Aktas Samur A, et al. Biallelic loss of BCMA as a resistance mechanism to CAR T cell therapy in a patient with multiple myeloma. Nat Commun. 2021;12:868.
17. Da Via MC, Dietrich O, Truger M, et al. Homozygous BCMA gene deletion in response to anti-BCMA CAR T cells in a patient with multiple myeloma. Nat Med. 2021;27:616–9.
18. Sotillo E, Barrett DM, Black KL, et al. Convergence of acquired mutations and alternative splicing of CD19 enables resistance to CART-19 immunotherapy. Cancer Discov. 2015;5:1282–95.
19. Pegram HJ, Lee JC, Hayman EG, et al. Tumor-targeted T cells modified to secrete IL-12 eradicate systemic tumors without need for prior conditioning. Blood. 2012;119:4133–41.
20. Jacoby E, Nguyen SM, Fountaine TJ, et al. CD19 CAR immune pressure induces B-precursor acute lymphoblastic leukaemia lineage switch exposing inherent leukaemic plasticity. Nat Commun. 2016;7:12320.
21. Lucero OM, Parker K, Funk T, et al. Phenotype switch in acute lymphoblastic leukaemia associated with 3 years of persistent CAR T cell directed-CD19 selective pressure. Br J Haematol. 2019;186:333–6.
22. Oberley MJ, Gaynon PS, Bhojwani D, et al. Myeloid lineage switch following chimeric antigen receptor T-cell therapy in a patient with TCF3-ZNF384 fusion-positive B-lymphoblastic leukemia. Pediatr Blood Cancer. 2018;65:e27265.
23. Rabilloud T, Potier D, Pankaew S, Nozais M, Loosveld M, Payet-Bornet D. Single-cell profiling identifies pre-existing CD19-negative subclones in a B-ALL patient with CD19-negative relapse after CAR-T therapy. Nat Commun. 2021;12:865.
24. Grupp SA, Kalos M, Barrett D, et al. Chimeric antigen receptor-modified T cells for acute lymphoid leukemia. N Engl J Med. 2013;368:1509–18.
25. le Viseur C, Hotfilder M, Bomken S, et al. In childhood acute lymphoblastic leukemia, blasts at different stages of immunophenotypic maturation have stem cell properties. Cancer Cell. 2008;14:47–58.
26. Hamieh M, Dobrin A, Cabriolu A, et al. CAR T cell trogocytosis and cooperative killing regulate tumour antigen escape. Nature. 2019;568:112–6.
27. Fry TJ, Shah NN, Orentas RJ, et al. CD22-targeted CAR T cells induce remission in B-ALL that is naive or resistant to CD19-targeted CAR immunotherapy. Nat Med. 2018;24:20–8.
28. Ruella M, Xu J, Barrett DM, et al. Induction of resistance to chimeric antigen receptor T cell therapy by transduction of a single leukemic B cell. Nat Med. 2018;24:1499–503.
29. Braig F, Brandt A, Goebeler M, et al. Resistance to anti-CD19/CD3 BiTE in acute lymphoblastic leukemia may be mediated by disrupted CD19 membrane trafficking. Blood. 2017;129:100–4.
30. Cheng J, Zhao L, Zhang Y, et al. Understanding the mechanisms of resistance to CAR T-cell therapy in malignancies. Front Oncol. 2019;9:1237.
31. Chen PH, Lipschitz M, Weirather JL, et al. Activation of CAR and non-CAR T cells within the tumor microenvironment following CAR T cell therapy. JCI Insight. 2020;5
32. Boulch M, Cazaux M, Loe-Mie Y, et al. A cross-talk between CAR T cell subsets and the tumor microenvironment is essential for sustained cytotoxic activity. Sci Immunol. 2021;6
33. van Bruggen JAC, Martens AWJ, Fraietta JA, et al. Chronic lymphocytic leukemia cells impair mitochondrial fitness in CD8(+) T cells and impede CAR T-cell efficacy. Blood. 2019;134:44–58.
34. Singh N, Perazzelli J, Grupp SA, Barrett DM. Early memory phenotypes drive T cell proliferation in patients with pediatric malignancies. Sci Transl Med. 2016;8:320ra3.
35. Das RK, Vernau L, Grupp SA, Barrett DM. Naive T-cell deficits at diagnosis and after chemotherapy impair cell therapy potential in pediatric cancers. Cancer Discov. 2019;9:492–9.
36. Cieri N, Camisa B, Cocchiarella F, et al. IL-7 and IL-15 instruct the generation of human memory stem T cells from naive precursors. Blood. 2013;121:573–84.
37. Buschle M, Campana D, Carding SR, Richard C, Hoffbrand AV, Brenner MK. Interferon gamma inhibits apoptotic cell death in B cell chronic lymphocytic leukemia. J Exp Med. 1993;177:213–8.
38. Dancescu M, Rubio-Trujillo M, Biron G, Bron D, Delespesse G, Sarfati M. Interleukin 4 protects chronic lymphocytic leukemic B cells from death by apoptosis and upregulates Bcl-2 expression. J Exp Med. 1992;176:1319–26.

39. Neelapu SS, Jacobson CA, Oluwole OO, et al. Outcomes of older patients in ZUMA-1, a pivotal study of axicabtagene ciloleucel in refractory large B-cell lymphoma. Blood. 2020;135:2106–9.
40. Sommermeyer D, Hudecek M, Kosasih PL, et al. Chimeric antigen receptor-modified T cells derived from defined CD8+ and CD4+ subsets confer superior antitumor reactivity in vivo. Leukemia. 2016;30:492–500.
41. Turtle CJ, Hanafi LA, Berger C, et al. Immunotherapy of non-Hodgkin's lymphoma with a defined ratio of CD8+ and CD4+ CD19-specific chimeric antigen receptor-modified T cells. Sci Transl Med. 2016;8:355ra116.
42. Stroncek DF, Lee DW, Ren J, et al. Elutriated lymphocytes for manufacturing chimeric antigen receptor T cells. J Transl Med. 2017;15:59.
43. Fraietta JA, Nobles CL, Sammons MA, et al. Disruption of TET2 promotes the therapeutic efficacy of CD19-targeted T cells. Nature. 2018;558:307–12.
44. Deng Q, Han G, Puebla-Osorio N, et al. Characteristics of anti-CD19 CAR T cell infusion products associated with efficacy and toxicity in patients with large B cell lymphomas. Nat Med. 2020;26:1878–87.
45. Wherry EJ, Kurachi M. Molecular and cellular insights into T cell exhaustion. Nat Rev Immunol. 2015;15:486–99.
46. Sen DR, Kaminski J, Barnitz RA, et al. The epigenetic landscape of T cell exhaustion. Science. 2016;354:1165–9.
47. Pauken KE, Sammons MA, Odorizzi PM, et al. Epigenetic stability of exhausted T cells limits durability of reinvigoration by PD-1 blockade. Science. 2016;354:1160–5.
48. Chen J, Lopez-Moyado IF, Seo H, et al. NR4A transcription factors limit CAR T cell function in solid tumours. Nature. 2019;567:530–4.
49. Liu X, Wang Y, Lu H, et al. Genome wide analysis identifies NR4A1 as a key mediator of T cell dysfunction. Nature. 2019;567:525–9.
50. Lynn RC, Weber EW, Sotillo E, et al. c-Jun overexpression in CAR T cells induces exhaustion resistance. Nature. 2019;576:293–300.
51. Sheih A, Voillet V, Hanafi LA, et al. Clonal kinetics and single-cell transcriptional profiling of CAR-T cells in patients undergoing CD19 CAR-T immunotherapy. Nat Commun. 2020;11:219.
52. Frigault MJ, Lee J, Basil MC, et al. Identification of chimeric antigen receptors that mediate constitutive or inducible proliferation of T cells. Cancer Immunol Res. 2015;3:356–67.
53. Long AH, Haso WM, Shern JF, et al. 4-1BB costimulation ameliorates T cell exhaustion induced by tonic signaling of chimeric antigen receptors. Nat Med. 2015;21:581–90.
54. de Larrea CF, Staehr M, Lopez AV, et al. Defining an optimal dual-targeted CAR T-cell therapy approach simultaneously targeting BCMA and GPRC5D to prevent BCMA escape-driven relapse in multiple myeloma. Blood Cancer Discov. 2020;1:146–54.
55. Tong C, Zhang Y, Liu Y, et al. Optimized tandem CD19/CD20 CAR-engineered T cells in refractory/relapsed B-cell lymphoma. Blood. 2020;136:1632–44.
56. Michie J, Beavis PA, Freeman AJ, et al. Antagonism of IAPs enhances CAR T-cell efficacy. Cancer Immunol Res. 2019;7:183–92.
57. Ma X, Shou P, Smith C, et al. Interleukin-23 engineering improves CAR T cell function in solid tumors. Nat Biotechnol. 2020;38:448–59.
58. Lange S, Sand LG, Bell M, Patil SL, Langfitt D, Gottschalk S. A chimeric GM-CSF/IL18 receptor to sustain CAR T-cell function. Cancer Discov. 2021;
59. Choi BD, Yu X, Castano AP, et al. CAR-T cells secreting BiTEs circumvent antigen escape without detectable toxicity. Nat Biotechnol. 2019;37:1049–58.
60. Choi BD, Yu X, Castano AP, et al. CRISPR-Cas9 disruption of PD 1 enhances activity of universal EGFRvIII CAR T cells in a preclinical model of human glioblastoma. J Immunother Cancer. 2019;7:304.
61. Weber EW, Parker KR, Sotillo E, et al. Transient rest restores functionality in exhausted CAR-T cells through epigenetic remodeling. Science. 2021;372

Part III
TIL

Tumor Infiltrating Lymphocytes (TIL): From Bench to Bedside

Jeffrey P. Ward

Abstract While the number of therapeutic options for patients with cancer have grown exponentially as the collective knowledge of cancer biology and genomics has improved, the fact remains that the majority of those with metastatic solid tumors will never be cured of their disease. With the development of targeted therapies that disrupt aberrant signaling pathways in cancer cells caused by distinct genetic alterations, the paradigm of "personalized therapy" has developed, with the goal of individualizing a patient's treatment to their own tumor's distinct mutational make-up. However, a truly personalized approach that takes advantage of the ability of the immune system to not only recognize and destroy tumor cells, but also to prevent recurrence through immune memory, has been successfully applied to patients with metastatic disease for more than 3 decades. Preclinical observations by many groups using mouse models beginning in the first half of the twentieth century led to pioneering work carried out by the group led by Steven A. Rosenberg at the Surgery Branch of the National Cancer Institute (NCI) that developed adoptive cellular therapy (ACT) with tumor infiltrating lymphocytes (TIL). Numerous clinical trials have now demonstrated the feasibility of generating large numbers of TIL from surgical biopsies which can be safely administered to patients to effectively treat multiple solid tumor histologies. The availability of TIL products has proven instrumental for the demonstration that tumor-specific T-cell populations are capable of inducing complete therapeutic responses lasting for decades. As our understanding of how the immune system recognizes pathogens and is regulated to prevent autoimmunity has grown, pharmacologic approaches utilizing antibody-mediated blockade of immunologic "checkpoint" molecules now provide additional treatment options for patients. This has led to the opening of a substantial gap in the treatment landscape of many solid tumors of patients that do not derive long-term benefit from currently available immunotherapies, and much ongoing work is directed at filling this gap with novel TIL approaches in the coming years. Here, we

J. P. Ward (✉)
Division of Oncology, Department of Medicine, Washington University School of Medicine, St. Louis, MO, USA
e-mail: jward2@wustl.edu

review the preclinical studies that served as the basis for human translation of TIL therapies, clinical trial data for TIL across tumor types, and discuss future developments in TIL therapy that seek to refine personalized treatments for patients directed at tumor-specific mutations.

Keywords Tumor infiltrating lymphocytes (TIL) · Adoptive cellular therapy (ACT) · Lymphokine-activated killer (LAK) cells · IL-2 · Melanoma · Renal cell carcinoma · Non-small cell lung cancer · Malignant gliomas · Gastrointestinal cancers · Gynecologic malignancies · Lifileucel · CD28 · CD27 · Tumor-associated antigens (TAA) · Cancer-germline/cancer testis antigens (CTA) · Tumor-specific antigens · Neoantigens

Preclinical Demonstration that Tumor Infiltrating Lymphocytes Have Therapeutic Potential

Using chemically induced sarcomas, it had become established by the 1940s that inbred mice immunized with small doses of tumor cells were resistant to a subsequent challenge of the same, but not an unrelated, tumor cell line [1]. In subsequent decades, preclinical mouse models became invaluable tools used by many groups to understand how the immune system could be harnessed therapeutically [2]. Single-cell suspensions of tumor draining lymph nodes from mice with progressively growing sarcomas were found to provide resistance to a subsequent sarcoma challenge after transfer, strongly suggesting that a cellular basis for mediating antitumor responses existed [3]. Further evidence that lymphocytes could demonstrate antitumor properties came with the finding that *in vitro* incubation of lymphocytes, but not serum, from preimmunized animals inhibited the establishment of a sarcoma challenge [4, 5]. However, while adoptive transfers of lymphocytes from immunized animals could provide prophylaxis against a tumor challenge, it soon became apparent that controlling the growth of established tumors was more difficult. Using a rat fibrosarcoma model, in 1964 Delorme and Alexander showed that adoptive transfer of lymphocytes isolated from the thoracic ducts and lymph nodes of rats previously immunized with the same tumor could slow, but not eliminate, the growth of previously implanted tumors [6]. Established methylcholanthrene-induced sarcomas could also be inhibited by transfer of lymphocytes isolated from the spleens of immunized syngeneic mice [7]. As these studies utilized the adoptive transfer of large numbers of fresh lymphocytes, further clinical translation would require the technical development of methods that would enable the culture of sufficient numbers of lymphocytes at clinical scale *in vitro* for infusion into patients.

The addition of growth factors that are not present in standard cell growth media are required for the long-term propagation of lymphocytes *in vitro*. By the late

1970's protocols had become available for the production of "T-cell growth factor" from cultures of activated lymphocytes that enabled long-term culture of both mouse and human T-cells, but the cloning of the gene for IL-2 would not be reported until years later [8, 9]. This innovation made it possible to isolate and amplify lymphocytes directly from tumor tissues in order to test their reactivity against autologous tumor cells [10]. In 1983, Eberlein et al. showed that adoptive transfer of lymphocytes from mice previously immunized with the FBL-3 lymphoma and cultured for more than 2 months *in vitro* were able to cure mice with disseminated disease [11]. Notably, adoptive transfer of lymphocytes with recombinant IL-2, which supported persistence of the transferred lymphocytes, was more effective at prolonging the survival of mice with disseminated lymphoma than IL-2 or cultured lymphocytes alone [12]. Administration of cyclophosphamide together with spleen cells from mice previously immunized with tumor cells could also improve therapeutic efficacy [13]. Efforts also focused on the use of ACT in solid tumor models. Adoptive transfer of spleen cells from mice previously immunized with sarcoma tumor cell lines could be utilized therapeutically, demonstrating the potential of cellular therapies to treat both hematologic and solid tumor malignancies [14]. For clinical translation for the treatment of human tumors, however, a cellular source with antitumor activity and which could be generated to large numbers was required. Efforts soon focused on preclinical studies utilizing murine lymphocytes generated from *in vitro* culture with IL-2, termed lymphokine-activated killer (LAK) cells. Upon transfer into tumor-bearing hosts, LAK cells slowed the growth of pulmonary metastases in sarcoma and B16 melanoma models, and their antitumor efficacy could be further improved by concomitant administration of IL-2, as well as by total body irradiation [15–17] Soon, techniques that enabled the culture of LAK cells from the peripheral blood of patients using purified preparations of IL-2 that were also able to lyse autologous tumor cells were reported [18, 19]. The stage was set for the first clinical trials of ACT in patients with metastatic disease.

Clinical Demonstration of Tumor Responses with Lymphokine Activated Killer Cells (LAK)

The initial clinical trial to utilize LAK cells in patients with metastatic cancers administered cultured cells alone. Four separate phase I studies were completed at the NCI and first reported in 1984 [20]. In the first 10 patients treated, lymphoid cells were obtained by leukopheresis and cultured for 48 h in medium containing the lectin phytohemagglutin. In this cohort, infusions of up to 1.7×10^{11} cells were well tolerated, with fevers being seen in all patients; however, no objective tumor regressions were noted Efforts to improve clinical efficacy with either pretreatment with cyclophosphamide, addition of activated macrophages into the infusion product, or activation of LAK cells with recombinant IL-2 ultimately proved unsuccessful [20]. As systemic administration of IL-2 together with LAK cells in preclinical models had markedly improved the antitumor efficacy, efforts were undertaken at the NCI to identify the maximum tolerated dose that could be safely administered in humans. In two pioneering studies, purified IL-2 was shown to have a short half-life of approximately 7 min and induce multiple dose-related toxicities, including fever and a capillary leak syndrome which resolved with discontinuation of therapy [21, 22]. Objective tumor responses were not seen on these early studies, which used lower doses than would be tested in subsequent larger trials. However, this expertise in the clinical administration of IL-2 would prove to be critical, and in 1985, Rosenberg et al. reported a small trial of 25 patients with refractory metastatic malignancies treated with autologous LAK cells and IL-2. Patients underwent multiple rounds of leukapheresis and received as many as 90 doses of IL-2 (in some cases well over a million units), together with as many as 14 infusions of LAK cells. Tumor regressions were seen in 11 of 25 patients, defined as at least 50 percent of tumor volume, including a complete response in a patient with melanoma. Responses were also seen in rectal, colon, renal cell, and lung carcinomas [23] Similar results were seen in a separate study which administered LAK cells with a constant infusion of IL-2 instead of repeat boluses [24]. While this therapeutic approach was able to reproduce the clinical activity seen in the earlier NCI studies, the high doses of IL-2 required to maintain LAK cell function remained a challenge to more widespread clinical use. Work soon turned to identifying alternative sources of tumor-specific immune cells suitable for ACT.

Identification and Purification of Tumor-Infiltrating Lymphocytes (TIL)

In 1986, the Rosenberg laboratory published their initial experience utilizing tumor-infiltrating lymphocytes (TIL) for the treatment of established tumors in multiple murine tumor models [25]. It was found that lymphocytes could be induced to egress from tumor fragments upon *in vitro* culture in high doses of IL-2 and subcultured for prolonged periods, allowing the generation of the large cell numbers required for ACT experiments [25]. When transferred into tumor-bearing hosts, TIL were found to be 50 to 100 times more potent on a per cell basis than LAK cells in curing mice of pulmonary metastases. While infusion of TIL alone or together with IL-2 was ineffective at curing mice of large, established lung or liver metastases, the addition of either cyclophosphamide or total body irradiation (TBI) to TIL and IL-2 was capable of inducing cures in the majority of mice. A subsequent report demonstrated the efficacy of murine TIL against preclinical models of sarcoma, melanoma, colon carcinoma and bladder carcinoma. The concomitant administration of systemic IL-2 with TIL was two- to five-fold more effective at eliminating pulmonary metastases than TIL alone [26]. Using antibody depletion studies, Thy-1-positive T-cells were demonstrated to be the precursor of TIL that mediated antitumor efficacy [26] A year later, a report demonstrated the successful isolation of TIL from a series of six patients with metastatic melanoma that were capable of lysing autologous tumor cells [27]. TIL from three of these patients had a limited ability to also recognize allogeneic melanoma cell lines, but the others did not, suggesting that TIL recognized tumor-specific antigens. Given the consistency that sufficient numbers of TIL could be generated for infusion into patients and the clear therapeutic benefit in preclinical models, clinical trials utilizing this approach in patients were soon initiated.

Initial Clinical Trials of TIL Therapies

In a small phase I trial reported in 1987, 7 patients with metastatic lung adenocarcinoma received TIL isolated from biopsy specimens that were cultured in IL-2 [28]. While infusions were safe, no objective responses were seen. Significant efforts were made by the Rosenberg group at the NCI to develop protocols for the expansion of the large numbers of TIL that would make clinical trials feasible. In initial studies, tumor fragments from 24 separate patients representing sarcomas, melanomas, and adenocarcinomas were cultured in high doses of IL-2, and TIL could be maintained over many weeks [29]. These methods were subsequently refined in an effort to expand TIL on a sufficient scale for clinical use, with 5 of 8 TIL cultures generating more than 10^{10} lymphocytes over a 3–6 week period [29]. With these methods in place, Topalian *et al* proceeded with a pilot study of 17 patients who underwent tumor resections to generate TIL cultures. TIL were successfully generated from 12 patients in sufficient numbers to allow infusion (six with melanoma, four with renal cell carcinoma, and one each with breast and colon carcinoma). The trial was designed to test a variety of treatment protocols and included escalating doses of cyclophosphamide and at least 1×10^{10} TIL together with IL-2 at one of three separate dose intensities. Two partial responses, defined as a decrease of at least 50% in the sum of the products of the perpendicular diameters of all measurable lesions for at least 1 month, were seen in one patient each with melanoma and renal cell carcinoma [30]. A larger study was subsequently undertaken in patients with metastatic melanoma at the NCI [31]. An initial cohort of 13 patients was treated with escalating doses of cyclophosphamide from 10–50 mg/kg followed 36 h later by boluses of IL-2 given at a dose of 100,000 IU/kg every 8 h. Two of the 13 patients achieved partial responses, which was concluded to be a response rate similar to what would be expected with IL-2 alone. An additional 20 patients were then treated on a defined protocol consisting of administration of a single 25 mg/kg dose of cyclophosphamide 36 h prior to the first infusion of TIL. IL-2 was then given at a dose of 100,000 IU/kg every 8 h beginning immediately following the first dose of TIL until dose-limiting toxicity occurred [31]. On this study, eleven of the 20 patients achieved a clinical response, including one patient with complete resolution of all subcutaneous sites of disease. Responses were seen across a wide variety of systemic sites, including the lungs, liver, spleen, lymph nodes, bone, and skin. The infused TIL products consisted of more than 90% CD3+ T-cells in all but 3 cases, with a wide range of CD4 to CD8 ratios, with some products containing more than 90% of either cell type.

Additional studies were subsequently completed at other centers that corrobo-rated the efficacy of TIL therapy when given together with IL-2. In a small trial of 28 patients from Massachusetts General Hospital, 3 of 13 patients with melanoma had a partial response (defined as reduction of more than 50% of the product of vertical and horizontal diameters of all measurable lesions), as did 2 of 7 patients with renal cell carcinoma [32]. Notably, cyclophosphamide was not part of this study's treatment regimen. Responding patients with subcutaneous melanoma were characterized histologically by lymphocytic infiltrates and tumor necrosis, which were not present in progressing lesions. Goedegebuure and colleagues reported a study of 26 patients (18 metastatic melanoma and 8 renal cell carcinoma) utilizing TIL expanded using the anti-CD3 antibody OKT3 together with moderate-dose IL-2 at a maximum dose of 30,000 IU/kg per injection given every 8 h for a total of 28 doses [33]. The overall response rate amongst melanoma patients was 19%, all with complete regressions of tumor, although one patient had a delayed response within a year of therapy.

Role of Nonmyeloablative Conditioning and Total Body Irradiation Prior to TIL Therapy

Early TIL studies utilized different nonmyeloablative chemotherapy regimens or eliminated this step altogether. Work in murine models had demonstrated that cyclo-phosphamide therapy prior to ACT improved therapeutic efficacy, which was hypothesized to be due to depletion of suppressive immune cell components [13, 25]. While CD4+ helper T-cells provide IL-2 that enables persistence of the CD8+ T-cells that mediate tumor cytotoxicity post transfer, CD4+ CD25+ regulatory T-cells, which are sensitive to depletion by cyclophosphamide, can prevent effective ACT responses [34]. An additional potential mechanism for the efficacy of nonmy-eloablative conditioning is the depletion of host cells that exhaust stores of IL-7 and IL-15, thereby increasing the amounts of these homeostatic cytokines available for adoptively transferred CD8+ T-cells [35]. Multiple clinical studies have subse-quently been undertaken in an effort to improve conditioning regimens for patients undergoing ACT.

Wallen et al. conducted a phase I trial of TIL therapy in patients with refractory metastatic melanoma that utilized an innovative design to assess the utility of the purine analog fludarabine for conditioning [36]. Patients received two infusions of a tumor-specific CTL clone; the second of these infusions was given after a course of 25 mg/m^2 fludarabine for a period of 5 days. In this study, 3 of 9 evaluable patients achieved stable disease, and fludarabine provided a 2.9 fold increase in the persistence of the adoptively transferred CTL, from a median of 4.5 days to 13.0 days [36].

In further optimization of the NCI protocol, nonmyeloablative conditioning with 2 days of cyclophosphamide at a dose of 60 mg/kg followed by 5 days of fludara-bine (25 mg/m^2) was trialed in 35 patients with metastatic melanoma prior to infusion of rapidly expanded TIL and high-dose IL-2 at 720,000 IU/kg every 8 h to tolerance [37]. There were 18 responses, for an ORR of 51%. Using this study as a baseline, follow-up protocols assessed the role of the addition of total body irradiation (TBI) as an adjunct. Administration of either 2 Gy or 12 Gy of TBI to cyclophosphamide/fludarabine conditioning increased the ORR to 52% and 72%, respectively [38]. Similar to data from murine studies, host lymphodepletion was associated with an increase in circulating IL-7 and IL-15 levels [38]. In three sequential clinical trials that enrolled 93 patients with metastatic melanoma who received autologous TIL and IL-2 after three different lymphodepletion regimens, the ORR was 49% for chemotherapy alone, 52% with chemotherapy plus 2 Gy TBI and 72% with chemotherapy plus 12 Gy TBI [39]. The CR rate was 22%, and in all but one patient who achieved a CR responses were ongoing at 3 years [39]. The role of TBI as part of the ideal nonmyeloablative conditioning regimen was definitively assessed in a randomized trial of 101 patients with metastatic melanoma who received one of two separate conditioning regimens consisting of cyclophosphamide/fludarabine with or without 2 Gy of TBI twice daily for 3 days [40]. Results were similar in the two groups, with an ORR of 45% in the chemotherapy alone arm and 62% in the arm with radiation. The CR rate was 24% in both arms. At a median follow up of 40.9 months, only one patient with a CR had recurred. In all of these trials, treatment toxicity was largely a result of the nonmyeloablative chemotherapy and high-dose IL-2 administration. Febrile neutropenia was reported in 25% of patients receiving chemotherapy alone and 36% of patients receiving chemotherapy and TBI [40]. TBI itself caused the late onset of thrombotic microangiopathy in 27% of patients and was the cause of death of one patient who had achieved a prior CR. The median ICU length of stay was 4 days in each arm, attributable to the administration of high-dose IL-2, and the median length of hospital admission was 18 days in the chemotherapy arm. Based on these results, a commonly utilized preparative regimen in NCI trials has remained cyclophosphamide 60 mg/kg/day on days −7 and − 6 and fludarabine 25 mg/m² per day given on days −5 to −1 prior to TIL infusion [41, 42].

Management of Side Effects of High Dose IL-2 Therapy

High-dose IL-2 (HD IL-2) administration has been utilized to induce durable complete responses, sometimes for decades, in metastatic renal cell carcinoma and melanoma, but due to it toxicity has largely lost favor with the introduction of checkpoint blockade immunotherapies and targeted therapies. The lessons learned from this experience, however, now has added importance with the routine introduction of HD IL-2 to TIL protocols. Prior HD IL-2 trials in solid tumors typically administered the maximum number of IL-2 doses as limited by toxicity in multiple courses, with patients often receiving a range of 16–20 doses in two prescribed cycles of treatment [43]. Currently ongoing TIL trials utilize differing doses of systemic IL-2 following TIL infusion, such as at the dose of 720,000 IU/kg every 8 h beginning

24 h post-TIL infusion for a maximum of 15 doses in NCI trials [41] and 600,000 IU/kg for up to 6 doses in commercial multicenter trials conducted by Iovance [42]. There are many management considerations for how HD IL-2 therapy is administered to maximize patient safety, and treatment guidelines are available [44]. HD IL-2 is typically given in the inpatient setting, either on specialized oncology or stem cell transplantation units, or in intensive care units. This is due to the requirement for frequent patient monitoring to manage multiple potential adverse events. Hypotension occurs in nearly all patients and is due to capillary leak and decreased peripheral vascular resistance with high cardiac output, similar to the systemic inflammatory response syndrome [44]. HD IL-2 induced hypotension is typically managed with intravenous fluids and/or vasopressors, the management of which requires substantial nursing support. High fevers with rigors, gastrointestinal complications, such as high-volume diarrhea, skin breakdown, infection, and neurologic toxicity are not infrequent. Other commonly observed laboratory abnormalities include hypoalbuminemia (secondary to both capillary leak and decreased synthesis), elevated bilirubin and hepatic enzymes, mild coagulopathy, thrombocytopenia, lymphopenia and rises in creatinine. While all of these events are promptly reversible with discontinuation of IL-2 therapy, substantial provider expertise is required to manage these complications and make decisions on when to safely administer subsequent doses in order to maintain therapeutic dose intensity.

Generation of TIL Products at Clinical Scale

While successful in most patients, the approach for isolation and expansion of TIL developed at the NCI is extremely laborious and can require up to 6 weeks to generate sufficient cells for infusion [29]. Patient age, history of prior therapy, and sex can all predict for the efficacy of the generation of TIL cultures [45]. Figure 1 outlines the logistics of manufacturing and administering TIL in the clinical setting. The protocol consists of cutting surgically resected tumors into small fragments that are cultured in high doses of IL-2 to allow TIL to egress from the tumor. High numbers of TIL can then be generated using a clinical-scale rapid expansion procedure in gas-permeable flasks by co-culture with allogeneic irradiated peripheral blood mononuclear cells and monoclonal anti-CD3 antibodies [41]. Prior to expansion, TIL can be first tested for reactivity against autologous cell lines or against individual peptides incubated with antigen-presenting cells, and only reactive lines expanded for use. Most patients will receive a single infusion of TIL following nonmyeloablative conditioning. While the exact number of TIL is specified by each individual protocol, it is often approximately 1×10^{10} cells, although it is also known that repeat infusions are safe and feasible [46].

Efficacy has also been reported utilizing protocols that culture TIL for a shorter duration of 10–18 days before rapid expansion and administration with nonmyeloablative chemotherapy and IL-2 [47]. The overall response rate of an early study was 29% (less than what has been reported in some NCI Surgery Branch studies)

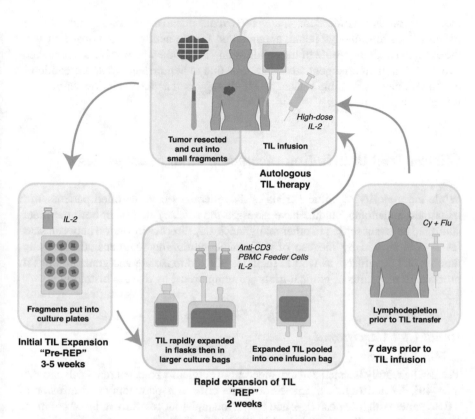

Fig. 1 Overall process for manufacturing and administration of TIL

with a median overall survival of 9.8 months, although responding patients had a 3 year OS of 78%. Lifileucel is a commercial TIL product developed by Iovance that is being tested in multiple ongoing multicenter clinical trials in different disease histologies. Lifileucel is manufactured using a rapid proprietary process over approximately 22 days [42]. Once approximately 10^9–10^{11} cells have been produced, the lifileucel product is harvested, washed, and may be cryopreserved to facilitate shipment and patient administration. In a recent single-arm phase II trial of patients with metastatic melanoma refractory to prior therapies, 66 patients received nonmyeloablative conditioning with cyclophosphamide 60 mg/kg for 2 days and fludarabine 25 mg/m2 daily for 5 days, followed 24 h later by a single infusion of previously cryopreserved lifileucel at a dose of 1×10^9 to 1.5×10^{11} cells [48]. Following TIL infusion, patients received bolus HD IL-2 at a dose of 600,000 IU/kg every 8–12 h for up to 6 doses. All patients had received prior anti-PD-1 or anti-PD-L1 therapy, and 80% had received prior anti-CTLA-4 therapy. The ORR was 36% with two CRs. The median progression free survival was 4.1 months and median overall survival 17.4 months. The duration of response had not been met at the time of the report. The median number of IL-2 doses given was 5.5, and the most common grade 3 or 4 adverse events occurring in more than 50% of patients were thrombocytopenia, anemia, and febrile neutropenia, consistent with the expected toxicity profile of the conditioning chemotherapy and IL-2. There were two fatal treatment emergent adverse events due to hemorrhage of an intraabdominal tumor that was possibly related to TIL therapy, and acute respiratory failure that was not felt to be related.

Clinical Trial Data in Non-melanoma Tumor Histologies

While the majority of clinical trials of TIL therapies have enrolled patients with metastatic melanoma, studies have assessed the efficacy of TIL in both the metastatic and adjuvant setting in other malignancies. A direct comparison between studies is complicated by the use of different conditioning regimens, IL-2 dosing, number of TIL infused, as well as methods utilized to isolate and generate the TIL product. Here, results of clinical trials are summarized by disease histology.

Renal Cell Carcinoma

TIL can be readily isolated and expanded from surgically resected renal cell carcinomas [49]. Administration of interferon alpha prior to nephrectomy and infusion of TIL together with low-dose IL-2 and interferon alpha successfully induced complete responses in a small trial published in 1993 [50]. These results, as well as those in other small trials eventually led to an international, multicenter trial that was reported in 1999 [51]. In a phase III design, 178 patients underwent nephrectomy and were randomized to receive either purified CD8+ TIL plus IL-2 for one to four cycles at a dose of five million IU/m^2 by continuous infusion daily for 4 days per week for 4 weeks or a placebo cell infusion plus IL-2 alone. Only 59% of patients randomized to the TIL group received a cell infusion due to difficulties with generation of suitable cell products, and the study was terminated early due to lack of efficacy.

Non-small Cell Lung Cancer

TIL products isolated from treatment-naïve NSCLC patients demonstrate reactivity against primary tumor digests [52]. An early trial of TIL therapy given with continuously-infused IL-2 enrolled 8 patients with NSCLC, without any clinical responses [32]. TIL were subsequently investigated as an adjuvant therapy to prevent recurrence after definitive surgical resection. In a randomized study, 113 patients received a TIL infusion 6–8 weeks post-operatively together with subcutaneous IL-2 or standard chemoradiotherapy [53]. The median survival was prolonged in the group that received TIL (22.4 months vs 14.1 months) and subgroup analysis demonstrate that the benefit was predominantly in patients with stage III disease. Studies are currently ongoing to test the efficacy of TIL therapy in patients with metastatic NSCLC who have failed checkpoint inhibitor therapies.

Gynecologic Malignancies

In an early study, 7 patients with advanced or recurrent ovarian cancer were treated with a regimen of TIL alone or in combination with cisplatin-containing chemotherapy [54]. Of seven patients treated with two to three infusions of TIL preceded by cyclophosphamide, there were 5 responses, one of them complete. Responses were seen at the primary tumor sites as well as in lung, liver, and lymph node metastases, although they were of short duration in all but one patient. An additional 10 patients were treated with TILs together with FCAP (cyclophosphamide, doxorubicin, 5-FU, and cisplatin) or the cisplatin analogue 254-S (for those with platinum-resistant disease). Nine of ten patients responded (7 complete), and three responses lasted more than 2 years. A later study assessed responses to TIL therapy in 13 patients with epithelial ovarian cancer who were disease-free following surgical resection and cisplatin-containing chemotherapy [55]. The estimated disease-free survival was 82.1%, compared to 54.5% in a historical control of 11 patients who were not treated with TIL infusion as a comparator arm.

Given the ability of T-cells to recognize cells infected with HPV, the causative agent of cervical cancer, TIL therapy has been investigated in this patient population. In an initial study of 9 patients with refractory metastatic cervical cancer, a single infusion of TIL selected for reactivity against HPV-16 or HPV-18 E6 and E7 resulted in two complete and one partial response, for an ORR of 33% [56] Reactivity against HPV antigens correlated with response. In a subsequent phase II study of patients with HPV-positive malignancies, 28% of patients with cervical cancer and 18% of patients with non-cervical cancer HPV-related tumors achieved a response. Two of the cervical cancer patients had CRs that were ongoing more than 4 years post-therapy [57]. Based on these results, a trial of checkpoint blockade naïve patients with advanced cervical cancer is ongoing where patients receive cyclophosphamide and fludarabine conditioning followed by a single infusion of TIL, followed by up to 6 doses of IL-2 (600,000 IU/kg) [105] . At the 2020 ESMO meeting, early results from this study reported an ORR of 44% with a disease control rate of 85%. Interestingly, TCR sequencing demonstrated that 47% of TIL products did not react with HPV, although clinical responses in this cohort were still seen [58].

Gastrointestinal Malignancies

A group from Yamanashi Medical University in Japan reported a protocol for the generation of TIL by repetitive stimulation *in vitro* with autologous tumor cells in 2002. Patients with metastatic gastric cancer were randomized to receive TIL expanded using this method in combination with cisplatin/5-FU chemotherapy or chemotherapy alone, with a small survival benefit of 3 months reported (11.5 vs 8.3 months) [59]. TIL therapy has also been assessed in the adjuvant setting in hepatocellular carcinoma (HCC). A small Chinese trial reported the successful generation of TIL cultures following surgical resection of HCC in 88% of patients, with 12 of 15 patients without evidence of recurrence after a median follow up of 14 months [60].

Malignant Gliomas

In 1999, a pilot study of 6 patients was reported by Quattrocchi et al. that assessed the safety of delivering TIL therapy to the intracranial tumor bed locally through an Ommaya reservoir. TIL were successfully expanded from tumor fragments from all six patients available in the presence of IL-2 and were infused twice, 14 days apart, together with intratumoral infusion of IL-2 three times weekly for 1 month. Three responses were seen, with one patient each with anaplastic astrocytoma and glioblastoma multiforme (GBM) achieving a partial response, and one additional patient with GBM achieving a complete response that lasted over 45 months [61].

Persistence of TIL Post-Infusion

During the initial clinical trials of TIL therapy, efforts were made to assess the ability of infused lymphocytes to traffic into tumor tissues. Using labeling with indium 111 (^{111}In), the Rosenberg group noted that TIL immediately localized to the lung, liver, and spleen within 2 h of infusion [62]. Using tumor biopsies as well as ^{111}In imaging, TIL could be identified having migrated into tumor tissues by 24 h. Cyclophosphamide conditioning increased the likelihood that TIL would traffic into tumors [63]. In 1990 five patients received TIL that had been modified with retroviral vectors expressing a neomycin resistance cassette [64]. Gene-marked TIL could be detected in the peripheral circulation in all five patients for 3 weeks and for up to 2 months in two patients. Notably, the gene-marked TIL could be recovered from tumor biopsies as long as 64 days following infusion. More than a decade later, using sequencing of TCR beta-chain variable regions, similar results were seen with a significant correlation between tumor regression and persistence of transferred TIL in peripheral blood [65].

Each time a cell divides, the repetitive sequences that make up telomeres at the ends of chromosomes shorten. TILs from responders to therapy have been shown to possess longer telomeres, as have individual clonotypes of TILs that persisted longer following transfer [66]. This observation contributed to the hypothesis that the ideal T-cell type to utilize for ACT exhibits a more naïve phenotype. It has been shown in murine models that while the acquisition of a terminal effector phenotype increases the efficacy of tumor cell killing *in vitro*, it impairs *in vivo* persistence and tumor clearance [67]. Attempts to insert IL-2 and IL-12 transcripts into TIL did not lead to improved persistence and resulted in unexpected toxicities [68, 69]. To investigate the phenotypes of TIL during the transition from *in vitro* cultured effector cells into memory cells that persist long-term *in vivo*, six patients with metastatic melanoma treated on NCI protocols were assessed with multiparameter flow cytometry [70]. TIL used for adoptive transfer had lower expression of the costimulatory molecules CD27 and CD28 as well as low expression of the IL-7 receptor. However, TIL that persisted in the circulation rapidly upregulated IL-7Ra, providing additional evidence for the requirement of IL-7 for long-term TIL persistence.

Determination of TIL Specificity

The efficacy of TIL therapy depends on the presence of T-cells capable of recognizing antigens expressed by tumor cells that are presented in the context of major histocompatibility complex (MHC) molecules; however, the results of early clinical trials had to be interpreted without a clear understanding of the antigen determinants that defined this reactivity. Methods were available to facilitate the culture of melanoma cells derived from clinical biopsies, and it was recognized that the majority of successful TIL products contained T-cells that could react against autologous tumor. An analysis of 860 attempted TIL cultures from 62 individual HLA-A*02 positive patients demonstrated reactivity against autologous melanoma cells in 29 of 36 patients screened (81%) [71]. Importantly, patients whose TIL cultures were capable of lysing autologous tumor cell lines were more likely to respond to ACT [72, 73]. Identifying the types of antigen determinants that were recognized by TIL became a priority for multiple groups by the mid-1990's.

Tumor antigens can be categorized into three broad classes: (1) tumor-associated antigens (TAA), (2) cancer-germline/cancer testis antigens (CTA) and (3) tumor-specific antigens or neoantigens (reviewed in [74, 75]). There is evidence for the presence of T-cells reactive with all three classes in TIL. TAA are proteins encoded in the normal genome that may be expressed aberrantly by tumor cells. Using classical cDNA expression cloning, CTL derived from the TIL of melanoma patients were found to recognize the glycoprotein gp100 [76], tyrosinase-related protein 1 [77] and melanocyte lineage-specific protein (MART-1) [78]in an MHC Class I restricted manner. All three of these transcripts were found to be highly expressed in melanoma cell lines but were also present in normal melanocytes or other tissues. CTA are expressed in germ cells (testis and ovary), and can also be overexpressed in cancer cells, often as a consequence of epigenetic mechanisms. The first human example was identified by the group of Thierry Boon in 1991 via screening of cDNA expression libraries with HLA-A*01 restricted CTL's derived from melanoma TIL [79]. Melanoma antigen family A1 (MAGE-A1), as this CTA is now known, belongs to a family of molecules with expression in multiple tumor types, as well as the testis. Another example of a CTA is NY-ESO-1, which was identified from a patient with an esophageal squamous carcinoma using serological analysis of recombinant cDNA expression library, or SEREX, in 1995 [80]. The experience and expertise developed in the TIL research field were also critical to the identification of the first human cancer neoantigens, which are aberrant proteins that are formed by nonsynonymous mutations that occur during cellular transformation. In 1995, Wolfel et al. reported the identification of a R24C mutation in CDK4 that was recognized by an HLA-A*02:01 restricted CTL line derived from a melanoma patient [81] and Coulie and colleagues also isolated a mutation at an intron/exon boundary that could be recognized by human CTL [82]. These studies clearly suggested the molecular basis for the antigen determinants expressed on melanoma cells and opened the door to refinements in TIL clinical protocols.

Clinical Studies of Tumor Antigen-Targeted TIL

Tumor-associated antigens clearly provide an attractive class of antigen targets for TIL therapy. Selective expansion of T-cells specific for gp100 and MART-1 was attempted in a small NCI trial reported in 2002 [83]. Of 7 patients identified whose cell products contained HLA-A*02-restricted CD8+ T-cells specific for MART-1 treated with T-cell transfer and IL-2 following nonmyeloablative chemotherapy, 3 had a tumor response. However, multiple autoimmune side effects were also seen in this cohort, including vitiligo and uveitis, raising concerns that even low expression of TAA molecules in normal tissues is sufficient to cause treatment limiting toxicities.

As cancer neoantigens are tumor-specific and therefore not expressed in normal tissues, additional studies have been undertaken to identify TIL products containing cancer neoantigen-specific T-cell clones. Lennerz et al. showed in 2005 that a single TIL product contained CD8+ T-cells specific for three separate TAAs and five neoantigens [84], and a separate study from the NCI identified two separate neoantigens in a patient who had experienced a CR to TIL therapy [85]. One challenge to be surmounted was that the cDNA expression library approaches utilized to identify the first cancer neoantigens in melanoma were extremely laborious. In 2012, an immunogenomics approach taking advantage of next generation sequencing and bioinformatic MHC Class I epitope prediction algorithms was reported that successfully identified a cancer neoantigen in a murine sarcoma [86]. A similar strategy was able to successfully identify neoantigens using TIL lines from three separate melanoma patients treated on NCI protocols [87].Multiple groups have since demonstrated that the presence of T-cells specific for cancer neoantigens in TIL products is a generalizable finding. Of three patients with melanoma who achieved a CR following TIL infusion that were assessed for neoantigen-specific CD8+ T-cell responses, the infusion products contained reactivities against 5, 4, and 1 neoantigens, respectively. One of these patient's products contained CD8+ T-cells specific for 5 separate antigens, with one specificity making up 29% of the total [88]. A single TIL product from a patient that induced a complete response for over 3 years recognized as many as 10 separate cancer neoantigens [89]. Interestingly, neoantigen-specific CD8+ T-cells are present in TIL products isolated from patients with HPV-positive malignancies, suggesting that tumor-specific mutations may be preferentially recognized by the immune system in comparison to viral-derived peptides [90]. MHC Class II restricted neoantigens that elicit CD4+ T-cell responses have also been identified in patient TIL products, strongly indicating that CD4+ T-cells play a significant role in TIL therapy mediated responses [91].

While these early studies focused on the identification of neoantigens in melanomas, the role of neoantigen-specific T-cell responses in other histologies were also investigated. In a pivotal case report, a 43-year-old female with metastatic cholangiocarcinoma who received TIL therapy derived from resected lung metastases on a clinical trial at the NCI initially achieved a partial response for 13 months [92]. Assessment of her TIL product demonstrated that approximately 25% of the 42.4 billion transferred cells were composed of three separate clones of CD4+ T-cells specific for a missense mutation in ERBB2IP. Following development of disease progression in the lungs, a second TIL infusion was administered, of which >95% was composed of a single clone of ERBB2IP-reactive CD4+ T-cells that induced a long-term tumor response. Subsequent work suggested that in gastrointestinal malignancies, approximately 80% of patients generate neoantigen-specific T-cell populations, although less than 2% of all missense mutations may encode immunogenic peptides [93]. The NCI group has also reported two additional case reports of responses to TIL therapy consisting of neoantigen specific T-cells: a 50 year old woman with metastatic colorectal carcinoma who achieved a response in lung metastases following infusion of HLA-C*08:02-restricted CD8+ T-cells specific for a G12D mutation in KRAS, as well as a 49 year old woman with metastatic estrogen-receptor positive, HER2 negative breast cancer who achieved a durable response in a chest wall mass and liver metastases after receiving a TIL product containing CD4+ and CD8+ T-cells specific for four separate neoantigens and the PD-1 blocking antibody pembrolizumab [41, 94]. These observations have led to the reassessment of TIL therapy in non-melanoma tumor histologies, and multiple clinical trials are currently in progress (Table 1).

Table 1 Active clinical trials of TIL therapies

Study title	Tumor type	Phase	Institution	Start date	Clinicaltrial.gov identifier
Adoptive transfer of tumor infiltrating lymphocytes for biliary tract cancers	Biliary tract cancer	2	University of Pittsburgh	19-Feb-19	NCT03801083
Adoptive transfer of tumor infiltrating lymphocytes for metastatic uveal melanoma	Uveal melanoma	2	University of Pittsburgh	14-May-18	NCT03467516
Adoptive transfer of tumor infiltrating lymphocytes for advanced solid cancers	Multiple solid tumors	2	University of Pittsburgh	3-Dec-19	NCT03935893

(continued)

Table 1 (continued)

Study title	Tumor type	Phase	Institution	Start date	Clinicaltrial. gov identifier
Autologous tumor infiltrating lymphocytes MDA-TIL in treating patients with recurrent or refractory ovarian cancer, colorectal cancer, or pancreatic ductal adenocarcinoma	Ovarian, colorectal and pancreatic cancer	2	MD Anderson	17-Aug-18	NCT03610490
Autologous tumor infiltrating lymphocytes in patients with pretreated metastatic triple negative breast cancer	Triple negative breast cancer	2	Yale university	23-Dec-19	NCT04111510
Adoptive cell transfer of autologous tumor infiltrating lymphocytes and high-dose interleukin 2 in select solid tumors	Melanoma, head and neck cancer	1	UC san Diego	7-Oct-20	NCT03991741
Nivolumab and tumor infiltrating lymphocytes (TIL) in advanced non-small cell lung cancer	NSCLC	1	Moffitt Cancer Center	11-Oct-17	NCT03215810
Tumor-infiltrating lymphocytes after combination chemotherapy in treating patients with metastatic melanoma	Melanoma	2	Fred hutch/ university of Washington	20-Aug-13	NCT01807182
A study of metastatic gastrointestinal cancers treated with tumor infiltrating lymphocytes in which the gene encoding the intracellular immune checkpoint CISH is inhibited using CRISPR genetic engineering	GI malignancies	1 + 2	University of Minnesota	15-May-20	NCT04426669
Lymphodepletion plus adoptive cell therapy with high dose IL-2 in adolescent and young adult patients with soft tissue sarcoma	Sarcoma	1	Moffitt Cancer Center	27-Aug-19	NCT04052334
Prospective randomized study of cell therapy for metastatic melanoma using short-term cultured tumor infiltrating lymphocytes plus IL-2 following either a non-Myeloablative lymphocyte depleting chemotherapy regimen alone or in conjunction w/1200 TBI	Melanoma	2	NCI	24-Mar-11	NCT01319565

(continued)

Table 1 (continued)

Study title	Tumor type	Phase	Institution	Start date	Clinicaltrial. gov identifier
Pembrolizumab, standard chemotherapy, tumor infiltrating lymphocytes, and high- or low-dose Aldesleukin in treating patients with metastatic melanoma	Melanoma	2	MD Anderson	7-Aug-15	NCT02500576
Immunotherapy using tumor infiltrating lymphocytes for patients with metastatic melanoma	Melanoma	2	NCI	12-Dec-13	NCT01993719
LN-145 or LN-145-S1 in treating patients with relapsed or refractory ovarian cancer, anaplastic thyroid cancer, osteosarcoma, or other bone and soft tissue sarcomas	Sarcomas	2	MD Anderson	27-Apr-18	NCT03449108
Autologous LN-145 in patients with metastatic non-small-cell lung cancer	NSCLC	2	Multicenter, sponsor Iovance	Mar-21	NCT04614103
A pilot study using short-term cultured anti-tumor autologous lymphocytes	Melanoma	1	Yale university	6-Feb-18	NCT03526185
Study of LN-145, autologous tumor infiltrating lymphocytes in the treatment of patients with cervical carcinoma	Cervical cancer	2	Multicenter, sponsor Iovance	22-Jun-17	NCT03108495
Study of LN-145/LN-145-S1 autologous tumor infiltrating lymphocytes in the treatment of squamous cell carcinoma of the Head & Neck	Head and neck cancer	2	Multicenter, sponsor Iovance	9-Jan-17	NCT03083873
Study of autologous tumor infiltrating lymphocytes in patients with solid tumors	Melanoma, head and neck cancer, NSCLC	2	Multicenter, sponsor Iovance	7-May-19	NCT03645928
Study of Lifileucel (LN-144), autologous tumor infiltrating lymphocytes, in the treatment of patients with metastatic melanoma (LN-144)	Melanoma	2	Multicenter, sponsor Iovance	Sep-15	NCT02360579
Lymphodepletion plus adoptive cell transfer with high dose IL-2 in patients with metastatic melanoma	Melanoma	Pilot	Moffitt Cancer Center	20-Oct-09	NCT01005745

(continued)

Table 1 (continued)

Study title	Tumor type	Phase	Institution	Start date	Clinicaltrial. gov identifier
Gene-modified T cells with or without Decitabine in treating patients with advanced malignancies expressing NY-ESO-1	Multiple tumor types	1 + 2a	Roswell Park	30-Jun-17	NCT02650986
Combining PD-1 blockade, CD137 Agonism and adoptive cell therapy for metastatic melanoma	Melanoma	1	Moffitt Cancer Center	8-Mar-16	NCT02652455
Vemurafenib with Lymphodepletion plus adoptive cell transfer & high dose IL-2 metastatic melanoma	Melanoma	2	Moffitt Cancer Center	26-Jul-12	NCT01659151
Genetically modified T-cells followed by Aldesleukin in treating patients with stage III-IV melanoma	Melanoma	1	MD Anderson	15-Oct-14	NCT01955460
Ipilimumab with Lymphodepletion plus adoptive cell transfer and high dose IL-2 in melanoma Mets pts	Melanoma	Pilot	Moffitt Cancer Center	9-Oct-12	NCT01701674
Genetically modified therapeutic autologous lymphocytes followed by Aldesleukin in treating patients with stage III or metastatic melanoma	Melanoma	1 + 2	MD Anderson	28-Jan-15	NCT01740557
Lymphodepletion plus adoptive cell transfer with or without dendritic cell immunization in patients with metastatic melanoma	Melanoma	2	MD Anderson	1-Feb-06	NCT00338377
Immunotherapy using tumor infiltrating lymphocytes for patients with metastatic cancer	Multiple tumor types	2	NCI	26-Aug-10	NCT01174121

Future Directions

The development and clinical application of TIL therapy is one of the most significant bench-to-bedside-and-back-again stories of the 20th and 21st centuries, spanning discoveries made in mouse models to the design and conduct of large clinical trials. Unlike commercially produced chimeric antigen receptor T-cell therapies, to date no TIL product has received FDA approval, although pivotal clinical trials are ongoing that may lead to this milestone in the years to come. While TIL therapies are currently utilized at experienced medical centers, the scientific observations that have been made from these studies have highly influenced the tumor immunology field. In the coming years, further advances that strive to address some key remaining questions will no doubt continue to push innovation forward.

Which Populations of TIL Have the Best Capacity for Therapeutic Efficacy?

As TIL products are isolated from tumor tissue, only lymphocytes that have migrated into the tumor are able to be selected. Besides this inherent selection, responses in clinical trials that selected TIL cultures prior to the rapid expansion step based on screening for reactivity against autologous tumor cells or individual antigens have successfully demonstrated the validity of these approaches. However, the best strategy for how to select TIL for infusion into patients is unclear. Recent reports of the efficacy of neoantigen-specific TIL with a stem-like phenotype make the identification of tumor-specific T-cells a priority; however, these approaches are time and labor-intensive [95]. Recent gene expression profiling studies of T-cell clones that persisted for more than 40 days following infusion have revealed expression changes in multiple transcripts, which may provide additional markers to facilitate the identification of TIL with therapeutic potential [96]. The ideal ratio of CD4+ and CD8+ T-cells for TIL therapy also remains undefined. While a large body of investigation has demonstrated that CD8+ T-cells are involved in TIL therapy responses, recent studies demonstrating that TIL products consisting almost exclusively of neoantigen-specific CD4+ T-cells can induce clinical responses has led to studies to better understand these mechanisms. Cytotoxic CD4+ T-cells with the capacity to destroy bladder cancer cells in an MHC Class II restricted manner have recently been described, leading to the possibility that future TIL therapy trials may benefit from identification of neoantigen-specific CD4+ T-cells for expansion as well [97, 98]. Finally, multiple studies have demonstrated that T-cell receptors (TCRs) isolated from CD8+ TIL can demonstrate reactivity against autologous cell lines when retrovirally transduced [99]. These findings lead to the possibility that TIL could be used as a source for the identification of TCRs that can be used for therapeutic purposes, even if antigen specificity is not available.

What Are the Ideal Conditions for the Generation of TIL Products?

The majority of TIL protocols continue to utilize similar techniques to those developed at the NCI Surgical Branch for the generation of cell products. The basic procedure is based on the *in vitro* expansion of TIL that are first allowed to egress from surgically excised tumor fragments in medium containing high-dose IL-2 before rapid expansion in the presence of irradiated allogeneic feeder cells, IL-2, and anti-CD3 antibody. This is a very time intensive process, and while total preparation times in excess of 6 weeks per patient have been reported in earlier clinical trials, shorter-duration protocols have been developed and are being assessed in ongoing studies.

Culturing techniques using preselection of TIL by flow cytometry with CD134, CD137 and/or PD-1 allowed detection of neoantigen-specific populations that were missed using conventional techniques utilizing culture of small tumor fragments, which suggests that further optimization of conditions has the potential to improve on therapeutic efficacy [100]. For example, the addition of agonistic anti-CD137 antibodies has been suggested to increase TIL yield and shorten production time, and further optimization of these processes are likely [101, 102].

Where Does TIL Therapy Fit into the Current Clinical Landscape?

Currently, TIL therapies have mostly been administered as part of clinical trials at highly experienced centers. Patients with solid tumors who have either not benefited from or progressed following treatment with checkpoint-blockade immunotherapies currently represent a major unmet need in clinical oncology and may prove to be a population who may benefit from TIL therapy. Early results suggest that TIL therapy is indeed effective in melanoma patients refractory to prior targeted therapy or checkpoint blockade, and cost-effectiveness analysis indicates that TIL therapy is expected to yield an improvement in quality adjusted life years vs ipilimumab as second line therapy in metastatic melanoma [48, 103]. While small studies suggest that TIL therapy can eliminate small brain metastases in patients with melanoma as well, further study will be necessary to validate this approach [104].

Decades of work utilizing preclinical model systems, clinical investigation, and correlative studies of patient samples has led to the current treatment landscape where a large fraction of patients with metastatic cancer will receive some form of checkpoint blockade immunotherapy during their treatment course. The recognition that multiple histologies of epithelial malignancies as well as melanoma contain tumor-specific T-cells with the capacity to effectively restrain tumor growth upon expansion and re-infusion provides hope that TIL therapy approaches may be beneficial for a wide range of tumor histologies. Within the next few years, the results from ongoing clinical trials and studies in development will further inform on the potential of TIL therapy to become a standard of care option for patients.

References

1. Gross L. Intradermal immunization of C3H mice against a sarcoma that originated in an animal of the same line. Cancer Res. 1943;3(5):326–33.
2. Rosenberg SA, Restifo NP, Yang JC, Morgan RA, Dudley ME. Adoptive cell transfer: a clinical path to effective cancer immunotherapy. Nat Rev Cancer. 2008;8(4):299–308.
3. Mitchison NA. Studies on the immunological response to foreign tumor transplants in the mouse i. the role of lymph node cells in conferring immunity by adoptive transfer. J Exp Med. 1955;102(2):157–77.
4. Klein G, Sjogren HO, Klein E, Hellstrom KE. Demonstration of resistance against methylcholanthrene-induced sarcomas in the primary autochthonous host. Cancer Res. 1960;20:1561–72.
5. Klein E, Sjogren HO. Humoral and cellular factors in homograft and isograft immunity against sarcoma cells. Cancer Res. 1960;20:452–61.
6. Delorme EJ, Alexander P. Treatment of primary fibrosarcoma in the rat with immune lymphocytes. Lancet. 1964;284(7351):117–20.
7. Borberg H, Oettgen HF, Choudry K, Beattie EJ. Inhibition of established transplants of chemically induced sarcomas in syngeneic mice by lymphocytes from immunized donors. Int J Cancer. 1972;10(3):539–47.
8. Rosenberg SA, Spiess PJ, Schwarz S. In vitro growth of murine T cells. I. Production of factors necessary for T cell growth. J Immunol Baltim Md 1950. 1978;121(5):1946–50.
9. Taniguchi T, Matsui H, Fujita T, et al. Structure and expression of a cloned cDNA for human interleukin-2. Nature. 1983;302(5906):305–10.
10. Yron I, Wood TA, Spiess PJ, Rosenberg SA, In Vitro Growth of Murine T Cells V. The isolation and growth of lymphoid cells infiltrating syngeneic solid tumors. J Immunol Baltim Md 1950. 1980;125(1):238–45.
11. Eberlein TJ, Rosenstein M, Spiess P, Wesley R, Rosenberg SA. Adoptive chemoimmunotherapy of a syngeneic murine lymphoma with long-term lymphoid cell lines expanded in T cell growth factor. Cancer Immunol Immunother. 1982;13(1):5–13.
12. Donohue JH, Rosenstein M, Chang AE, Lotze MT, Robb RJ, Rosenberg SA. The systemic administration of purified interleukin 2 enhances the ability of sensitized murine lymphocytes to cure a disseminated syngeneic lymphoma. J Immunol Baltim Md 1950. 1984;132(4):2123–8.
13. Cheever MA, Greenberg PD, Fefer A. Specificity of adoptive chemoimmunotherapy of established syngeneic tumors. J Immunol Baltim Md 1950. 1980;125(2):711–4.
14. Shu SY, Rosenberg SA. Adoptive immunotherapy of newly induced murine sarcomas. Cancer Res. 1985;45(4):1657–62.
15. Mazumder A, Rosenberg SA. Successful immunotherapy of natural killer-resistant established pulmonary melanoma metastases by the intravenous adoptive transfer of syngeneic lymphocytes activated in vitro by interleukin 2. J Exp Med. 1984;159(2):495–507.
16. Mule J, Shu S, Schwarz S, Rosenberg S. Adoptive immunotherapy of established pulmonary metastases with LAK cells and recombinant interleukin-2. Science. 1984;225(4669):1487–9.
17. Mulé JJ, Shu S, Rosenberg SA. The anti-tumor efficacy of lymphokine-activated killer cells and recombinant interleukin 2 in vivo. J Immunol Baltim Md 1950. 1985;135(1):646–52.
18. Grimm EA, Mazumder A, Zhang HZ, Rosenberg SA. Lymphokine-activated killer cell phenomenon. Lysis of natural killer-resistant fresh solid tumor cells by interleukin 2-activated autologous human peripheral blood lymphocytes. J Exp Med. 1982;155(6):1823–41.
19. Lotze MT, Grimm EA, Mazumder A, Strausser JL, Rosenberg SA. Lysis of fresh and cultured autologous tumor by human lymphocytes cultured in T-cell growth factor. Cancer Res. 1981;41(11 Pt 1):4420–5.
20. Rosenberg SA. Immunotherapy of cancer by systemic administration of lymphoid cells plus interleukin-2. J Biol Resp Modif. 1984;3(5):501–11.

21. Lotze MT, Frana LW, Sharrow SO, Robb RJ, Rosenberg SA. In vivo administration of puri-
    fied human interleukin 2. I. Half-life and immunologic effects of the Jurkat cell line-derived
    interleukin 2. J Immunol Baltim Md 1950. 1985;134(1):157–66.
22. Lotze MT, Matory YL, Ettinghausen SE, et al. In vivo administration of purified human
    interleukin 2. II. Half life, immunologic effects, and expansion of peripheral lymphoid cells
    in vivo with recombinant IL 2. J Immunol Baltim Md 1950. 1985;135(4):2865–75.
23. Rosenberg SA, Lotze MT, Muul LM, et al. Observations on the systemic administration of
    autologous lymphokine-activated killer cells and recombinant interleukin-2 to patients with
    metastatic cancer. N Engl J Med. 1985;313(23):1485–92.
24. West WH, Tauer KW, Yannelli JR, et al. Constant-infusion recombinant Interleukin-2 in
    adoptive immunotherapy of advanced cancer. N Engl J Med. 1987;316(15):898–905.
25. Rosenberg S, Spiess P, Lafreniere R. A new approach to the adoptive immunotherapy of
    cancer with tumor-infiltrating lymphocytes. Science. 1986;233(4770):1318–21.
26. Spiess PJ, Yang JC, Rosenberg SA. In vivo antitumor activity of tumor-infiltrating lympho-
    cytes expanded in recombinant interleukin-2. JNCI J Natl Cancer Inst. 1987;79(5):1067–75.
27. Muul LM, Spiess PJ, Director EP, Rosenberg SA. Identification of specific cytolytic immune
    responses against autologous tumor in humans bearing malignant melanoma. J Immunol
    Baltim Md 1950. 1987;138(3):989–95.
28. Kradin RL, Boyle LA, Preffer FI, et al. Tumor-derived interleukin-2-dependent lymphocytes
    in adoptive immunotherapy of lung cancer. Cancer Immunol Immunother. 1987;24(1):76–85.
29. Topalian SL, Muul LM, Solomon D, Rosenberg SA. Expansion of human tumor infiltrating
    lymphocytes for use in immunotherapy trials. J Immunol Methods. 1987;102(1):127–41.
30. Topalian SL, Solomon D, Avis FP, et al. Immunotherapy of patients with advanced can-
    cer using tumor-infiltrating lymphocytes and recombinant interleukin-2: a pilot study. J Clin
    Oncol. 1988;6(5):839–53.
31. Rosenberg SA, Packard BS, Aebersold PM, et al. Use of tumor-infiltrating lymphocytes and
    Interleukin-2 in the immunotherapy of patients with metastatic melanoma. N Engl J Med.
    1988;319(25):1676–80.
32. Kradin Richard L, Lazarus David S, Dubinett Steven M, et al. Tumour-infiltrating lympho-
    cytes and interleukin-2 in treatment of advanced cancer. Lancet. 1989;333(8638):577–80.
33. Goedegebuure PS, Douville LM, Li H, et al. Adoptive immunotherapy with tumor-infiltrating
    lymphocytes and interleukin-2 in patients with metastatic malignant melanoma and renal cell
    carcinoma: a pilot study. J Clin Oncol. 1995;13(8):1939–49.
34. Antony PA, Piccirillo CA, Akpinarli A, et al. CD8+ T cell immunity against a tumor/self-
    antigen is augmented by CD4+ T helper cells and hindered by naturally occurring T regula-
    tory cells. J Immunol. 2005;174(5):2591–601.
35. Gattinoni L, Finkelstein SE, Klebanoff CA, et al. Removal of homeostatic cytokine sinks
    by lymphodepletion enhances the efficacy of adoptively transferred tumor-specific CD8+ T
    cells. J Exp Med. 2005;202(7):907–12.
36. Wallen H, Thompson JA, Reilly JZ, Rodmyre RM, Cao J, Yee C. Fludarabine modulates
    immune response and extends in vivo survival of adoptively transferred CD8 T cells in
    patients with metastatic melanoma. PLoS One. 2009;4(3):e4749.
37. Dudley ME, Wunderlich JR, Yang JC, et al. Adoptive cell transfer therapy following non-
    myeloablative but lymphodepleting chemotherapy for the treatment of patients with refrac-
    tory metastatic melanoma. J Clin Oncol. 2005;23(10):2346–57.
38. Dudley ME, Yang JC, Sherry R, et al. Adoptive cell therapy for patients with metastatic mela-
    noma: evaluation of intensive myeloablative chemoradiation preparative regimens. J Clin
    Oncol. 2008;26(32):5233–9.
39. Rosenberg SA, Yang JC, Sherry RM, et al. Durable complete responses in heavily pretreated
    patients with metastatic melanoma using T-cell transfer immunotherapy. Clin Cancer Res.
    2011;17(13):4550–7.
40. Goff SL, Dudley ME, Citrin DE, et al. Randomized, prospective evaluation comparing
    intensity of lymphodepletion before adoptive transfer of tumor-infiltrating lymphocytes for
    patients with metastatic melanoma. J Clin Oncol 2016;34(20):2389-2397.

41. Tran E, Robbins PF, Lu Y-C, et al. T-cell transfer therapy targeting mutant KRAS in cancer. N Engl J Med. 2016;375(23):2255–62.
42. Fardis M, Fardis M, DiTrapani K, Finckenstein FG, Chartier C. Current and future directions for tumor infiltrating lymphocyte therapy for the treatment of solid tumors. Cell Gene Ther Insights. 2020;6(6):855–63.
43. Dandamudi UB, Ghebremichael M, Sosman JA, et al. A phase II study of bevacizumab and high-dose Interleukin-2 in patients with metastatic renal cell carcinoma. J Immunother. 2013;36(9):490–5.
44. Dutcher JP, Schwartzentruber DJ, Kaufman HL, et al. High dose interleukin-2 (Aldesleukin) - expert consensus on best management practices-2014. J Immunother Cancer. 2014;2(1):26.
45. Joseph RW, Peddareddigari VR, Liu P, et al. Impact of clinical and pathologic features on tumor-infiltrating lymphocyte expansion from surgically excised melanoma metastases for adoptive T-cell therapy. Clin Cancer Res. 2011;17(14):4882–91.
46. Ravaud A, Legrand E, Delaunay M, et al. A phase I trial of repeated tumour-infiltrating lymphocyte (TIL) infusion in metastatic melanoma. Br J Cancer. 1995;71(2):331–6.
47. Besser MJ, Shapira-Frommer R, Treves AJ, et al. Clinical responses in a phase II study using adoptive transfer of short-term cultured tumor infiltration lymphocytes in metastatic melanoma patients. Clin Cancer Res. 2010;16(9):2646–55.
48. Sarnaik AA, Hamid O, Khushalani NI, et al. Lifileucel, a tumor-infiltrating lymphocyte therapy, in metastatic melanoma. J Clin Oncol. 2021;39(24):2656–66.
49. Belldegrun A, Muul LM, Rosenberg SA. Interleukin 2 expanded tumor-infiltrating lymphocytes in human renal cell cancer: isolation, characterization, and antitumor activity. Cancer Res. 1988;48(1):206–14.
50. Belldegrun A, Pierce W, Kaboo R, et al. Interferon-α primed tumor-infiltrating lymphocytes combined with Interleukin-2 and interferon-α as therapy for metastatic renal cell carcinoma. J Urol. 1993;150(5):1384–90.
51. Figlin RA, Thompson JA, Bukowski RM, et al. Multicenter, randomized, phase III trial of CD8 + tumor-infiltrating lymphocytes in combination with recombinant Interleukin-2 in metastatic renal cell carcinoma. J Clin Oncol. 1999;17(8):2521.
52. Groot RD, Loenen MMV, Guislain A, et al. Polyfunctional tumor-reactive T cells are effectively expanded from non-small cell lung cancers, and correlate with an immune-engaged T cell profile. Onco Targets Ther. 2019;8(11):1–14.
53. Ratto GB, Zino P, Mirabelli S, et al. A randomized trial of adoptive immunotherapy with tumor-infiltrating lymphocytes and interleukin-2 versus standard therapy in the postoperative treatment of resected nonsmall cell lung cancer. Cancer. 1996;78(2):244–51.
54. Aoki Y, Takakuwa K, Kodama S, et al. Use of adoptive transfer of tumor-infiltrating lymphocytes alone or in combination with cisplatin-containing chemotherapy in patients with epithelial ovarian cancer. Cancer Res. 1991;51(7):1934–9.
55. Fujita K, Ikarashi H, Takakuwa K, et al. Prolonged disease-free period in patients with advanced epithelial ovarian cancer after adoptive transfer of tumor-infiltrating lymphocytes. Clin Cancer Res Off J Am Assoc Cancer Res. 1995;1(5):501–7.
56. Stevanović S, Draper LM, Langhan MM, et al. Complete regression of metastatic cervical cancer after treatment with human papillomavirus-targeted tumor-infiltrating T cells. J Clin Oncol. 2015;33(14):1543–50.
57. Stevanović S, Helman SR, Wunderlich JR, et al. A phase II study of tumor-infiltrating lymphocyte therapy for human papillomavirus–associated epithelial cancers. Clin Cancer Res. 2018;25(5):1486–93.
58. Jazaeri A, Gontcharova V, Blaskovich M, et al. In vivo persistence of Iovance tumour-infiltrating lymphocytes LN-145 in cervical cancer patients. Ann Oncol. 2020;31:S642.
59. Kono K, Takahashi A, Ichihara F, et al. Prognostic significance of adoptive immunotherapy with tumor-associated lymphocytes in patients with advanced gastric cancer: a randomized trial. Clin Cancer Res Official J Am Assoc Cancer Res. 2002;8(6):1767–71.
60. Jiang S-S, Tang Y, Zhang Y-J, et al. A phase I clinical trial utilizing autologous tumor-infiltrating lymphocytes in patients with primary hepatocellular carcinoma. Oncotarget. 2015;6(38):41339–49.

61. Quattrocchi KB, Miller CH, Cush S, et al. Pilot study of local autologous tumor infiltrating lymphocytes for the treatment of recurrent malignant gliomas. J Neuro-Oncol. 1999;45(2):141–57.

62. Fisher B, Packard BS, Read EJ, et al. Tumor localization of adoptively transferred indium-111 labeled tumor infiltrating lymphocytes in patients with metastatic melanoma. J Clin Oncol. 1989;7(2):250–61.

63. Pockaj BA, Sherry RM, Wei JP, et al. Localization of 111Indium-labeled tumor infiltrating lymphocytes to tumor in patients receiving adoptive immunotherapy. Augmentation with cyclophosphamide and correlation with response. Cancer. 1994;73(6):1731–7.

64. Rosenberg SA, Aebersold P, Cornetta K, et al. Gene transfer into humans — immunotherapy of patients with advanced melanoma, using tumor-infiltrating lymphocytes modified by retroviral gene transduction. N Engl J Med. 1990;323(9):570–8.

65. Robbins PF, Dudley ME, Wunderlich J, et al. Cutting edge: persistence of transferred lymphocyte Clonotypes correlates with cancer regression in patients receiving cell transfer therapy. J Immunol. 2004;173(12):7125–30.

66. Zhou J, Shen X, Huang J, Hodes RJ, Rosenberg SA, Robbins PF. Telomere length of transferred lymphocytes correlates with in vivo persistence and tumor regression in melanoma patients receiving cell transfer therapy. J Immunol. 2005;175(10):7046–52.

67. Gattinoni L, Klebanoff CA, Palmer DC, et al. Acquisition of full effector function in vitro paradoxically impairs the in vivo antitumor efficacy of adoptively transferred CD8+ T cells. J Clin Invest. 2005;115(6):1616–26.

68. Heemskerk B, Liu K, Dudley Mark E, et al. Adoptive cell therapy for patients with melanoma, using tumor-infiltrating lymphocytes genetically engineered to secrete Interleukin-2. Hum Gene Ther. 2008;19(5):496–510.

69. Zhang L, Morgan RA, Beane JD, et al. Tumor-infiltrating lymphocytes genetically engineered with an inducible gene encoding Interleukin-12 for the immunotherapy of metastatic melanoma. Clin Cancer Res. 2015;21(10):2278–88.

70. Powell DJ, Dudley ME, Robbins PF, Rosenberg SA. Transition of late-stage effector T cells to CD27+ CD28+ tumor-reactive effector memory T cells in humans after adoptive cell transfer therapy. Blood. 2005;105(1):241–50.

71. Dudley ME, Wunderlich JR, Shelton TE, Even J, Rosenberg SA. Generation of tumor-infiltrating lymphocyte cultures for use in adoptive transfer therapy for melanoma patients. J Immunother. 2003;26(4):332–42.

72. Aebersold P, Hyatt C, Johnson S, et al. Lysis of autologous melanoma cells by tumor*infiltrating lymphocytes: association with clinical response. JNCI J Natl Cancer Inst. 1991;83(13):932–7.

73. Schwartzentruber DJ, Hom SS, Dadmarz R, et al. In vitro predictors of therapeutic response in melanoma patients receiving tumor-infiltrating lymphocytes and interleukin-2. J Clin Oncol. 1994;12(7):1475–83.

74. Coulie PG, den Eynde BJV, van der Bruggen P, Boon T. Tumour antigens recognized by T lymphocytes: at the core of cancer immunotherapy. Nat Rev Cancer. 2014;14(2):135–46.

75. Heemskerk B, Kvistborg P, Schumacher TNM. The cancer antigenome. Embo J. 2013;32(2):194–203.

76. Bakker AB, Schreurs MW, de Boer AJ, et al. Melanocyte lineage-specific antigen gp100 is recognized by melanoma-derived tumor-infiltrating lymphocytes. J Exp Med. 1994;179(3):1005–9.

77. Wang RF, Robbins PF, Kawakami Y, Kang XQ, Rosenberg SA. Identification of a gene encoding a melanoma tumor antigen recognized by HLA-A31-restricted tumor-infiltrating lymphocytes. J Exp Med. 1995;181(2):799–804.

78. Kawakami Y, Eliyahu S, Delgado CH, et al. Cloning of the gene coding for a shared human melanoma antigen recognized by autologous T cells infiltrating into tumor. Proc Natl Acad Sci U S A. 1994;91(9):3515–9.

79. van der Bruggen P, Traversari C, Chomez P, et al. A gene encoding an antigen recognized by cytolytic T lymphocytes on a human melanoma. Science. 1991;254(5038):1643–7.

80. Chen Y-T, Scanlan MJ, Sahin U, et al. A testicular antigen aberrantly expressed in human cancers detected by autologous antibody screening. Proc Natl Acad Sci U S A. 1997;94(5):1914–8.
81. Wolfel T, Hauer M, Schneider J, et al. A p16INK4a-insensitive CDK4 mutant targeted by cytolytic T lymphocytes in a human melanoma. Science. 1995;269(5228):1281–4.
82. Coulie PG, Lehmann F, Lethé B, et al. A mutated intron sequence codes for an antigenic peptide recognized by cytolytic T lymphocytes on a human melanoma. Proc Natl Acad Sci U S A. 1995;92(17):7976–80.
83. Dudley ME, Wunderlich JR, Robbins PF, et al. Cancer regression and autoimmunity in patients after clonal repopulation with antitumor lymphocytes. Science. 2002;298(5594):850–4.
84. Lennerz V, Fatho M, Gentilini C, et al. The response of autologous T cells to a human melanoma is dominated by mutated neoantigens. Proc Natl Acad Sci U S A. 2005;102(44):16013–8.
85. Zhou J, Dudley ME, Rosenberg SA, Robbins PF. Persistence of multiple tumor-specific T-cell clones is associated with complete tumor regression in a melanoma patient receiving adoptive cell transfer therapy. J Immunother. 2005;28(1):53–62.
86. Matsushita H, Vesely MD, Koboldt DC, et al. Cancer exome analysis reveals a T-cell-dependent mechanism of cancer immunoediting. Nature. 2012;482(7385):400–4.
87. Robbins PF, Lu Y-C, El-Gamil M, et al. Mining exomic sequencing data to identify mutated antigens recognized by adoptively transferred tumor-reactive T cells. Nat Med. 2013;19(6):747–52.
88. van den Berg JH, Heemskerk B, van Rooij N, et al. Tumor infiltrating lymphocytes (TIL) therapy in metastatic melanoma: boosting of neoantigen-specific T cell reactivity and long-term follow-up. J Immunother Cancer. 2020;8(2):e000848.
89. Prickett TD, Crystal JS, Cohen CJ, et al. Durable complete response from metastatic melanoma after transfer of autologous T cells recognizing 10 mutated tumor antigens. Cancer Immunol Res. 2016;4(8):669–78.
90. Stevanović S, Pasetto A, Helman SR, et al. Landscape of immunogenic tumor antigens in successful immunotherapy of virally induced epithelial cancer. Science. 2017;356(6334):200–5.
91. Linnemann C, van Buuren MM, Bies L, et al. High-throughput epitope discovery reveals frequent recognition of neo-antigens by CD4+ T cells in human melanoma. Nat Med. 2014;21(1):81–5.
92. Tran E, Turcotte S, Gros A, et al. Cancer immunotherapy based on mutation-specific CD4+ T cells in a patient with epithelial cancer. Science. 2014;344(6184):641–5.
93. Parkhurst MR, Robbins PF, Tran E, et al. Unique neoantigens arise from somatic mutations in patients with gastrointestinal cancers. Cancer Discov. 2019;9(8):1022–35.
94. Zacharakis N, Chinnasamy H, Black M, et al. Immune recognition of somatic mutations leading to complete durable regression in metastatic breast cancer. Nat Med. 2018;24(6):724–30.
95. Krishna S, Lowery FJ, Copeland AR, et al. Stem-like CD8 T cells mediate response of adoptive cell immunotherapy against human cancer. Science. 2020;370(6522):1328–34.
96. Lu Y-C, Jia L, Zheng Z, Tran E, Robbins PF, Rosenberg SA. Single-cell transcriptome analysis reveals gene signatures associated with T-cell persistence following adoptive cell therapy. Cancer Immunol Res. 2019;7(11):1824–36.
97. Leko V, McDuffie LA, Zheng Z, et al. Identification of neoantigen-reactive tumor-infiltrating lymphocytes in primary bladder cancer. J Immunol. 2019;202(12):3458–67.
98. Oh DY, Kwek SS, Raju SS, et al. Intratumoral CD4+ T cells mediate anti-tumor cytotoxicity in human bladder cancer. Cell. 2020;181(7):1612–1625.e13.
99. Turcotte S, Gros A, Tran E, et al. Tumor-reactive CD8+ T cells in metastatic gastrointestinal cancer refractory to chemotherapy. Clin Cancer Res. 2014;20(2):331–43.
100. Yossef R, Tran E, Deniger DC, et al. Enhanced detection of neoantigen-reactive T cells targeting unique and shared oncogenes for personalized cancer immunotherapy. JCI Insight. 2018;3(19):e122467.
101. Tavera RJ, Forget M-A, Kim YU, et al. Utilizing T-cell activation signals 1, 2, and 3 for tumor-infiltrating lymphocytes (TIL) expansion. J Immunother. 2018;41(9):399–405.

102. Chacon JA, Sarnaik AA, Chen JQ, et al. Manipulating the tumor microenvironment ex vivo for enhanced expansion of tumor-infiltrating lymphocytes for adoptive cell therapy. Clin Cancer Res. 2015;21(3):611–21.
103. Retèl VP, Steuten LMG, Foppen MHG, et al. Early cost-effectiveness of tumor infiltrating lymphocytes (TIL) for second line treatment in advanced melanoma: a model-based economic evaluation. BMC Cancer. 2018;18(1):895.
104. Mehta GU, Malekzadeh P, Shelton T, et al. Outcomes of adoptive cell transfer with tumor-infiltrating lymphocytes for metastatic melanoma patients with and without brain metastases. J Immunother. 2018;41(5):241–7.
105. Jazaeri AA, Zsiros E, Amaria RN, et al. Safety and efficacy of adoptive cell transfer using autologous tumor infiltrating lymphocytes (LN-145) for treatment of recurrent, metastatic, or persistent cervical carcinoma. J Clin Oncol. 2019;37(15_suppl):2538.

Part IV
TCR

T-Cell Receptor (TCR) Engineered Cells and Their Transition to the Clinic

Mateusz Opyrchal

Abstract Immune-modulatory treatments have shown a great promise in treating patients with advanced or metastatic disease. Currently approved immunotherapy approaches target PD1/PDL1 pathway or use specific autologous T-cells genetically modified to express a chimeric antigen receptor (CAR). Although promising, in most patients with solid malignancies these approaches either do not work or the disease becomes resistant to treatment. Unlike CAR-T cell therapy, genetically modifying T cell receptor T cells (TCR-T) have an advantage of targeting intracellular proteins and expanding number of potential targets. These approaches are limited by recognition of peptides bound to specific MHC molecules. There are currently no approved TCR-T cell products but increasing number of clinical trials are providing us with preliminary efficacy and toxicity data. Encouraging results in reported clinical trials show the potential for impressive and durable responses, but also highlights the challenges of on-target off-tumor toxicities. Current research is focusing on improving efficacy, expanding targets and limiting toxicities. Continual development of multiple products holds a great promise and new technologies aim to improve efficacy, identify novel targets and streamline production to allow larger number of patients to be eligible to be treated with TCR-T cell approaches in the future.

Keywords T cell receptor (TCR) · MHC · HLA · CEA · MART-1 · NY-ESO-1 · gp100 · Mage-A3 · Mage-A4 · Neurotoxicity · Cardiotoxicity

Introduction

The immune system has been shown to play an ever-increasing role in tumorigenesis, metastasis, and response to treatments. It is increasingly clear that in order to have a robust anti-tumor response there needs to be recognition, infiltration,

M. Opyrchal (✉)
Department of Medicine, Washington University School of Medicine, St. Louis, MO, USA
e-mail: m.opyrchal@wustl.edu

© Springer Nature Switzerland AG 2022
A. Ghobadi, J. F. DiPersio (eds.), *Gene and Cellular Immunotherapy for Cancer*, Cancer Drug Discovery and Development,
https://doi.org/10.1007/978-3-030-87849-8_14

activation, and continued stimulation of the lymphocytic component of the immune system. Innate infiltrating tumor lymphocytes (TILs) have been recognized as strongly correlating with clinical outcomes in many malignancies [1–3]. TILs are often addressed as single subset, but they are not a uniform entity and specific subtypes are more prognostic correlating with their function [4, 5]. CD8⁺ T cells have the best described direct anti-tumor effect and can produce high levels of known anti-tumor cytokines [6]. One of the limitations of effective CD8⁺ T cell response is T cell exhaustion after persistent antigen stimulation resulting in decreased anti-tumor activity [7, 8]. The exhaustion results in upregulation of multiple inhibitory signals [9, 10]. Immune checkpoint inhibitors currently target the PD1/PDL1 pathway and their successes in multiple tumors show the importance of the pathway in tumor immunotherapy [11–16]. Unfortunately, despite multiple approvals in many cancer diagnoses most patients never respond or become resistant to these approaches [17–20]. Manufacturing of TILs is challenging as it requires isolation and expansion of TILs from surgically removed tumor. T cell receptor (TCR) gene modified T cells (TCR T) are generated by transduction of T cells isolated from peripheral blood of patients with TCR specific to a tumor associated antigen being presented in the context of a specific HLA (usually class I). T cells are unique due to their specific TCR which was first identified in 1980s [21, 22]. TCRs enables T cells to recognize and bind to specific peptides/antigens presented in the context of specific HLA. Binding of TCR to the antigen/HLA complex triggers a signaling cascade which results in activation of T cell and cell lysis. TCR (CD3) is a complicated multimeric complex consisting of polymorphic α and β chains, gamma and delta chains, two monomorphic epsilon chains and a signaling zeta chain. Approximately 1–5% of T cells have TCR constructed of γ and δ chains (without surface expression of α and β chains or have an invariant TCR recognizing glycolipids bound to CD1d on antigen presenting cells.

Tumor Infiltrating Lymphocytes

TILs are presented in detail in chapter "Tumor Infiltrating Lymphocytes (TIL): From Bench to Bedside" but described briefly as relevant to this topic. The autologous transfer of *ex vivo* expanded non-specific T lymphocytes has shown limited clinical efficacy in treatment of cancers as these cells often lack specificity. Expanding TILs and infusing them after pre-conditioning regimen improved response rates [23–25]. These approaches have allowed investigators to identify and clone specific TCR genes which recognized specific cancer antigens [26]. These genes were the first examples of identifying specific cancer directed TCR. Unfortunately, tumor specific T cells are not identified in most patients therefore these approaches were limited to only a few diseases. Another approach for identifying cancer antigens in other tumor types was to use allogenic T cells or T cells from transgenic mice that express human MHC. These cells are incubated with tumor cells and activated T cells are identified and their TCRs cloned [27, 28]. Further refinement of the receptor can be done once cancer antigens have been identified resulting in optimization of binding, optimizing of codon sequences and humanization of TCRs to minimize eventual immunologic rejection by the host innate immune system. TCR phage library can be established to screen for TCRs that have increased affinity and specificity [29–31]. TCR can be further modified to improve its clinical performance. Amino acids in the antigen binding region can be changed to increase binding and sensitivity of TCR [32].

TCR Receptor

Unlike CAR-Ts, which are engineered with an antibody fragments (scFvs) that recognizes specific membrane antigens on surface of cancer cells, TCRs recognized peptides presented on the surface of cells when bound to specific MHC molecules (Fig. 1). Most current engineered TCRs are restricted to peptides bound to HLA-A*02. Because the engineered TCR contains all of the other components of the multimeric TCR (CD3) complex, TCR-T cells can be activated and induce strong anti-tumor effects even when target antigen (peptide) is expressed in small amounts on target cells. Another advantage of TCR in addition to recognizing shared tumor associated antigens (TAA) that are differentially expressed on tumor cells is their ability to also recognize mutated peptides (neoantigens) that are unique to cancers and not expressed in normal cells [33].

Manufacturing of TCR Gene Modified T (TCR-T) Cells

Limitation of large-scale treatment of patients with engineered TCR T cells is the labor-intensive manufacturing process. Peripheral blood mononuclear cells (PBMCs) are collected from patients through leukapheresis. The cells are cultured

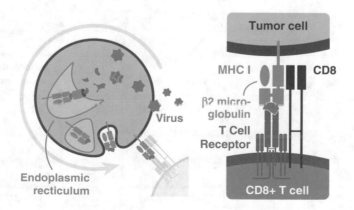

Fig. 1 Representation of T cell receptor interacting with tumor antigen

in medium containing IL2 and stimulated with a mitogeneic anti-CD3 epsilon antibody. 24–48 h after stimulation the cells are transduced with, most commonly, viral vectors containing transgenes composed of cloned TCR α and β chains. Recently other techniques are being explored including the use of sleeping beauty transposons and minicircle transposons. After effective transduction, the cells are expanded with IL-2 for additional 3–6 days to achieve the desired yield and administered fresh or thawed after cryopreservation. Each step requires spinning, washing and transfer of cells which increases risk of contamination (Fig. 2). Therefore, multiple checks are employed throughout the process to assure safety to patients and accurate calculation of viable, transfected cells [34]. The process is moving toward automation and several modular closed or semi-closed systems are being tested. The sufficient yields have been a bigger challenge as compared to CAR-T cell production. This transition will be another step in making these therapies a more viable option in clinic through decentralizing production and reducing costs.

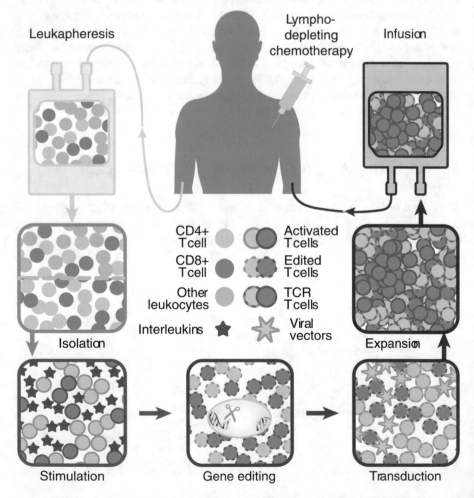

Fig. 2 Outline of the manufacturing process and administration of TCR-T cell therapy

Clinical TCR Targets

There is no approved TCR-T cell product. The number of clinical trials using this platform is rapidly increasing each year ([35, 36] and Table 1). Here we present results of a few clinical trials using this platform.

Table 1 Summary of actively recruiting TCR cell therapies

Target	NCT identifier	Cancer type	Phase
MC2	NCT04729543	Melanoma Melanoma, uveal Head and neck cancer	1
LMP2	NCT03925896	Nasopharyngeal carcinoma	1
LMP1, LMP2 and EBNA1	NCT03648697	Nasopharyngeal carcinoma	2
HBV antigen	NCT03899415	Hepatocellular carcinoma	1
AFP	NCT03971747	Hepatocellular carcinoma	1
EBV antigen Secreted PD1 antagonist	NCT04139057	Head and neck squamous cell carcinoma	1
AFP	NCT04368182	Hepatocellular carcinoma	1
Tumor specific antigens	NCT03891706	Solid tumor	1
HPV E6 antigen Secreted PD1 antagonist	NCT03578406	Cervical cancer Head and neck squamous cell carcinoma	1
LMP2- IL12-secreting	NCT04509726	Nasopharyngeal carcinoma	1/2
NY-ESO-1	NCT03462316	Bone sarcoma Soft tissue sarcoma	1
Mutant KRAS G12V	NCT04146298	Pancreatic cancer Solid tumors	1/2
HBV	NCT04745403	Hepatocellular carcinoma	1
Mesothelin	NCT04809766	Pancreatic ductal adenocarcinoma	1
NY-ESO-1 DR5 EGFR VIII Mesothelin	NCT03941626	Esophagus cancer Hepatoma Glioma, hepatoma Gastric cancer	1/2
MCPyV With anti-PD1/PDL1	NCT03747484	Merkel cell	1/2
E7	NCT02858310	Cervical, vulvar, vaginal, penilc, anal, or oropharyngeal	1/2
MAGE-A1 With PD1 inhibitor	NCT04639245	Triple negative breast cancer, urothelial cancer, or non-small cell lung cancer	1/2
PRAME	NCT03503968	High risk myeloid and lymphoid neoplasms	1/2
NY-ESO-1	NCT03240861	Solid tumors/sarcoma	1
NY-ESO-1	NCT04878484	Solid tumors	1
HERV-E	NCT03354390	Kidney cancer	1
Up to 5 tumor specific antigens With CDX-1140 And Pembrolizumab	NCT04520711	Solid tumors	1

(continued)

Table 1 (continued)

Target	NCT identifier	Cancer type	Phase
NY-ESO-1	NCT02869217	Solid tumors	1
NY-ESO-1	NCT02774291	Solid tumors	1
MAGE-A1	NCT03441100	Solid tumors	1
MAGEA-4/8	NCT03247309	Solid tumors	1
PRAME	NCT03686124	Solid tumors	1
MAGE-A3/A6	NCT03139370	Solid tumors	1
Neo-antigens With nivolumab	NCT03970382	Solid tumors	1
NY-ESO-1/LAGE-1a With pembrolizumab	NCT03709706	Solid tumors	1
Melanoma antigen tyrosinase	NCT02870244	Melanoma	1
gp100	NCT03649529	Melanoma	1
NY-ESO-1 LAGE-1a	NCT04526509	Solid tumors	1
E7	NCT03912831	Human papillomavirus (HPV) 16+ relapsed/refractory cancer	1
AFP	NCT03132792	Hepatocellular cancer AFP expressing tumors	1
NY-ESO-1	NCT04318964	Soft tissue sarcoma	1
HBV	NCT03634683	Hepatocellular carcinoma	1/2
PRAME With anti-PD1	NCT04262466	Solid tumors	1
MAGE-A4	NCT03132922	Urinary bladder cancer Melanoma Head and neck cancer Ovarian cancer Non-small cell lung cancer Esophageal cancer Gastric cancer Synovial sarcoma Myxoid round cell Liposarcoma Gastroesophageal junction	1
NY-ESO-1 LAGE-1a	NCT03967223	Solid tumors	2
HA-1	NCT03326921	Relapsed leukemia	1

MART1

The first trial to demonstrate safety, feasibility and early clinical activity of this approach was a clinical trial of using anti–MART-1 TCR for treatment of patients with metastatic melanoma. The trial treated 17 patients with metastatic melanoma who also had HLA-A*0201 phenotype. The investigators were able to achieve transfection efficiencies of 17–62% and demonstrated relative safety of this approach with no major autoimmune toxicities. Two out of 17 patients experienced disease regression and prolonged clinical benefit. These patients had transfected cells that could be detected in the peripheral blood for up to 1 year after infusion [37]. A follow-up clinical trial (NCT00910650) tested targeting MART-1 through engineered TCR-T cell in patients with metastatic melanoma in a larger cohort of patients. Fourteen patients were tested with all eligible patients being HLA-A*0201 by HLA genotyping. Thirteen patients received treatment and nine demonstrated objective responses. The treatment was combined with DC vaccination with an observation of increased in vivo number of MART-1-specific T cells suggesting increased expansion. The trial also tested cryopreserved cells but demonstrated lower in vivo expansion of these cells and that these cryopreserved TCR-T cells were also found to be unresponsive to DC vaccination. The transfected T cells persisted in the peripheral blood for up 100 days [38].

A high affinity MART-1 TCR was developed and tested in 20 patients with MRT-1 expressing metastatic melanoma with HLA-A*02 (NCT00509288). Compared to previous MART-1 TCR-T trials increased INF-γ was detected in serum peaking at day 3–5 after cell infusion. There was noted to be on target off-tumor toxicity in majority of patients with evidence of anterior uveitis. Patients' symptoms resolved after ocular administration of steroid eyedrops. 10/20 50% developed hearing loss with 7 requiring intratympanic steroid injections with improvement and resolution of symptoms (two patients died from progressive disease prior to retesting). Six of the twenty treated patients (30%) showed objective tumor response. There was no correlation between responses and total number of cells infused but there was correlation between response and persistence of cells at 1 month and INF-γ and IL-2 detection. One patient had pre- and serial post-treatment biopsies of the subcutaneous lesion which showed T cell infiltration 5 days after cell infusion with evidence of progressive necrosis in subsequent biopsies correlating with partial response. Most of the T cell infiltrate was shown to be MART-1 tetramer-positive demonstrating treatment effect [39].

gp100

Phase II clinical trial, NCT00509288, evaluated the anti-gp100 TCR-T cell in 16 patients with metastatic melanoma HLA-A*02 restricted. Patients tolerated treatment relatively well but 13/16 81% developed skin erythema, 4/16 25% experienced anterior uveitis and 5/16 31% developed hearing loss. All of the toxicities resolved with minimal intervention with two patients requiring steroid eyedrops and one patients intratympanic steroid injection. Three out of sixteen (19%) of patients showed objective tumor responses. The trial demonstrated potential of the treatment with evidence of manageable predicted toxicities in tissues with known melanocytes [39].

CEA

TCR-T targeting CEA was tested in patients with metastatic colorectal cancer. CEA decrease was observed in all three treated patients and one patient demonstrated a partial response. All three patients experienced severe colitis and the clinical trial was stopped. This toxicity highlighted the potential for on target, but off-tumor antigen recognition expressed in normal tissues [27].

NY-ESO-1

Next strategy was to target the cancer testis antigen NY-ESO-1. NCT00670748 trial was targeting patients with NY-ESO-1 expressing metastatic synovial cell sarcoma and metastatic melanoma patients. Four out of six patients with synovial cell sarcoma who had NY-ESO-1 expression had documented partial responses. In one patient the response persisted for 18 months. Two patients with metastatic melanoma had complete responses with three of eleven patients having partial responses. The CRs persisted for over 1 year. There was no documented on- target off-tumor toxicities [40]. In an expansion cohort, patients also received a recombinant APIPOX oncolytic viral treatment which encoded the NY-ESO-1 HLA-A*0201 T cell epitope. There were no documented differences in toxicities or clinical responses between TCR or combination with virally treated groups. Eleven out of eighteen (61%) synovial cell sarcoma patients and eleven out of twenty (55%) melanoma patients demonstrated objective clinical responses. For synovial sarcoma cohort, one patient received two additional infusions of cells with documented responses after each treatment. In melanoma cohort, two patients received a second infusion without any evidence of responses. The responses did not correlate with persistence of TCR-T in the peripheral blood. Despite small numbers of patients, the treatment was felt to be safe and exhibiting promising clinical benefit [41].

A follow-up trial with engineered NY-ESO-1 TCR-T cells targeting HLA-A2–restricted NY-ESO-1 expressing synovial cell sarcomas was performed. It used an affinity enhanced TCR without IL2. Fifteen patients were deemed eligible but only twelve underwent treatment. The overall response rate (ORR) was 50% (six out of twelve) with one CR. Median time to response was 6.2 weeks with median duration of response of 30.9 weeks (13–72 weeks). Most grade 3 toxicities were due to chemotherapy treatment, but two patients had grade 3 CRS. There was no documented neurotoxicity. The cells were detectable in all transfused patients but were significantly higher in documented responders. The cells were also detectable in all six responders at 6 months as opposed to two out six non-responders. The results provided evidence for clinical activity with clinically meaningful response rate and disease control [42]. Next trial used a transfected T cells with TCR recognizing peptide shared by the cancer-testis antigens NY-ESO-1 and LAGE-1 in patients with multiple myeloma (MM). Twenty patients were treated with cell infusion

2 days after autologous bone marrow transplant. The median survival was 19.1 months with evidence of clinical response in 16 out of 20 patients. The continued clinical benefit was related to evidence of persistent transfected cells and persistence of antigen expression on the MM cells [43].

MAGE-A3

Clinical trial, NCT01273181, evaluated the safety and efficacy of anti-MAGE-A3 TCR engineered T cells. All patients had tumors which were expressing MAGE-A3 by IHC or RT-PCR and were HLA-A*0201. Nine patients were treated, most with metastatic melanoma, one with synovial cell sarcoma and one with esophageal cancer in a dose escalation schema from 5×10^9 to 1×10^{11} cells infused. Five out of nine patients demonstrated response with one CR and four PRs. Two of the responders (CR and PR) were in the initial, lower dose cohort. In higher dose cohort three patients experienced neurotoxicity leading to death in two of them. This result again highlights the promise of the engineered TCR T cell but also dangers and challenges of making the therapy safe for patients [44].

Two other trials tested targeting MAGE-A3 NCT01350401 and NCT01352286 targeting patients with melanoma and multiple myeloma, respectively. Patients had to have documented tumor expression of MAGE-A3 and HLA-A*01 allele. Unfortunately, the first two patients enrolled developed fever, hypoxia, and hypotension five to 7 days after the cell infusion. Both patients died and extensive analysis showed that TCR T-cell mediated cardiac injury was the likely cause and the testing was stopped [45].

MAGE-A4

A trial in patients with esophageal cancer used TCR targeting MAGE-A4 (UMIN000002395). The engineered TCR T cell therapy was combined with a peptide vaccination. The additional difference was that the treatment did not include a preconditioning regimen. Ten patients were treated in three dose cohorts. All patients had squamous cell esophageal cancer with MAGE4 expression confirmed by PCR for nine and one by IHC. Three patients had day 35 tumor biopsy, in one out of these three there were detectable TCR-T cells which accounted for 10% of all PBMCs. Five patients had established persistence of transfected cells for at least 200 days with one for a period of 800 days. Administration of the peptide vaccine had no measurable effect on transfected T cell numbers. Out of seven patients with evaluable responses best response obeserved was stable disease. The three patients without RECIST criteria for measurable disease had no evidence of progression for over 1 year. There was no correlation between persistence of transfected cells and tumor responses. There were no high grade TCR-T cell related toxicities observed [46].

Toxicities

Treatment with TCT-T cells holds a promise of effective anti-cancer therapy but there is also potential for severe toxicities. Most toxicities reported in clinical trials are associated with the preconditioning lymphodepleting chemotherapy regimen which can be difficult to administer in highly pre-treated patient population. Neutropenic fever and infections are more common in the period immediately following the chemotherapy. The diagnosis is often more difficult due to TCR-T cell infusion during this period with subsequent initiation of IL2 treatment. The experience with CAR-T cell treatments has taught us many valuable clinical lessons resulting in improved safety for patients.

There are also more specific toxicities related to TCR-T cell themselves. Most tumor associated antigens are also expressed on normal cells at lower levels which can lead to on target off-tumor toxicity. The transfected T cells continue to have endogenous T cell receptor. Transfection of TCR gene may disrupt function of the endogenous T cell receptor leading to increased response to self-antigens causing autoimmune reaction. Also, transduced TCR can form dimers with endogenous TCR resulting in loss of tumor specificity and potential for autoimmune toxicity [47]. TCR-T cell therapy can most likely be safely administered even when transfecting T cells recognizing self-antigen as long as the level of the antigen is relatively low [48]. Transfecting TCR gene to more monoclonal population of T cells decreases the risk of unanticipated autoimmune response [49].

Transfection of TCR gene product often is achieved through use of viral vector. There is a theoretical danger of the viral vector achieving ability to self-replicate. Analysis of patient samples post infusion of the cell product did not show any evidence of self-replicating virus [50, 51]. This theoretical toxicity is further attenuated by novel, non-viral means of transfecting the TCR gene.

Off-tumor on-target or cross-reactivity of TCR remains a major potential for autoimmune toxicity in treatment with TCR-T cell therapies. The experience with targeting MAGE-A3 showed that the neurotoxicity that developed in three patients was most likely a result of the transfected cell. In the two deceased patients there was necrotic brain tissue with lymphocytic infiltration. Further analysis showed expression of MAGE-A12 in the brains of these patients [44]. Subsequent attempt with targeting different epitope of MAGE-A3 resulted in deaths in the first two patients. Both cases underwent extensive investigation, and both were found to be related to TCR-T cell infusion. There was evidence of lymphocytic infiltrates in the cardiac tissues. Further analysis discovered that the MAGE-A3 TCR can cross react to epitope of titin protein found in cardiac smooth muscles [45].

In the trial targeting CEA in patients with metastatic colorectal cancer all three patients developed severe colitis leading to early termination of the trial. The colon samples showed large infiltration of CD3+ T cells. With known expression of CEA in small intestine and colon cells this was an example of off-tumor on target toxicity [27].

Targeting MART-1 with a high affinity TCR resulted in increased off-tumor toxicities when compared to previous studies. Patients experienced skin erythema

(70% 14/20), anterior uveitis (55% 11/20) and ototoxicity (50% 10/20). Fortunately, all the toxicities were temporary. Skin biopsies showed CD3+ T lymphocyte infiltrate with evidence of destruction of epidermal melanocytes. These patients eventually developed vitiligo. The rash resolved in all patients without intervention. Interestingly, in two patients who had pre-existing vitiligo the rash only developed in pigmented skin areas, further providing evidence of on-target off-tumor toxicity. Melanocytes are found in the eye which is the explanation for the finding of anterior uveitis. One patient had sampling of the eye anterior chamber fluid which demonstrated MART-1 tetramer-positive T cells. Melanocytes also exist in the striae vascularis of the inner ear which explains the hearing loss in these patients. The increase in on-target off-tumor toxicities was most likely the result of increased affinity to MART-1 of modified TCR resulting in TCR-T cell activation at lower level of MART-1 expression [39].

Strategies to Enhance TCR-T Efficacy

There are potential resistance mechanisms that tumors employ to develop resistance to T cell therapies. The cancer cells can downregulate processing and expression of antigens or MHC proteins preventing T cell recognition [52]. One strategy to overcome MHC pairing limitations and downregulation of MHC expression is using TCRs that are MHC independent (reviewed [53, 54]). HLA independent TCRs can target multiple tumor specific antigens, pathogen derived lipids, metabolites, phospho-antigens and stress-ligands and they offer an attractive modality to overcome limitation and resistance to TCR therapies. Another strategy is to redirect the TCR to cell surface antigens by engineering an antibody-derived specific recognition domain. Using T cell antigen coupler (TAC) results in efficient TCR signaling while targeting MHC independent surface antigens which may have theoretical advantages over CAR-T cell approaches targeting the same surface proteins in an MHC independent fashion [55, 56].

The tumor microenvironment can support tumor growth and shield them from therapies with TCR engineered T cells and other immunotherapies [57]. The tumor stroma made up of predominantly tumor associated cells can limit T cells from interacting with tumor cells directly [58]. Often tumors downregulate expression of molecules that serve as homing signals for T cells thus preventing migration and infiltration of TCR engineered cells [59] . Once T cells are able to overcome these barriers and come into direct contact with tumor cells there still may be other limitations for optimal TCR-T cell anti tumor effects including the lack of stimulatory cytokines and over expression of suppressive molecules that reduce their function [60]. Newer approaches are addressing potential resistance mechanisms to cellular therapy. Several approaches are being investigated to improve TCR T cell infiltration through expression of cytokine and growth factor receptors [61–64]. Introduction of positive co-stimulatory molecules or deletion of negative co-stimulatory molecules in CAR-T cells have been extensively studies and these approaches are being investigated clinically with TCR engineered cells. MAGE-A3 cells transduced with CXCR2 had increased infiltration into tumors in mouse models [65]. There are several approaches of directing T cells to the stroma component which led to increased tumor infiltration of T cells. Fibroblast activation protein (FAP) targeting lead to increased infiltration of EphA2+ tumor cells [66]. FAP CAR-T cells led to increase in tumor infiltration of CD8+ cells with increased anti-tumor responses [67]. FAP directed cells led to increased survival of mice in pancreatic model [68]. Therefore, targeting the tumor stroma may result in increased tumor associated T cell infiltration and may represent a viable combination strategy to increase efficacy of TCR engineered T cells.

In the context of many clinical trials the persistence of transfected TCR-T cells was correlated with enhanced clinical responses. Groups are testing additional T cell modifications to enhance T cell persistence by decreasing apoptosis signals [69–72]. Reduced expansion of T cells after infusion can also lead to decreased clinical responses. Researchers are also working to enhance engineered T cell proliferation often by adding growth factor receptors whose ligands are expressed in the tumor microenvironment [73–75]. There are also several approaches being tested to overcome tumor immune-suppressive microenvironment by targeting AKT or TGFβ or through adding positive co-stimulatory stimulatory molecules to TCR-T and to CART [76–78].

Conclusion

Although adoptive cellular therapy approaches using engineered TCR-T cells show considerable promise for the treatment of solid tumors there continues to be challenges in making them widely available in clinic. Genomic and phenotypic heterogeneity of solid tumors may lead to different levels of neoantigen expression making effective anti-tumor activity of TCR-T even more challenging. In mouse models it has been shown that neoantigen expression can change under selective pressure and a broad neoantigen targeting approach might be necessary for higher and more persistent anti-tumor responses [79, 80]. Identification of more tumor-specific antigens continues to expand the list of potential targets for both TCR-T and CAR-T therapies. Improved sequencing techniques and algorithms hold promise for identification of specific, shared tumor associated antigens and neoantigens. There are currently over 100 active protocols using various TCR-T cell approaches in United States and over 200 around the world [35, 36] with actively recruiting trials shown in Table 1. Majority of the trials target solid tumor malignancies and are in the early stages of investigation. Cost, limited patient selection, time of manufacturing and requirement for hospital administration continue to be barriers to clinical translation. Increasingly, protocols include combinatorial approaches to enhance activity, infiltration, and persistence of engineered T cells. Improved targeting, antigen selection and toxicity profile together with better understanding of mechanisms of resistance will expand the promise of this therapeutic approach to more patients.

References

1. García-Teijido P, Cabal ML, Fernández IP, Pérez YF. Tumor-infiltrating lymphocytes in triple negative breast cancer: the future of immune targeting. Clin Med Insights Oncol. 2016;10:31–9.
2. Paijens ST, Vledder A, de Bruyn M, Nijman HW. Tumor-infiltrating lymphocytes in the immunotherapy era. Cell Mol Immunol. 2021;18:842–59.
3. Mardanpour K, Rahbar M, Mardanpour S, Mardanpour N, Rezaei M. CD8+ T-cell lymphocytes infiltration predict clinical outcomes in Wilms' tumor. Tumour Biol. 2020;42:1010428320975976.
4. Zloza A, Al-Harthi L. Multiple populations of T lymphocytes are distinguished by the level of CD4 and CD8 coexpression and require individual consideration. J Leukoc Biol. 2006;79:4–6.
5. Parrot T, Oger R, Allard M, et al. Transcriptomic features of tumour-infiltrating CD4(low) CD8(high) double positive alphabeta T cells in melanoma. Sci Rep. 2020;10:5900.
6. Hamann D, Baars PA, Rep MH, et al. Phenotypic and functional separation of memory and effector human CD8+ T cells. J Exp Med. 1997;186:1407–18.
7. Jiang Y, Li Y, Zhu B. T-cell exhaustion in the tumor microenvironment. Cell Death Dis. 2015;6:e1792.
8. Xia A, Zhang Y, Xu J, Yin T, Lu X-J. T cell dysfunction in cancer immunity and immunotherapy. Front Immunol. 2019;10:1719.
9. Egelston CA, Avalos C, Tu TY, et al. Human breast tumor-infiltrating CD8(+) T cells retain polyfunctionality despite PD-1 expression. Nat Commun. 2018;9:4297.
10. Pauken KE, Wherry EJ. Overcoming T cell exhaustion in infection and cancer. Trends Immunol. 2015;36:265–76.
11. Topalian SL, Hodi FS, Brahmer JR, et al. Safety, activity, and immune correlates of anti-PD-1 antibody in cancer. N Engl J Med. 2012;366:2443–54.
12. Topalian SL, Sznol M, McDermott DF, et al. Survival, durable tumor remission, and long-term safety in patients with advanced melanoma receiving nivolumab. J Clin Oncol. 2014;32:1020–30.
13. Shitara K, Van Cutsem E, Bang YJ, et al. Efficacy and safety of Pembrolizumab or Pembrolizumab plus chemotherapy vs chemotherapy alone for patients with first-line, advanced gastric cancer: the KEYNOTE-062 phase 3 randomized clinical trial. JAMA Oncol. 2020;6:1571–80.
14. Maubec E, Boubaya M, Petrow P, et al. Phase II study of Pembrolizumab as first-line, single-drug therapy for patients with unresectable cutaneous squamous cell carcinomas. J Clin Oncol. 2020;38:3051–61.
15. Burtness B, Harrington KJ, Greil R, et al. Pembrolizumab alone or with chemotherapy versus cetuximab with chemotherapy for recurrent or metastatic squamous cell carcinoma of the head and neck (KEYNOTE-048): a randomised, open-label, phase 3 study. Lancet (London, England). 2019;394:1915–28.
16. Hodi FS, Chiarion-Sileni V, Gonzalez R, et al. Nivolumab plus ipilimumab or nivolumab alone versus ipilimumab alone in advanced melanoma (CheckMate 067): 4-year outcomes of a multicentre, randomised, phase 3 trial. Lancet Oncol. 2018;19:1480–92.
17. Schmid P, Adams S, Rugo HS, et al. Atezolizumab and nab-paclitaxel in advanced triple-negative breast cancer. N Engl J Med. 2018;379:2108–21.
18. Robert C, Schachter J, Long GV, et al. Pembrolizumab versus Ipilimumab in Advanced Melanoma. N Engl J Med. 2015;372:2521–32.
19. Mok TSK, Wu YL, Kudaba I, et al. Pembrolizumab versus chemotherapy for previously untreated, PD-L1-expressing, locally advanced or metastatic non-small-cell lung cancer (KEYNOTE-042): a randomised, open-label, controlled, phase 3 trial. Lancet (London, England). 2019;393:1819–30.
20. Garassino MC, Gadgeel S, Esteban E, et al. Patient-reported outcomes following pembrolizumab or placebo plus pemetrexed and platinum in patients with previously untreated, metastatic, non-squamous non-small-cell lung cancer (KEYNOTE-189): a multicentre, double-blind, randomised, placebo-controlled, phase 3 trial. Lancet Oncol. 2020;21:387–97.

21. Hedrick SM, Cohen DI, Nielsen EA, Davis MM. Isolation of cDNA clones encoding T cell-specific membrane-associated proteins. Nature. 1984;308:149–53.
22. Yanagi Y, Yoshikai Y, Leggett K, Clark SP, Aleksander I, Mak TW. A human T cell-specific cDNA clone encodes a protein having extensive homology to immunoglobulin chains. Nature. 1984;308:145–9.
23. Dudley ME, Wunderlich JR, Robbins PF, et al. Cancer regression and autoimmunity in patients after clonal repopulation with antitumor lymphocytes. Science. 2002;298:850–4.
24. Ahmadzadeh M, Johnson LA, Heemskerk B, et al. Tumor antigen-specific CD8 T cells infiltrating the tumor express high levels of PD-1 and are functionally impaired. Blood. 2009;114:1537–44.
25. Rosenberg SA, Packard BS, Aebersold PM, et al. Use of tumor-infiltrating lymphocytes and interleukin-2 in the immunotherapy of patients with metastatic melanoma. A preliminary report. N Engl J Med. 1988;319:1676–80.
26. Rosenberg SA, Restifo NP, Yang JC, Morgan RA, Dudley ME. Adoptive cell transfer: a clinical path to effective cancer immunotherapy. Nat Rev Cancer. 2008;8:299–308.
27. Parkhurst MR, Yang JC, Langan RC, et al. T cells targeting carcinoembryonic antigen can mediate regression of metastatic colorectal cancer but induce severe transient colitis. Mol Ther. 2011;19:620–6.
28. Stanislawski T, Voss RH, Lotz C, et al. Circumventing tolerance to a human MDM2-derived tumor antigen by TCR gene transfer. Nat Immunol. 2001;2:962–70.
29. Gehring AJ, Xue SA, Ho ZZ, et al. Engineering virus-specific T cells that target HBV infected hepatocytes and hepatocellular carcinoma cell lines. J Hepatol. 2011;55:103–10.
30. Scholten KB, Turksma AW, Ruizendaal JJ, et al. Generating HPV specific T helper cells for the treatment of HPV induced malignancies using TCR gene transfer. J Transl Med. 2011;9:147.
31. Jurgens LA, Khanna R, Weber J, Orentas RJ. Transduction of primary lymphocytes with Epstein-Barr virus (EBV) latent membrane protein-specific T-cell receptor induces lysis of virus-infected cells: a novel strategy for the treatment of Hodgkin's disease and nasopharyngeal carcinoma. J Clin Immunol. 2006;26:22–32.
32. Robbins PF, Li YF, El-Gamil M, et al. Single and dual amino acid substitutions in TCR CDRs can enhance antigen-specific T cell functions. J Immunol (Baltimore, Md : 1950). 2008;180:6116–31.
33. Pleasance ED, Cheetham RK, Stephens PJ, et al. A comprehensive catalogue of somatic mutations from a human cancer genome. Nature. 2010;463:191–6.
34. Johnson LA, Heemskerk B, Powell DJ, Jr., et al. Gene transfer of tumor-reactive TCR confers both high avidity and tumor reactivity to nonreactive peripheral blood mononuclear cells and tumor-infiltrating lymphocytes. J Immunol (Baltimore, Md : 1950) 2006;177:6548–59.
35. Oppermans N, Kueberuwa G, Hawkins RE, Bridgeman JS. Transgenic T-cell receptor immunotherapy for cancer: building on clinical success. Ther Adv Vacc Immunother. 2020;8:2515135520933509.
36. Cancer Cell Therapy Landscape. 2021. https://www.cancerresearch.org/scientists/immuno-oncology-landscape/cancer-cell-therapy-landscape. Accessed 14 June 2021
37. Morgan RA, Dudley ME, Wunderlich JR, et al. Cancer regression in patients after transfer of genetically engineered lymphocytes. Science. 2006;314:126–9.
38. Chodon T, Comin-Anduix B, Chmielowski B, et al. Adoptive transfer of MART-1 T-cell receptor transgenic lymphocytes and dendritic cell vaccination in patients with metastatic melanoma. Clin Cancer Res. 2014;20:2457–65.
39. Johnson LA, Morgan RA, Dudley ME, et al. Gene therapy with human and mouse T-cell receptors mediates cancer regression and targets normal tissues expressing cognate antigen. Blood. 2009;114:535–46.
40. Robbins PF, Morgan RA, Feldman SA, et al. Tumor regression in patients with metastatic synovial cell sarcoma and melanoma using genetically engineered lymphocytes reactive with NY-ESO-1. J Clin Oncol. 2011;29:917–24.
41. Robbins PF, Kassim SH, Tran TLN, et al. A pilot trial using lymphocytes genetically engineered with an NY-ESO-1-reactive T-cell receptor: long-term follow-up and correlates with response. Clin Cancer Res. 2015;21:1019–27.

42. D'Angelo SP, Melchiori L, Merchant MS, et al. Antitumor activity associated with prolonged persistence of adoptively transferred NY-ESO-1 (c259)T cells in synovial sarcoma. Cancer Discov. 2018;8:944–57.
43. Rapoport AP, Stadtmauer EA, Binder-Scholl GK, et al. NY-ESO-1–specific TCR–engineered T cells mediate sustained antigen-specific antitumor effects in myeloma. Nat Med. 2015;21:914–21.
44. Morgan RA, Chinnasamy N, Abate-Daga D, et al. Cancer regression and neurological toxicity following anti-MAGE-A3 TCR gene therapy. J Immunother. 2013;36:133–51.
45. Linette GP, Stadtmauer EA, Maus MV, et al. Cardiovascular toxicity and titin cross-reactivity of affinity-enhanced T cells in myeloma and melanoma. Blood. 2013;122:863–71.
46. Kageyama S, Ikeda H, Miyahara Y, et al. Adoptive transfer of MAGE-A4 T-cell receptor gene-transduced lymphocytes in patients with recurrent esophageal cancer. Clin Cancer Res. 2015;21:2268–77.
47. Bendle GM, Linnemann C, Hooijkaas AI, et al. Lethal graft-versus-host disease in mouse models of T cell receptor gene therapy. Nat Med. 2010;16:565–70; 1p following 70
48. Weinhold M, Sommermeyer D, Uckert W, Blankenstein T. Dual T cell receptor expressing CD8+ T cells with tumor- and self-specificity can inhibit tumor growth without causing severe autoimmunity. J Immunol (Baltimore, Md : 1950). 2007;179:5534–42.
49. Heemskerk MH, Hoogeboom M, Hagedoorn R, Kester MG, Willemze R, Falkenburg JH. Reprogramming of virus-specific T cells into leukemia-reactive T cells using T cell receptor gene transfer. J Exp Med. 2004;199:885–94.
50. Cornetta K, Duffy L, Turtle CJ, et al. Absence of replication-competent lentivirus in the clinic: analysis of infused T cell products. Mol Ther. 2018;26:280–8.
51. Marcucci KT, Jadlowsky JK, Hwang W-T, et al. Retroviral and lentiviral safety analysis of gene-modified T cell products and infused HIV and oncology patients. Mol Ther. 2018;26:269–79.
52. Restifo NP, Marincola FM, Kawakami Y, Taubenberger J, Yannelli JR, Rosenberg SA. Loss of functional beta 2-microglobulin in metastatic melanomas from five patients receiving immunotherapy. J Natl Cancer Inst. 1996;88:100–8.
53. Mori L, Lepore M, De Libero G. The immunology of CD1- and MR1-restricted T cells. Annu Rev Immunol. 2016;34:479–510.
54. Godfrey DI, Uldrich AP, McCluskey J, Rossjohn J, Moody DB. The burgeoning family of unconventional T cells. Nat Immunol. 2015;16:1114–23.
55. Curtsinger JM, Lins DC, Mescher MF. CD8+ memory T cells (CD44high, Ly-6C+) are more sensitive than naive cells to (CD44low, Ly-6C-) to TCR/CD8 signaling in response to antigen. J Immunol (Baltimore, Md : 1950). 1998;160:3236–43.
56. Baeuerle PA, Ding J, Patel E, et al. Synthetic TRuC receptors engaging the complete T cell receptor for potent anti-tumor response. Nat Commun. 2019;10:2087.
57. Motz GT, Coukos G. The parallel lives of angiogenesis and immunosuppression: cancer and other tales. Nat Rev Immunol. 2011;11:702–11.
58. Lanitis E, Dangaj D, Irving M, Coukos G. Mechanisms regulating T-cell infiltration and activity in solid tumors. Ann Oncol. 2017;28:xii18–32.
59. Nagarsheth N, Wicha MS, Zou W. Chemokines in the cancer microenvironment and their relevance in cancer immunotherapy. Nat Rev Immunol. 2017;17:559–72.
60. Binnewies M, Roberts EW, Kersten K, et al. Understanding the tumor immune microenvironment (TIME) for effective therapy. Nat Med. 2018;24:541–50.
61. Craddock JA, Lu A, Bear A, et al. Enhanced tumor trafficking of GD2 chimeric antigen receptor T cells by expression of the chemokine receptor CCR2b. J Immunother. 2010;33:780–8.
62. Chinnasamy D, Yu Z, Kerkar SP, et al. Local delivery of Interleukin-12 using T cells targeting VEGF Receptor-2 eradicates multiple vascularized tumors in mice. Clin Cancer Res. 2012;18:1672.
63. Buckanovich RJ, Facciabene A, Kim S, et al. Endothelin B receptor mediates the endothelial barrier to T cell homing to tumors and disables immune therapy. Nat Med. 2008;14:28–36.
64. Legler DF, Johnson-Léger C, Wiedle G, Bron C, Imhof BA. The α vβ 3 integrin as a tumor homing ligand for lymphocytes. Eur J Immunol. 2004;34:1608–16.

65. Idorn M, Skadborg SK, Kellermann L, et al. Chemokine receptor engineering of T cells with CXCR2 improves homing towards subcutaneous human melanomas in xenograft mouse model. Onco Targets Ther. 2018;7:e1450715.
66. Kakarla S, Chow KK, Mata M, et al. Antitumor effects of chimeric receptor engineered human T cells directed to tumor stroma. Mol Ther. 2013;21:1611–20.
67. Wang LC, Lo A, Scholler J, et al. Targeting fibroblast activation protein in tumor stroma with chimeric antigen receptor T cells can inhibit tumor growth and augment host immunity without severe toxicity. Cancer Immunol Res. 2014;2:154–66.
68. Schuberth PC, Hagedorn C, Jensen SM, et al. Treatment of malignant pleural mesothelioma by fibroblast activation protein-specific re-directed T cells. J Transl Med. 2013;11:187.
69. Emtage PCR, Lo ASY, Gomes EM, Liu DL, Gonzalo-Daganzo RM, Junghans RP. Second-generation anti–carcinoembryonic antigen designer T cells resist activation-induced cell death, proliferate on tumor contact, secrete cytokines, and exhibit superior antitumor activity in vivo: a preclinical evaluation. Clin Cancer Res 2008;14:8112.
70. Dotti G, Savoldo B, Pule M, et al. Human cytotoxic T lymphocytes with reduced sensitivity to Fas-induced apoptosis. Blood. 2005;105:4677–84.
71. Lei X-Y, Xu Y-M, Wang T, et al. Knockdown of human bid gene expression enhances survival of CD8+ T cells. Immunol Lett. 2009;122:30–6.
72. Charo J, Finkelstein SE, Grewal N, Restifo NP, Robbins PF, Rosenberg SA. Bcl-2 overexpression enhances tumor-specific T-cell survival. Cancer Res. 2005;65:2001–8.
73. Lo ASY, Taylor JR, Farzaneh F, Kemeny DM, Dibb NJ, Maher J. Harnessing the tumour-derived cytokine, CSF-1, to co-stimulate T-cell growth and activation. Mol Immunol. 2008;45:1276–87.
74. Stromnes IM, Fowler C, Casamina CC, et al. Abrogation of Src homology region 2 domain-containing phosphatase 1 in tumor-specific T cells improves efficacy of adoptive immunotherapy by enhancing the effector function and accumulation of short-lived effector T cells in vivo. J Immunol. 2012;189:1812.
75. Cooper LJN, Al-Kadhimi Z, Serrano LM, et al. Enhanced antilymphoma efficacy of CD19-redirected influenza MP1–specific CTLs by cotransfer of T cells modified to present influenza MP1. Blood. 2005;105:1622–31.
76. Koehler H, Kofler D, Hombach A, Abken H. CD28 Costimulation overcomes transforming growth factor-β–mediated repression of proliferation of redirected human CD4+ and CD8+ T cells in an antitumor cell attack. Cancer Res. 2007;67:2265–73.
77. Sun J, Dotti G, Huye LE, et al. T cells expressing constitutively active Akt resist multiple tumor-associated inhibitory mechanisms. Mol Ther. 2010;18:2006–17.
78. Bollard CM, Rössig C, Calonge MJ, et al. Adapting a transforming growth factor β–related tumor protection strategy to enhance antitumor immunity. Blood. 2002;99:3179–87.
79. Verdegaal EME, de Miranda NFCC, Visser M, et al. Neoantigen landscape dynamics during human melanoma–T cell interactions. Nature. 2016;536:91–5.
80. Matsushita H, Vesely MD, Koboldt DC, et al. Cancer exome analysis reveals a T-cell-dependent mechanism of cancer immunoediting. Nature. 2012;482:400–4.

Part V
Viral CTLs

Viral Cytotoxic T Lymphocytes (CTLs): From Bench to Bedside

Susan E. Prockop and Sanam Shahid

Abstract It was first demonstrated almost three decades ago that adoptive transfer of viral-specific T cells could prevent or eradicate viral disease in immune-compromised recipients of allogeneic hematopoetic stem cell transplant (HCT). Since then, advances in our understanding of cellular therapy products as well as in production methods have led to progress in this field now on the brink of having FDA-approved products available for treatment of patients in need. This chapter will highlight some of those advances, as well as the clinical experience to date in the use of these products.

Keywords Viral-specific T cells · Viral cytotoxic T lymphocytes (CTLs) · PTLD · CMV · EBV · BK · Adenovirus · HHV6 · GVHD · Latent membrane protein (LMP) · CMVpp65 · MHC · HLA

History

Unlike other arenas of cellular and gene therapy, few of the advances in the field of viral-specific T cell therapies have been established in pre-clinical animal models prior to first-in-human studies. This is in large part due to a paucity of good models for the human infectious diseases that occur in the immune-compromised recipients of HCT. In 1985, Reddehase and colleagues described the population of T cells mediating control of murine CMV pneumonitis [1] and demonstrated that transfer of syngeneic, polyclonal CD8+ T cells, but not CD4+ T cells, from immune-competent mice could protect immunosuppressed mice from LCMV infection [2]. Subsequent advances in our understanding of viral-specific T cell responses [3–5] increased interest in this approach, and a decade later, it was demonstrated that in humans, bulk populations of lymphocytes from seropositive HCT donors contained sufficient numbers of polyclonal viral-specific T cells to successfully control adenovirus [6],

S. E. Prockop (✉) · S. Shahid
Department of Pediatrics, Memorial Sloan Kettering Cancer Center, New York, NY, USA
e-mail: prockops@mskcc.org

© Springer Nature Switzerland AG 2022
A. Ghobadi, J. F. DiPersio (eds.), *Gene and Cellular Immunotherapy for Cancer*, Cancer Drug Discovery and Development,
https://doi.org/10.1007/978-3-030-87849-8_15

HHV6 [7] and Epstein-Barr virus (EBV) lymphoproliferative disease arising after HCT [8] even in the CNS, although with the potential risk of graft-versus-host disease (GVHD). At the same time, several groups were establishing in vitro culture methods to enrich for either clonal [9] or polyclonal [10] viral-specific cytotoxic T cells and demonstrating the in vivo efficacy of these populations [11–13].

These early studies led to multiple reports, primarily in small cohorts of patients enrolled on Phase I and Phase II trials. Subsequent advances included techniques for more rapid generation and selection, identification of the immunodominance of certain viral antigens and HLA presentation of these antigens, characterization of the phenotype and function of T cells for adoptive transfer, and the expansion of these therapies to target other viruses. Finally, the use of banked, third-party viral-specific T cells extends the potential of this therapy beyond what can be offered by a few specialized centers. Trials have now been reported using these approaches, and adoptive T cell therapy for viral infections and virally driven malignancy in immunocompromised hosts is more broadly applicable and available.

Simultaneously, investigators have continued to explore whether these approaches can be expanded to immunocompetent individuals with virus-bearing tumors.

Generation

The first products for adoptive T cell therapy targeted CMV and were generated using anti-CD3 and CD28 monoclonal antibodies to clone cytotoxic T lymphocytes (CTLs) generated against CMV-infected fibroblasts from normal CMV-seropositive donors [14]. The clones were assayed for CMV-specific cytotoxicity in a chromium-release assay [15]. In these early studies, clones that lysed more than 30% of CMV-positive target cells and less than 5% of control target cells at an effector:target (E:T) ratio of 5:1 were characterized for their antigen recognition. The predominant specificity of these clones was for the CMV structural proteins pp65 and pp150, as demonstrated by coculture with daptomycin [15], establishing that the pp65 protein is immunogenic [16].

The first polyclonal viral-specific CTLs for use in clinical trials were generated against EBV [10, 13] using a method initially developed by Rickinson et al [17]. Lymphoblastoid cell lines (BLCLs) were generated by infection of donor PBMCs with a laboratory strain of the EBV virus, B95.8. These BLCLs present both latent and lytic EBV viral antigens with the most immunogenic proteins including EBNA 3a, 3b, and 3c, BLZF1, BMLF1, BRLF1, and BMRF1. Donor PBMCs were co-cultured with irradiated BLCLs, re-stimulated with IL-2 weekly at an E:T ratio of 4:1, then transduced with a G1Na retroviral vector with an efficacy of 1–10%. These EBV-CTLs were characterized for EBV specificity, immunophenotype, HLA typing, sterility, and absence of competent retrovirus.

The most formidable limitation of these early approaches was the 12–15 weeks it took to generate each line. Given that patients diagnosed with EBV PTLD typically receive first line therapy with a month of rituximab, and those with disease that is refractory to rituximab have a median overall survival as short as 13–31 days [18–20], a two-plus month process cannot start only when disease is diagnosed. Thus, it was necessary to generate lines in advance of patient need, but for rare indications this proved impractical. Two major advances have circumvented this issue: (1) methods for rapid expansion and selection of viral-specific T cells (Fig. 1)

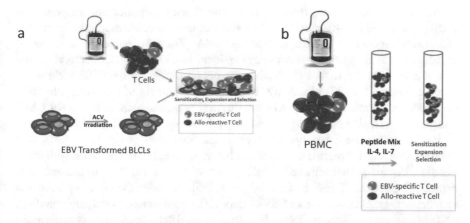

Fig. 1 Generation of viral-specific CTLs using (**a**) cultured professional antigen presenting cells. These cultured professional antigen presenting cells can be EBV transformed BLCLs (as depicted) or monocyte-derived DCs and can be transduced to present other viral antigens or pulsed with peptides from other viral antigens or (**b**) avoiding the use of cultured antigen presenting cells. PBMCs can be stimulated with immunogenic viral peptides and selected immediately based on IFNg or Streptamer/Tetramer binding or, as depicted, expanded in a peptide and cytokine cocktail

and (2) established banks of well-characterized viral-specific T cells, allowing use of third-party, partially HLA-matched lines.

The first advance in generating populations of viral-specific CTLs more rapidly was the use of monocyte-derived dendritic cells (Mo-DC) as the initial antigen presenting cells (APCs). This approach requires genetic modification with recombinant adenoviral or lentiviral vectors encoding, e.g., latent membrane protein (LMP) or other viral antigens [21, 22]. However, limitations in generating sufficient numbers of mo-DCs meant that this approach initially required a second round of stimulation with the more time-consuming BLCLs [23–25]. Alternatively, other sources of mo-DCs were also explored, including isolation of PBMCs from leukoreduction chambers [26]. Alternative sources of APCs included activated monocytes [27], artificial APCs [28], or viral antigen mRNA-electroporated CD40-B cells that could induce virus-specific CD8+ T cell responses after 7 days of co-culture [29]. Ultimately the introduction of gas-permeable systems and optimized cytokine cocktails eliminated the need for the second stimulation and decreased production time to 10–14 days [30].

In addition to a more rapid generation timeline, this system also allowed expansion of LMP2-directed and even LMP1-directed EBV CTLs, which could be preferentially used in targeting tumors expressing the less immunogenic EBV antigens such as the LMP proteins expressed by Hodgkin Lymphomas. As intracellular LMP1 is toxic, this system was optimized with an inactive but still immunogenic vector [31]. Similarly, other methods for improving antigenic stimulation have been introduced [32], including the addition of inhibitors of the potent anti-inflammatory protein A20. Monocyte-derived DCs can also be transduced with adenoviral vectors expressing other viral antigens such as CMVpp65 [33] or with HIV viral vectors to stimulate HIV-directed T cells. This system can generate clonal [34] as well as polyclonal [23] populations sufficient for clinical use in a 3–5 week period.

Advances in identifying the immunodominant viral peptides and responses to these peptides led investigators to use a variety of more specific methods for ex vivo stimulation, including electroporation of DNA plasmids encoding a range of immunodominant and subdominant viral antigens into DCs [35]. Concern about the risk of using intact virus as well as advances in optimizing the cytokine cocktail for T cell expansion [36, 37] ultimately led to the abandonment of this system in favor of broader adoption of pulsing APCs with viral peptides such as those for CMV antigen [38–41], also potentially shortening production to a 12–14 day period [42].

Finally, systems were developed that eliminated the need for professional APCs, with improved methods for peptide stimulation either independent of or combined with direct isolation. Peptide pulsed-activated T cells grown with IL-4 and IL-7 in a G-rex flask expands viral-specific T cells in a 10 day period [35]. However, the same approach was insufficient to generate autologous EBV-specific CTLs from patients with lymphoma [43].

Direct selection of specific T cells is another method that allows for very rapid availability of viral-specific T cells. These are based on either viral peptide multimers conjugated to magnetic beads to select highly pure cytotoxic T cells or stimulation with viral peptides followed by IFN-gamma capture with magnetic beads [44]. Limitations of these methods include generation of only CD8+ T cells and relatively limited numbers of viral-specific T cells, limiting the extent to which they can be further characterized prior to infusion. No studies have directly compared clinical responses or toxicity using these approaches, but overall responses are summarized in Table 1.

Multi-Viral Targeted Cells

The second advance that has substantially expanded the application of viral-specific, T cells is the targeting of viral infections beyond EBV and CMV, such that viral-specific CTLs are now part of the armamentarium for adenovirus, BK viral infection, and HHV6. Most recently, investigators are exploring the treatment of acquired viral infections such as Respiratory Syncytial Virus and even Sars-COV-2 with adoptive T cell therapy.

Genetic modification of EBV-BLCLs and Mo-DC APCs were the first modifications leading to multi-viral directed CTLs [23]. EBV+ BLCLs transduced with adenoviral vectors encoding CMVpp65 generated CTL lines with T cells specific to all three viruses. Electroporation of DNA plasmids with a range of viral peptides into the DCs similarly presents multiple viral antigens to T cells in culture. Subsequent advances introduced the use of peptide-pulsed APCs, enabling the expansion of T cell populations recognizing specific antigens of CMV or EBV. In addition to allowing the generation of T cells recognizing multiple different viral epitopes, this approach also enables expansion of T cells recognizing only specific viral epitopes. For example, it allows recognition of EBV disease expressing a more restricted set of EBV latency proteins. Finally, the need for professional APCs can be eliminated completely by culturing PBMCs with cytokines and peptide mixes [35]. In this approach, the PBMCs themselves serve as APCs. This approach also allows the

Table 1 Experience using EBV CTLs

A. Autologous EBV CTLs

Study	Method of selection	Treatment setting	N	Response (CR + PR)
Khanna et al., Proc Natl Acad Sci USA, 1999	EBV-BLCL sensitized EBV-CTL	PTLD after SOT	1	1/1 (100%)
Babel et al., Dtsch Med Wochenschr, 2003	Not documented	Chronic active EBV infection	1	1/1 (100%)
Sherritt et al., Transplant, 2003	EBV-BLCL sensitized EBV-CTL	PTLD after SOT	1	1/1 (100%)
Bollard et al., J Exp Med, 2004	EBV-BLCL sensitized EBV-CTL	Hodgkin's disease	14	6/11 (55%)
Straathof et al., Blood, 2005	EBV-BLCL sensitized EBV-CTL	NPC	6	3/6 (50%)
Savoldo et al., Blood, 2006	EBV-BLCL sensitized EBV-CTL	PTLD after SOT	2	2/2 (100%)
Louis et al., Blood, 2010	EBV-BLCL sensitized EBV-CTL	NPC	15	7/15 (49%)
Secondino et al., Ann Oncol, 2012	EBV-BLCL sensitized EBV-CTL	NPC	11	3/11 (27%)
Bollard et al., J Clin Oncol, 2014	EBV-BLCL sensitized EBV-CTL	EBV-associated lymphoma	21	13/21 (62%)
Pender et al., JCI Insight, 2018	AdE1-LMPpoly & IL-2	Multiple sclerosis	10	7/10 (70%)
Perna et al., Haematologica, 2014	Pepmix-pulsed and irradiated K562s	EBV-associated lymphoma	5	1/5 (20%)
Huang et al., Cancer, 2017	EBV-BLCL sensitized EBV-CTL	NPC	21	1/21 (%)
Secondino et al., Bone Marrow Transplant, 2019	EBV-BLCL sensitized EBV-CTL	NPC	12	7/12 (58%)

(continued)

Table 1 (continued)

B. Donor-derived EBV CTLs

Study	Method of selection	Treatment setting	N	Response (CR + PR)	Acute GVHD
Rooney et al., Lancet 1995, Blood, 1998 Heslop et al., Blood, 2010	EBV-BLCL sensitized	PTLD	13	11/13	8%
Lucas et al., Blood, 1996	EBV-BLCL sensitized	PTLD	1	1/1	100%
Imashuku et al., BMT, 1997	EBV-BLCL sensitized	PTLD	1	0/1	0%
Gottschalk et al., Blood, 2001	EBV-BLCL sensitized	PTLD	1	0/1	Not documented
Comoli et al., Blood Cells Mol Dis, 2008	EBV-BLCL sensitized	PTLD	5	5/5	0%
Leen et al., Blood, 2009	Ad5f35null vector infection and LCL stimulation	Post-HCT viremia	3	3/3	100%
Moosman et al., Blood, 2010	Peptide stimulation IFNγ capture	PTLD	6	3/6	0%
Doubrovina et al., Blood, 2012	EBV-BLCL sensitized	PTLD	19	13/19	0%
Icheva et al., JCO, 2013	EBNA-1 peptide stimulation IFNγ capture	PTLD Viremia	8 2	6/8 1/2	13% 0%
Gerdemann et al., Mol Ther, 2013	DC nucleofection viral plasmids	PTLD	1	1/1	100%
Papadopoulou et al., Sci Transl Med, 2014	Peptide-stimulated	PTLD	1	1/1	0%
Wang et al., Blood, 2016	Not documented	Post-HCT EBV viremia	15	13/15	Not documented

(continued)

C. Third-party EBV CTLs

Study	Method of selection	Treatment setting	Prior therapy	N	HLA	Response (CR + PR)
Alabama Sun et al., Br J Haematol, 2002	EBV-BLCL sensitized EBV-CTL	PTLD SOT Hodgkin's disease	RT Rituximab/C	1 1	4/6 6/6	1/1 (100%) 1/1 (100%)
Lucas et al., Cancer, 2004		AIDS-related NHL	C C	6 1	3–6/6 6/6	5/6 (83%) 0/1 (0%)
Cho et al., Int J Hematol, 2006	EBV-BLCL sensitized EBV-CTL	Natural killer (NK)/T-cell non-Hodgkin's lymphoma	RT	2	6/6	0/2 (0%)
Edinburgh Haque et al., Blood, 2007	EBV-BLCL sensitized EBV-CTL	PTLD HCT SOT	RIS Rituximab/C	2 31	2–5/6 2–5/6	2/2 (100%) 19/31 (61%)
Australia Gandhi et al., Am J Transplant, 2007	EBV-BLCL sensitized EBV-CTL	PTLD SOT	RIS Rituximab/C	3	≥ 3/6	2/3 (66%)
Baylor Leen et al., Blood, 2013	Transduced multivirus	PTLD HCT	Rituximab	9	≥ 1	6/9 (67%)
Inserm Gallot et al., J Immunother, 2014	EBV-BLCL sensitized EBV- CTL	PTLD HCT SOT NHL Lymphoproliferative syndrome	Rituximab/C Rituximab/C C Rituximab/C	6 3 1 1	≥ 2 ≥ 2 3/6 5/6	3/6 (50%) 1/3 (30%) 0/1 (0%) 0/1 (0%)
UK Chiou et al., Pediatric Transplant 2018	EBV-BLCL stimulated EBV-CTL	PTLD SOT	Rituximab RIS	10	Not specified	8/10 (80%)
Aberdeen Vickers et al., Br J Haematol, 2019	EBV-BLCL stimulated EBV-CTL	PTLD HCT SOT EBV-associated sarcoma	N/A N/A	6 4 1	≥ 3 ≥ 3 ≥ 3	4/6 (67%) 4/4 (80%) 1/1 (100%)
Baylor Tzannou et al., J Clin Oncol, 2017	Peptide stimulated	PTLD HCT Post-HCT viremia	None None	1 1	3/8 5/8	1/1 (100%) 1/1 (100%)
MSK Prockop et al., J Clin Invest, 2019	EBV-BLCL sensitized T-cell line	PTLD HCT SOT	Rituximab/C Rituximab/C	33 13	2–5/10 2–4/10	22/33 (68%) 7/13 (54%)
Spain Alonso et al., Bone Marrow Transplant, 2019	Not specified	PTLD HCT Post-HCT viremia EBV chronic active disease	Not documented	1 4 1	Not documented	0/1 (0%) 2/4 (50%) 0/1 (0%)
Gandhi et al., Hematol Oncol, 2019	Not specified	EBV+ lymphoma in immunosuppressed patients	Not documented	3	Not documented	3/3 (100%)
Rubinstein et al., Pediatr Blood Cancer, 2020	Peptide stimulated	EBV+ lymphoma in primary immunodeficiency patients	Rituximab/C Brentuximab/ nivolumab/C	1 1	6/10 3–4/10	2/2 (100%)

expansion of T cells recognizing a broader array of viruses generated from both donors and patients themselves, including varicella, HHV6, and BK [45–47].

One concern related to T cell products generated against multiple viruses simultaneously is whether antigen competition could impair the expansion of T cells with one viral specificity in favor of another [48]. Indeed, it was demonstrated that cultures generated against EBV, adenovirus, and CMV were dominated by CMV-specific T cells, and that eliminating the CMV stimulation increased the proportion of adenovirus-specific T cells [49]. These studies also revealed that in vivo expansion of adenovirus-specific T cells depends on viral reactivation in a way that expansion of EBV- and CMV-specific populations does not [50]. However, even in the absence of transduced or pulsed professional APCs, antigenic competition has been demonstrated to control the cell product [51].

It is likely that approaches for expansion of viral-specific CD3 T cells can benefit from improved culture conditions. A rapid throughput system for identifying the optimal cytokine cocktail recently demonstrated the superiority of specific combinations of IL-15/IL-6 and IL-4/IL-7 [52].

Lymphocyte Source

Regardless of the method of generation or selection, the use of donor-derived viral-specific CTLs is associated with several limitations. As discussed, one is the time it can take to generate an appropriately specific T cell line that lacks allo-reactivity. However, even with more rapid methods for generation, limitations still exist.

Though serologic typing may not fully identify those individuals from whom viral-specific CTLs can easily be generated [53], the generation of viral-specific T cells has typically involved the expansion of populations from immune individuals. Thus, for example, CMV seropositive recipients of transplants from CMV seronegative donors or of cord blood are at increased risk of CMV reactivation, persistent viremia, and even disease. The groups at Children's National and MD Anderson have demonstrated that T cell lines can be made from cord blood-derived, seronegative PMBCs, but it is yet to be demonstrated whether these can be as clinically effective as T cell lines from seropositive individuals [54]. In fact, the epitopes recognized by the T cell lines generated from seronegative individuals and cord blood are atypical and may not recapitulate the immunodominance demonstrated for recognition of these infections.

Another limitation is that in the HLA-disparate donor/recipient setting, donor-derived viral-specific T cells may be restricted in recognition and cytotoxicity through an HLA allele not shared by the recipient. Thus, if the virally infected target or reservoir is of host origin, the donor-derived viral-specific T cells may fail to recognize the target. This issue becomes more complex in the setting of multi-viral targeted T cells, where recognition of each virus can be through the same or different HLA alleles, making a given donor-derived line effective for some but not all infections.

Finally, viral-specific CTLs generated in vitro recognize viral epitopes presented in these culture systems. Mutations in endogenous viruses can mean that viral epitopes are not presented or fail to be recognized by the adoptively transferred T cells. This has been demonstrated by several different investigators in evaluating the reasons for failure of adoptively transferred EBV CTLs to mediate responses [55, 56], and has been addressed by investigators exploring the use of banked or third-party viral-specific CTLs (as reviewed in [57]). Third-party refers to T cells generated from someone other than the patient/recipient or the stem cell/solid organ donor.

It was first demonstrated by Dorothy Crawford and her group in Edinburgh that third-party EBV CTLs could clear EBV PTLD in solid organ transplant (SOT) recipients [58, 59], and was subsequently demonstrated in HCT recipients [56, 60]. These and a few other initial reports [61, 62] led to the development of banks of third-party virus-specific T cells. Published results in the largest trials found 60–80% efficacy [63–66] with a relatively low burden of GvHD, but signaled caution about the potential for triggering bystander GvHD [62]. Importantly, the use of third-party viral-specific T cells allows selection of CTL lines restricted by an HLA allele shared by the recipient, and for "switch therapy" to enable secondary therapy for those with disease refractory to a first cycle of therapy. The principle of switch therapy is that a secondary CTL line restricted by a different HLA allele presumably recognizes or can be demonstrated to recognize a different viral epitope [65, 67]. The initially reported successes have led more centers to establish banks of viral-specific T cell lines available for off-the-shelf use [64]. Questions of persistence of third-party donor viral-specific T cells remain, though durable responses have been demonstrated [65, 68].

Characterization of T Cells

The T cell products generated with different methods and used in adoptive therapy for viral infections have been characterized for their phenotype, antigen specificity, and HLA restriction. To date, none of the characteristics have defined a uniformly effective T cell product, though multiple investigators have identified the need for products that contain both CD8+ and CD4+ populations.

The early Baylor studies characterized EBV CTLs as having a majority of CD8+ T cells (71%) (range 3–99%) and median specific lysis of 40% (12–88%). The addition of adenoviral vectors into transduced APCs increased the proportion of CD4+ T cells to a mean of CD4+ 61.2% and a mixed population of Tem (CD45RA− CD62L−) and Tcm(CD45RA− CD62L+) cells [69]. Since that time, the variability demonstrated in these early studies of cultured viral-specific CTLs has been reported by other groups [39, 56]. For example, the multi-viral targeted products produced by pulsed mo-DCs [70] resulted in mean CD4+ of 55% with 75% Tem and 20% Tcm. Careful assessment of the response demonstrates preservation of diversity [71]. Selection by tetramer/streptamer or interferon gamma eliminates the need for prolonged culture, but results in a less phenotypically diverse product [72, 73].

Concern about the potential exhaustion of T cell populations cultured for prolonged periods is one of the factors that initially drove the desire to isolate viral-specific T cells with shorter culture periods and enhanced cytokine mixes [27, 52]. Subsequently, memory T cells with stem cell-like properties (Tscm) including the capacity of self-renewal and differentiation have been identified and defined by $CD8^+$ $CD45RA^+$ $CCR7^+$ $CD127^+$ $CD95^+$. Fewer than 1% of CMV-specific T cells express the Tscm phenotype and they do not appear to expand with current isolation approaches. Methods to expand this population have been developed [74], though not explored in clinical trials yet.

Antigen specificity of clinical grade products measured by Cr release, MHC tetramer, and IFNg production typically demonstrates ~20–40% cytotoxicity. Antigen specificity has been characterized by cytotoxicity using Cr release with an E:T ratio of 40:1, 20:1, 10:1, and 5:1 in targets including BLCLs, retroviral-transduced LCLs, and mo-DCs [10]. This system can be adapted to quantitatively assess the number of viral-specific CTL precursors by limiting dilution analysis [75]. Alternatively, characterization of IFNg release by enzyme-linked immunospot (ELIspot) assay has been used to characterize donor CTL lines prior to infusion, as well as patient responses before and after infusion [76]. As previously discussed, antigen competition can shape the relative proportions of viral specific CTLs generated in culture. In multi-viral cultures, responses to CMV predominate, with more viability in responses to adenovirus, BK, and EBV [70, 77].

Identifying the specific viral epitope(s) recognized by each T cell line is also important, especially in the context of multi-viral targeting. In addition to shaping the T cell repertoire expanded during the culture system, viral peptides representing immunogenic antigens for each virus being targeted can be used to identify the viral epitope recognized. Evaluating cytotoxicity against targets pulsed with a checkerboard created from overlapping penta-decapeptides spanning the sequence of immunodominant antigens is a powerful method to identify specific epitopes presented by specific HLA alleles [40].

In addition to validating antigen specificity, using third-party banked viral-specific T cells requires identification of the HLA allele through which each T cell line mediates viral-specific cytotoxicity. This has been done with both the use of predictive algorithms [30, 45, 50, 78] as well as by directly demonstrating HLA-specific cytotoxicity [79]. The careful characterization of HLA-specific cytotoxicity has led to an emerging understanding of a hierarchy of immune dominance of responses [80, 81] as well as realization that T cells restricted by certain HLA alleles may be less effective in the context of specific viral infections, as exemplified by responses to CMV [80] and SARS-Cov-2 [82].

Pre-Clinical Models

As mentioned, few studies of adoptive therapy with viral-specific T cells have been validated in preclinical models. That said, the first demonstration of adoptive transfer of CMV clones was in mice with LCMV. Subsequent murine studies demonstrated the HLA- and epitope-specificity of luciferase-expressing T cells in homing to tumors bearing the targeted HLA/epitope complex but not to other targets [79]. Preclinical models of nasopharyngeal carcinoma have targeted Latency II by EBV CTLs [83]. More recently, in vitro models for latency switch have demonstrated that increased expression of Latency II and III antigens can be induced by decitabine, leading to improved trafficking and cytotoxicity by EBV-specific CTLs in a murine PDX Burkitt Lymphoma model [84].

CTL Persistence

In initial studies of adoptively transferred CMV CTLs, persistence was detected in a dose-dependent manner by the in vivo presence of CMV-CTLs with the same constant sequences of Vα and Vβ usage [12], but CMV-specific CD4$^+$ populations were not found.

The polyclonal and gene-modified CTL populations infused by the group at Baylor allowed them to specifically identify the infused CTLs and demonstrate long-term in vivo persistence by PCR [13, 85]. This group evaluated cytotoxicity against [51] Cr-labeled autologous BLCLs using limiting dilution analysis (LDA) to calculate the EBV-specific precursor frequency, and demonstrated in vivo persistence for over 10 years. In addition, the use of gene-marked CTLs demonstrated these CTLs in the tumor of a treated patient [69].

Subsequent studies used ELISpot assays as well as LDA analysis to evaluate in vivo persistence demonstrated long-term persistence of transplant donor- and autologous donor-derived populations. In contrast, third-party origin viral-specific T cells persist for just days to months [63, 65, 66, 86]. Importantly, in the setting of third-party adoptive transfer of viral-specific CTLs, correlation between persistence and response has been difficult to establish [65].

Clinical Experience

Overall responses to donor-derived viral CTLs have been demonstrated across multiple production methods as summarized in Tables 1, 2, 3, 4, 5, and 6. The response rate in these reports ranges from ~70–90%. Comparison of results across studies is limited by a lack of consistency in the generation of viral CTLs, patient cohorts, and defined endpoints used for response assessment.

Banks of well-characterized populations of viral CTLs generated for off the shelf use have been established by a number of centers. Third party-derived viral CTLs have shown efficacy (Table 2) and eliminated some of the limitations of using donor-derived viral CTLs.

There are few predictors of response to viral CTLs. In uncontrolled experiments, several lines of evidence point to the importance of CD4$^+$ immunity for successful adoptive T cell immunotherapy. These include (1) persistence of CD8$^+$ clones in patients with concurrent reconstitution of CD4$^+$ responses [12], (2) polyclonal CD4$^+$

T cell populations leading to more robust in vivo expansion and longer persistence, and (3) recipient CD4[+] T cells predicting response to adoptive T cell therapy for refractory CMV [87]. This is consistent with our early understanding of the role of CD4[+] T cells in maintaining immune memory [88], and the viral-specific transcriptional matrix required for helper T cell responses (reviewed in [89]). Another early predictor of response was recently introduced by using mass cytometry in patients with CMV reactivation to identify an immune response signature associated with

Table 2 Experience using CMV CTLs

Study	CTL source	Method of selection	Treatment setting	N	Response (CR + PR)
Numazaki et al., Clin Infect Dis, 1997	Autologous	Co-culture with immobilized monoclonal antibody to CD3 cells and human rIL-2	Interstitial pneumonia	1	100%
Einsele et al., Blood, 2002	Donor-derived	CMV antigen stimulation	Post-HCT viremia	8	88%
Cobbold et al., J Exp Med, 2005	Donor-derived	CMVpp65 tetramer isolation	Post-HCT viremia	9	100%
Brestrich et al., Am J Transplant, 2009	Autologous	CMVpp65 peptide IFNγ capture	Post-SOT pneumonia	1	100%
Feuchtinger et al., Blood, 2010	Donor-derived	CMVpp65 peptide IFNγ capture	Post-HCT viremia	18	83%
Dong et al., J Pediatr Hematol Oncol, 2010	Donor-derived	EBV/CMV peptide pulsed DCs	Post-HCT viremia	2	100%
Schmitt et al., Transfusion, 2011	Donor-derived	CMVpp65 streptamers	Post-HCT viremia	2	100%
Uhlin et al., Clin Infect Dis, 2012	Donor-derived or third-party	CMVpp65 peptide pentamers	Post-HCT infection or disease or SCID infection	6	83%
Meij et al., J Immunother, 2012	Donor-derived or autologous	CMVpp65 peptide IFNγ capture	Post-HCT viremia	6	100%
Bao et al., J Immunother, 2012	Donor-derived	Pooled CMV overlapping peptide mixes	Post-HCT viremia	7	86%
Crough et al., Immunol Cell Biol, 2012	Autologous	CMV peptide epitopes in the presence of γC cytokine	GBM	1	100%

(continued)

Table 2 (continued)

Study	CTL source	Method of selection	Treatment setting	N	Response (CR + PR)
Leen et al., Blood, 2013	Third-party donor	Stimulated by BLCLs then transduced with an Ad5f35 vector encoding the CMV-derived pp65 antigen	Post-HCT viremia or disease	23	74%
Koehne et al., Biol Blood Marrow Transplant, 2015	Donor-derived	Monocyte-derived DCs loaded with a pool of peptides CMVpp65	Post-HCT viremia	16	94%
Holmes-Liew et al., Respirology, 2015	Autologous	Peptide stimulated	Post-SOT viremia	1	100%
Macesic et al., Am J Transplant, 2015	Third-party donor	Pooled CMV overlapping peptide mixes	Post-SOT disease	1	100%
Wang et al., Blood, 2016	Donor-derived	Not documented	Post-HCT viremia	15	87%
Neuenhahn et al., Leukemia, 2017.	Donor-derived or third-party donor	CMVpp65 streptamers	Post-HCT viremia	16	69%
Prockop et al., Blood, 2017	Third-party donor	CMVpp65 stimulated	Post-HCT disease or viremia	50	64%
Tzannou et al., Blood, 2017	Third-party donor	Peptide stimulated	Post-HCT disease or viremia	19	95%
Pei et al., J Infect Dis, 2017	Donor-derived	CMVpp65 peptide and cytokine stimulation	Post-HCT viremia	32	84%
Withers et al., Blood Adv, 2017	Third-party	CMVpp65 peptide	Post-HCT CMV viremia and/or disease	28	96%
Kallay et al., J Immunother, 2018	Donor-derived	CMVpp65 peptide IFNγ capture	Post-HCT viremia	3	67%
Lindemann et al., Bone Marrow Transplant, 2018	Third-party donor	CMVpp65 peptide IFNγ capture	Post-HCT viremia	1	100%
Alonso et al., Bone Marrow Transplant, 2019	Donor-derived or third-party donor	Not documented	Post-HCT infection or immunodeficiency-associated infection	10	60%
Seo et al., Blood Adv, 2019	Donor-derived	Peptide stimulated	Post-HCT CMV retinitis	1	100%

(continued)

Table 2 (continued)

Study	CTL source	Method of selection	Treatment setting	N	Response (CR + PR)
Smith et al., Clinical Infect Dis, 2019	Autologous	Peptide stimulated	Post-SOT CMV infection	13	84%
Fabrizio et al., Bone Marrow Transplant, 2020	Donor-derived, third-party, or both	Peptide stimulated	Post-HCT CMV viremia and/or disease	85	71%

Table 3 Experience using adenovirus CTLs

Study	CTL source	Method of selection	Treatment setting	N	Response (CR + PR)
Feuchtinger et al., Br J Haematol, 2006	Donor-derived	AdV antigen type C IFNγ capture	Post-HCT systemic infection	9	56%
Leen et al., Blood, 2009	Donor-derived	Ad5f35null vector infection and LCL stimulation	Post-HCT systemic infection	2	100%
Opherk et al., Blood, 2009	Donor-derived	Hexon-specific T-cell isolated by IFNγ secretion system	Post-HCT systemic infection	40	70%
Budig et al., Bone Marrow Transplant, 2012	Donor-derived	IFNγ secretion system	Post-HCT systemic infection	1	100%
Leen et al., Blood, 2013	Third-party donor	Stimulated by BLCLs transduced with an Ad5f35 vector encoding the CMV-derived pp65 antigen	Post-HCT viremia or disease	18	78%
DiNardo et al., Pediatr Blood Cancer, 2014	Donor-derived	Adeno peptide IFNγ capture	Post-HCT severe respiratory failure	1	100%
Papadopoulou et al., Sci Transl Med, 2014	Donor-derived	Peptide stimulated	Post-HCT viremia	1	100%
Feucht et al., Blood, 2015	Donor-derived	AdV hexon protein IFNγ capture	Post-HCT disease or viremia	30	70%
Qian et al., J Hematol Oncol, 2017	Donor-derived or third-party donor	Pepmix IFNγ capture	Post-HCT infection or disease	11	91%
Tzannou et al., Blood, 2017	Third-party donor	Peptide stimulated	Post-HCT viremia or disease	9	78%
Ip et al., Cytotherapy, 2018	Donor-derived	Peptide stimulated	Post-HCT viremia	8	100%
Alonso et al., Bone Marrow Transplant, 2019	Donor-derived or third-party donor	Not documented	Post-HCT viremia or disease	2	50%

Table 4 Experience using BK virus CTLs

Study	CTL source	Method of selection	Treatment setting	N	Response (CR + PR)
Tzannou et al., Blood, 2017	Third-party donor	Peptide stimulated	Post-HCT viremia or disease	19	100%
Pello et al., Eur J Hematol, 2017	Donor-derived	Pepmix stimulated IFNγ capture	Post-HCT BK virus associated hemorrhagic cystitis	1	100%
Eduwu et al., Am J Kidney Dis, 2019	Not documented	Not documented	BK virus nephropathy	1	100%
Olson et al., Blood, 2019	Third-party donor	Not documented	BK virus associated hemorrhagic cystitis	31	87%
Nelson et al., Blood Adv, 2020	Donor-derived or third-party donor	Pepmix stimulated	Post-HCT or post-SOT viremia and/or hemorrhagic cystitis	38	86%

Table 5 Experience using HHV6 CTLs

Study	CTL source	Method of selection	Treatment setting	N	Response (CR + PR)
Tzannou et al., Blood, 2017	Third-party donor	Peptide stimulated	Post-HCT	4	100%

Table 6 Experience using JC virus CTLs

Study	CTL source	Method of selection	Treatment Setting	N	Response (CR + PR)
Numazaki et al., Clinical Infect Dis, 1997	Autologous	Co-culture with immobilized monoclonal antibody to CD3 cells and human rIL-2	Interstitial pneumonia	1	100%
Balduzzi et al., Bone Marrow Transplant, 2011	Donor-derived	Stimulation with 15-mer peptides derived from VP1 and large T viral proteins	Post-HCT PML	1	100%
Muftuoglu et al., NEJM, 2019	Third-party donor	Pepmix stimulated (BK specific)	HIV, HCT, Ruxolitinib	3	100%
Berzero et al., Ann Neurol, 2021	Autologous or donor-derived	Peptide stimulated	HIV-negative PML	9	67%

Abbreviations: *EBV* Epstein Barr virus, *CMV* cytomegalovirus, *HHV6* human herpes virus 6, *CTLs* cytotoxic T cell lines, *BLCL* B cell lymphoblastoid cell line, Pepmix (peptide mixture), *NHL* non-Hodgkin lymphoma, *PTLD* post-transplant lymphoproliferative disorder, *NPC* nasopharyngeal carcinoma, *SOT* solid organ transplant, *HCT* hematopoietic stem cell transplant, *AdE1* adenoviral vector, *LMP* latent membrane protein

CMV control. This signature can be documented both in HCT recipients controlling CMV as well as those responding to adoptive CMV T cell therapy [90].

Future Directions

Accessibility

The use of adoptive therapy with viral-specific T cells is on the brink of becoming more broadly available. There are currently multi-center trials in progress (Table 7) already expanding access to these therapies to patients in multiple centers. Two of these trials are Phase 3 registration trials, and if successful, will lead to FDA approval of T cell products for EBV and BK viral infections after both allogeneic HCT and SOT.

Applicability

Applying adoptive viral CTLs to a broader array of viral infections has already been demonstrated, and current approaches being explored include generation of HIV-specific [91], PML-specific [92, 93], and SARs-COV-2-specific viral CTLs [94]. In addition, a better understanding of the best methods for manufacturing, the epitopes and HLA alleles associated with best clinical responses, and the ability to shape the repertoire of T cells expanded for infusion will improve responses, even in patients with more refractory disease.

Table 7 Multicenter clinical trials of viral CTLs

Multi-center trials	
Pilot study haploidentical donor CMV CTLs in SOT and HCT; (Ohio state)	NCT03665675
Therapeutic infusion of partially HLA matched third party donor derived virus and fungus specific T cells in patients after HCT or SOT, (Westmead)	NCT02779439
Pilot study of rituximab and third party LMP specific T cells in treating pediatric solid organ recipients with EBV+ CD20+ PTLD, 3 arms. (COG)	NCT02900976
Immunotherapy with tacrolimus resistant EBV CTL for lymphoproliferative disease after SOT, (great Ormond street)	NCT03131934
Phase 3 trial of Tabelecleucel for EBV-PTLD after failure of rituximab or rituximab and chemotherapy; (Atara biotherapeutics)	NCT03394365
Multivirus-specific T-cell transfer post SCT vs AdV, CMV and EBV infections - TRACE (European Commission)	NCT04832607
Virus-specific activated T lymphocytes from a donor in hematopoietic progenitor transplanted patients (Vall d'Hebron Institute of Oncology)	NCT04018261
Study of Viralym-M (ALVR105) in transplant patients with BK viremia (AlloVir)	NCT04605484

Finally, the transduction of off-the-shelf viral CTLs with chimeric antigen receptors [95, 96] or transgenic T cell receptors are examples of the potential ways to expand the use of viral CTL platforms for a broad range of disorders.

References

1. Reddehase MJ, Weiland F, Münch K, Jonjic S, Lüske A, Koszinowski UH. Interstitial murine cytomegalovirus pneumonia after irradiation: characterization of cells that limit viral replication during established infection of the lungs. J Virol. 1985;55:264–73.
2. Reddehase MJ, Mutter W, Münch K, Bühring HJ, Koszinowski UH. CD8-positive T lymphocytes specific for murine cytomegalovirus immediate-early antigens mediate protective immunity. J Virol. 1987;61:3102–8.
3. Zinkernagel RM, Pircher HP, Schulz M, Leist T, Oehen S, Hengartner H. Reactivity and tolerance of virus-specific T cells. Cold Spring Harb Symp Quant Biol. 1989;54(Pt 2):843–51.
4. Melief CJ, Kast WM. Efficacy of cytotoxic T lymphocytes against virus-induced tumors. Cancer Cells. 1990;2:116–20.
5. Liu Y, Janeway CA Jr. Microbial induction of co-stimulatory activity for CD4 T-cell growth. Int Immunol. 1991;3:323–32.
6. Hromas R, Cornetta K, Srour E, Blanke C, Broun ER. Donor leukocyte infusion as therapy of life-threatening adenoviral infections after T-cell-depleted bone marrow transplantation. Blood. 1994;84:1689–90.
7. Yoshihara S, Kato R, Inoue T, et al. Successful treatment of life-threatening human herpesvirus-6 encephalitis with donor lymphocyte infusion in a patient who had undergone human leukocyte antigen-haploidentical nonmyeloablative stem cell transplantation. Transplantation. 2004;77:835–8.
8. Papadopoulos EB, Ladanyi M, Emanuel D, et al. Infusions of donor leukocytes to treat Epstein-Barr virus-associated lymphoproliferative disorders after allogeneic bone marrow transplantation. N Engl J Med. 1994;330:1185–91.
9. Riddell SR, Rabin M, Geballe AP, Britt WJ, Greenberg PD. Class I MHC-restricted cytotoxic T lymphocyte recognition of cells infected with human cytomegalovirus does not require endogenous viral gene expression. J Immunol. 1991;146:2795–804.
10. Smith CA, Ng CY, Heslop HE, et al. Production of genetically modified Epstein-Barr virus-specific cytotoxic T cells for adoptive transfer to patients at high risk of EBV-associated lymphoproliferative disease. J Hematother. 1995;4:73–9.
11. Riddell SR, Watanabe KS, Goodrich JM, Li CR, Agha ME, Greenberg PD. Restoration of viral immunity in immunodeficient humans by the adoptive transfer of T cell clones. Science. 1992;257:238–41.
12. Walter EA, Greenberg PD, Gilbert MJ, et al. Reconstitution of cellular immunity against cytomegalovirus in recipients of allogeneic bone marrow by transfer of T-cell clones from the donor. N Engl J Med. 1995;333:1038–44.
13. Rooney CM, Smith CA, Ng CY, et al. Use of gene-modified virus-specific T lymphocytes to control Epstein-Barr-virus-related lymphoproliferation. Lancet. 1995;345:9–13.
14. Riddell SR, Greenberg PD. The use of anti-CD3 and anti-CD28 monoclonal antibodies to clone and expand human antigen-specific T cells. J Immunol Methods. 1990;128:189–201.
15. Reusser P, Riddell SR, Meyers JD, Greenberg PD. Cytotoxic T-lymphocyte response to cytomegalovirus after human allogeneic bone marrow transplantation: pattern of recovery and correlation with cytomegalovirus infection and disease. Blood. 1991;78:1373–80.
16. McLaughlin-Taylor E, Pande H, Forman SJ, et al. Identification of the major late human cytomegalovirus matrix protein pp65 as a target antigen for CD8+ virus-specific cytotoxic T lymphocytes. J Med Virol. 1994;43:103–10.

17. Rickinson AB, Moss DJ, Allen DJ, Wallace LE, Rowe M, Epstein MA. Reactivation of Epstein-Barr virus-specific cytotoxic T cells by in vitro stimulation with the autologous lymphoblastoid cell line. Int J Cancer. 1981;27:593–601.
18. Choquet S, Mamzer BM, Hermine O, et al. Identification of prognostic factors in post-transplant lymphoproliferative disorders. Recent Results Cancer Res. 2002;159:67–80.
19. Fox CP, Burns D, Parker AN, et al. EBV-associated post-transplant lymphoproliferative disorder following in vivo T-cell-depleted allogeneic transplantation: clinical features, viral load correlates and prognostic factors in the rituximab era. Bone Marrow Transplant. 2014;49:280–6.
20. Pagliuca S, Bommier C, Michonneau D, et al. Epstein-Barr virus-associated post-transplantation lymphoproliferative disease in patients who received anti-CD20 after hematopoietic stem cell transplantation. Biol Blood Marrow Transplant. 2019;25:2490–500.
21. Gahn B, Siller-Lopez F, Pirooz AD, et al. Adenoviral gene transfer into dendritic cells efficiently amplifies the immune response to LMP2A antigen: a potential treatment strategy for Epstein-Barr virus--positive Hodgkin's lymphoma. Int J Cancer. 2001;93:706–13.
22. Gruber A, Kan-Mitchell J, Kuhen KL, Mukai T, Wong-Staal F. Dendritic cells transduced by multiply deleted HIV-1 vectors exhibit normal phenotypes and functions and elicit an HIV-specific cytotoxic T-lymphocyte response in vitro. Blood. 2000;96:1327–33.
23. Sili U, Huls MH, Davis AR, et al. Large-scale expansion of dendritic cell-primed polyclonal human cytotoxic T-lymphocyte lines using lymphoblastoid cell lines for adoptive immunotherapy. J Immunother. 2003;26:241–56.
24. Zhu F, Ramadan G, Davies B, Margolis DA, Keever-Taylor CA. Stimulation by means of dendritic cells followed by Epstein-Barr virus-transformed B cells as antigen-presenting cells is more efficient than dendritic cells alone in inducing Aspergillus f16-specific cytotoxic T cell responses. Clin Exp Immunol. 2008;151:284–96.
25. Hanley PJ, Shaffer DR, Cruz CR, et al. Expansion of T cells targeting multiple antigens of cytomegalovirus, Epstein-Barr virus and adenovirus to provide broad antiviral specificity after stem cell transplantation. Cytotherapy. 2011;13:976–86.
26. Boudreau G, Carli C, Lamarche C, et al. Leukoreduction system chambers are a reliable cellular source for the manufacturing of T-cell therapeutics. Transfusion. 2019;59:1300–11.
27. Leen A, Ratnayake M, Foster A, et al. Contact-activated monocytes: efficient antigen presenting cells for the stimulation of antigen-specific T cells. J Immunother. 2007;30:96–107.
28. Sasawatari S, Tadaki T, Isogai M, Takahara M, Nieda M, Kakimi K. Efficient priming and expansion of antigen-specific CD8+ T cells by a novel cell-based artificial APC. Immunol Cell Biol. 2006;84:512–21.
29. Van den Bosch GA, Ponsaerts P, Nijs G, et al. Ex vivo induction of viral antigen-specific CD8 T cell responses using mRNA-electroporated CD40-activated B cells. Clin Exp Immunol. 2005;139:458–67.
30. Gerdemann U, Vera JF, Rooney CM, Leen AM. Generation of multivirus-specific T cells to prevent/treat viral infections after allogeneic hematopoietic stem cell transplant. J Vis Exp. 2011;
31. Gottschalk S, Edwards OL, Sili U, et al. Generating CTLs against the subdominant Epstein-Barr virus LMP1 antigen for the adoptive immunotherapy of EBV-associated malignancies. Blood. 2003;101:1905–12.
32. Hong B, Peng G, Berry L, et al. Generating CTLs against the subdominant EBV LMP antigens by transient expression of an A20 inhibitor with EBV LMP proteins in human DCs. Gene Ther. 2012;19:818–27.
33. Forsberg O, Carlsson B, Tötterman TH, Essand M. Strategic use of an adenoviral vector for rapid and efficient ex vivo-generation of cytomegalovirus pp65-reactive cytolytic and helper T cells. Br J Haematol. 2008;141:188–99.
34. Fonteneau JF, Larsson M, Somersan S, et al. Generation of high quantities of viral and tumor-specific human CD4+ and CD8+ T-cell clones using peptide pulsed mature dendritic cells. J Immunol Methods. 2001;258:111–26.
35. Gerdemann U, Keirnan JM, Katari UL, et al. Rapidly generated multivirus-specific cytotoxic T lymphocytes for the prophylaxis and treatment of viral infections. Mol Ther. 2012;20:1622–32.

36. Chamucero-Millares JA, Bernal-Estévez DA, Parra-López CA. Usefulness of IL-21, IL-7, and IL-15 conditioned media for expansion of antigen-specific CD8+ T cells from healthy donor-PBMCs suitable for immunotherapy. Cell Immunol. 2021;360:104257.
37. Luo XH, Meng Q, Liu Z, Paraschoudi G. Generation of high-affinity CMV-specific T cells for adoptive immunotherapy using IL-2, IL-15, and IL-21. Clin Immunol. 2020;217:108456.
38. Peggs K, Verfuerth S, Mackinnon S. Induction of cytomegalovirus (CMV)-specific T-cell responses using dendritic cells pulsed with CMV antigen: a novel culture system free of live CMV virions. Blood. 2001;97:994–1000.
39. Foster AE, Gottlieb DJ, Marangolo M, et al. Rapid, large-scale generation of highly pure cytomegalovirus-specific cytotoxic T cells for adoptive immunotherapy. J Hematother Stem Cell Res. 2003;12:93–105.
40. Trivedi D, Williams RY, O'Reilly RJ, Koehne G. Generation of CMV-specific T lymphocytes using protein-spanning pools of pp65-derived overlapping pentadecapeptides for adoptive immunotherapy. Blood. 2005;105:2793–801.
41. Kleihauer A, Grigoleit U, Hebart H, et al. Ex vivo generation of human cytomegalovirus-specific cytotoxic T cells by peptide-pulsed dendritic cells. Br J Haematol. 2001;113:231–9.
42. Grau-Vorster M, López-Montañés M, Cantó E, et al. Characterization of a cytomegalovirus-specific T lymphocyte product obtained through a rapid and scalable production process for use in adoptive immunotherapy. Front Immunol. 2020;11:271.
43. Ngo MC, Ando J, Leen AM, et al. Complementation of antigen-presenting cells to generate T lymphocytes with broad target specificity. J Immunother. 2014;37:193–203.
44. Pello OM, Innes AJ, Bradshaw A, et al. BKV-specific T cells in the treatment of severe refractory haemorrhagic cystitis after HLA-haploidentical haematopoietic cell transplantation. Eur J Haematol. 2017;98:632–4.
45. Blyth E, Clancy L, Simms R, et al. BK virus-specific T cells for use in cellular therapy show specificity to multiple antigens and polyfunctional cytokine responses. Transplantation. 2011;92:1077–84.
46. Lamarche C, Orio J, Georges-Tobar V, et al. Clinical-scale rapid autologous BK virus-specific T cell line generation from kidney transplant recipients with active viremia for adoptive immunotherapy. Transplantation. 2017;101:2713–21.
47. Ma CK, Blyth E, Clancy L, et al. Addition of varicella zoster virus-specific T cells to cytomegalovirus, Epstein-Barr virus and adenovirus tri-specific T cells as adoptive immunotherapy in patients undergoing allogeneic hematopoietic stem cell transplantation. Cytotherapy. 2015;17:1406–20.
48. Garcia Z, Pradelli E, Celli S, Beuneu H, Simon A, Bousso P. Competition for antigen determines the stability of T cell-dendritic cell interactions during clonal expansion. Proc Natl Acad Sci U S A. 2007;104:4553–8.
49. Leen AM, Christin A, Myers GD, et al. Cytotoxic T lymphocyte therapy with donor T cells prevents and treats adenovirus and Epstein-Barr virus infections after haploidentical and matched unrelated stem cell transplantation. Blood. 2009;114:4283–92.
50. Leen AM, Myers GD, Sili U, et al. Monoculture-derived T lymphocytes specific for multiple viruses expand and produce clinically relevant effects in immunocompromised individuals. Nat Med. 2006;12:1160–6.
51. Roubalová K, Němečková Š, Kryštofová J, Hainz P, Pumannová M, Hamšíková E. Antigenic competition in the generation of multi-virus-specific cell lines for immunotherapy of human cytomegalovirus, polyomavirus BK, Epstein-Barr virus and adenovirus infection in haematopoietic stem cell transplant recipients. Immunol Lett. 2020;228:64–9.
52. Lazarski CA, Datar AA, Reynolds EK, Keller MD, Bollard CM, Hanley PJ. Identification of new cytokine combinations for antigen-specific T-cell therapy products via a high-throughput multi-parameter assay. Cytotherapy. 2021;23:65–76.
53. Savoldo B, Cubbage ML, Durett AG, et al. Generation of EBV-specific CD4+ cytotoxic T cells from virus naive individuals. J Immunol. 2002;168:909–18.

54. Hanley PJ, Melenhorst JJ, Nikiforow S, et al. CMV-specific T cells generated from naïve T cells recognize atypical epitopes and may be protective in vivo. Sci Transl Med. 2015;7:285ra63.
55. Gottschalk S, Ng CY, Perez M, et al. An Epstein-Barr virus deletion mutant associated with fatal lymphoproliferative disease unresponsive to therapy with virus-specific CTLs. Blood. 2001;97:835–43.
56. Doubrovina E, Oflaz-Sozmen B, Prockop SE, et al. Adoptive immunotherapy with unselected or EBV-specific T cells for biopsy-proven EBV+ lymphomas after allogeneic hematopoietic cell transplantation. Blood. 2012;119:2644–56.
57. O'Reilly RJ, Prockop S, Hasan A, Doubrovina E. Therapeutic advantages provided by banked virus-specific T-cells of defined HLA-restriction. Bone Marrow Transplant. 2019;54:759–64.
58. Haque T, Wilkie GM, Taylor C, et al. Treatment of Epstein-Barr-virus-positive post-transplantation lymphoproliferative disease with partly HLA-matched allogeneic cytotoxic T cells. Lancet. 2002;360:436–42.
59. Haque T, Taylor C, Wilkie GM, et al. Complete regression of posttransplant lymphoprolif-erative disease using partially HLA-matched Epstein Barr virus-specific cytotoxic T cells. Transplantation. 2001;72:1399–402.
60. Barker JN, Doubrovina E, Sauter C, et al. Successful treatment of EBV-associated posttrans-plantation lymphoma after cord blood transplantation using third-party EBV-specific cytotoxic T lymphocytes. Blood. 2010;116:5045–9.
61. Uhlin M, Okas M, Gertow J, Uzunel M, Brismar TB, Mattsson J. A novel haplo-identical adoptive CTL therapy as a treatment for EBV-associated lymphoma after stem cell transplanta-tion. Cancer Immunol Immunother. 2010;59:473–7.
62. Qasim W, Derniame S, Gilmour K, et al. Third-party virus-specific T cells eradicate adenovi-raemia but trigger bystander graft-versus-host disease. Br J Haematol. 2011;154:150–3.
63. Tzannou I, Papadopoulou A, Naik S, et al. Off-the-shelf virus-specific T cells to treat BK virus, human herpesvirus 6, cytomegalovirus, Epstein-Barr virus, and adenovirus infections after allogeneic hematopoietic stem-cell transplantation. J Clin Oncol. 2017;35:3547–57.
64. Withers B, Clancy L, Burgess J, et al. Establishment and operation of a third-party virus-specific T cell bank within an allogeneic stem cell transplant program. Biol Blood Marrow Transplant. 2018;24:2433–42.
65. Prockop S, Doubrovina E, Suser S, et al. Off-the-shelf EBV-specific T cell immunotherapy for rituximab-refractory EBV-associated lymphoma following transplantation. J Clin Invest. 2020;130:733–47.
66. Leen AM, Bollard CM, Mendizabal AM, et al. Multicenter study of banked third-party virus-specific T cells to treat severe viral infections after hematopoietic stem cell transplantation. Blood. 2013;121:5113–23.
67. Di Ciaccio PR, Avdic S, Sutrave G, et al. Successful treatment of CMV, EBV, and adenovi-rus tissue infection following HLA-mismatched allogeneic stem cell transplant using infusion of third-party T cells from multiple donors in addition to antivirals, rituximab, and surgery. Transpl Infect Dis. 2020:e13528.
68. Withers B, Blyth E, Clancy LE, et al. Long-term control of recurrent or refractory viral infections after allogeneic HSCT with third-party virus-specific T cells. Blood Adv. 2017;1:2193–205.
69. Rooney CM, Smith CA, Ng CY, et al. Infusion of cytotoxic T cells for the prevention and treatment of Epstein-Barr virus-induced lymphoma in allogeneic transplant recipients. Blood. 1998;92:1549–55.
70. Gottlieb DJ, Clancy LE, Withers B, et al. Prophylactic antigen-specific T-cells targeting seven viral and fungal pathogens after allogeneic haemopoietic stem cell transplant. Clin Transl Immunol. 2021;10:e1249.
71. Hamel Y, Rohrlich P, Baron V, et al. Characterization of antigen-specific repertoire diversity following in vitro restimulation by a recombinant adenovirus expressing human cytomegalo-virus pp65. Eur J Immunol. 2003;33:760–8.
72. Casalegno-Garduño R, Schmitt A, Yao J, et al. Multimer technologies for detection and adop-tive transfer of antigen-specific T cells. Cancer Immunol Immunother. 2010;59:195–202.

73. Kelleher AD, Rowland-Jones SL. Functions of tetramer-stained HIV-specific CD4(+) and CD8(+) T cells. Curr Opin Immunol. 2000;12:370–4.
74. Schmueck-Henneresse M, Sharaf R, Vogt K, et al. Peripheral blood-derived virus-specific memory stem T cells mature to functional effector memory subsets with self-renewal potency. J Immunol. 2015;194:5559–67.
75. Lucas KG, Small TN, Heller G, Dupont B, O'Reilly RJ. The development of cellular immunity to Epstein-Barr virus after allogeneic bone marrow transplantation. Blood. 1996;87:2594–603.
76. Meij P, Leen A, Rickinson AB, et al. Identification and prevalence of CD8(+) T-cell responses directed against Epstein-Barr virus-encoded latent membrane protein 1 and latent membrane protein 2. Int J Cancer 2002;99:93–9.
77. Papadopoulou A, Gerdemann U, Katari UL, et al. Activity of broad-spectrum T cells as treatment for AdV, EBV, CMV, BKV, and HHV6 infections after HSCT. Sci Transl Med. 2014;6:242ra83.
78. Feucht J, Opherk K, Lang P, et al. Adoptive T-cell therapy with hexon-specific Th1 cells as a treatment of refractory adenovirus infection after HSCT. Blood. 2015;125:1986–94.
79. Koehne G, Doubrovin M, Doubrovina E, et al. Serial in vivo imaging of the targeted migration of human HSV-TK-transduced antigen-specific lymphocytes. Nat Biotechnol. 2003;21:405–13.
80. Hyun SJ, Sohn HJ, Lee HJ, et al. Comprehensive analysis of cytomegalovirus pp65 antigen-specific CD8(+) T cell responses according to human leukocyte antigen class I allotypes and intraindividual dominance. Front Immunol. 2017;8:1591.
81. Lacey SF, Diamond DJ, Zaia JA. Assessment of cellular immunity to human cytomegalovirus in recipients of allogeneic stem cell transplants. Biol Blood Marrow Transplant. 2004;10:433–47.
82. Habel JR, Nguyen THO, van de Sandt CE, et al. Suboptimal SARS-CoV-2-specific CD8(+) T cell response associated with the prominent HLA-A*02:01 phenotype. Proc Natl Acad Sci U S A. 2020;117:24384–91.
83. Yang D, Shao Q, Sun H, et al. Evaluation of Epstein-Barr virus latent membrane protein 2 specific T-cell receptors driven by T-cell specific promoters using lentiviral vector. Clin Dev Immunol. 2011;2011:716926.
84. Dalton T, Doubrovina E, Pankov D, et al. Epigenetic reprogramming sensitizes immunologically silent EBV+ lymphomas to virus-directed immunotherapy. Blood. 2020;135:1870–81.
85. Heslop HE, Slobod KS, Pule MA, et al. Long-term outcome of EBV-specific T-cell infusions to prevent or treat EBV-related lymphoproliferative disease in transplant recipients. Blood. 2010;115:925–35.
86. Naik S, Nicholas SK, Martinez CA, et al. Adoptive immunotherapy for primary immunodeficiency disorders with virus-specific T lymphocytes. J Allergy Clin Immunol. 2016;137:1498–505.e1.
87. Fabrizio VA, Rodriguez-Sanchez MI, Mauguen A, et al. Adoptive therapy with CMV-specific cytotoxic T lymphocytes depends on baseline CD4+ immunity to mediate durable responses. Blood Adv. 2021;5:496–503.
88. Matloubian M, Concepcion RJ, Ahmed R. CD4+ T cells are required to sustain CD8+ cytotoxic T-cell responses during chronic viral infection. J Virol. 1994;68:8056–63.
89. Sheikh AA, Groom JR. Transcription tipping points for T follicular helper cell and T-helper 1 cell fate commitment. Cell Mol Immunol. 2021;18:528–38.
90. McGuire HM, Rizzetto S, Withers BP, et al. Mass cytometry reveals immune signatures associated with cytomegalovirus (CMV) control in recipients of allogeneic haemopoietic stem cell transplant and CMV-specific T cells. Clin Transl Immunol. 2020;9:e1149.
91. Zhou Y, Maldini CR, Jadlowsky J, Riley JL. Challenges and opportunities of using adoptive T-cell therapy as part of an HIV cure strategy. J Infect Dis. 2021;223:38–45.
92. Muftuoglu M, Olson A, Marin D, et al. Allogeneic BK virus-specific T cells for progressive multifocal leukoencephalopathy. N Engl J Med. 2018;379:1443–51.
93. Berzero G, Basso S, Stoppini L, et al. Adoptive transfer of JC virus-specific T lymphocytes for the treatment of progressive multifocal leukoencephalopathy. Ann Neurol. 2021;89(4):769–79.

290 S. E. Prockop and S. Shahid

94. Keller MD, Harris KM, Jensen-Wachspress MA, et al. SARS-CoV-2-specific T cells are rapidly expanded for therapeutic use and target conserved regions of the membrane protein. Blood. 2020;136:2905–17.
95. Lapteva N, Gilbert M, Diaconu I, et al. T-cell receptor stimulation enhances the expansion and function of CD19 chimeric antigen receptor-expressing T cells. Clin Cancer Res. 2019;25:7340–50.
96. Watanabe N, Mamonkin M. Off-the-shelf chimeric antigen receptor T cells: how do we get there? Cancer J. 2021;27:176–81.

Part VI
NK Cell

Biology of NK Cells and NK Cells in Clinic

Grace C. Birch, Todd F. Fehniger, and Rizwan Romee

Abstract Natural killer (NK) cells are innate lymphoid cells with the capacity to detect and destroy malignant cells without requiring prior sensitization. As a result of their innate ability to target malignant cells, these cells are an attractive candidate for immune therapies for cancer. Initial studies following hematopoietic cell transplants for cancer therapy illuminated a potential role for NK cells in exerting a graft versus leukemia effect without initiating graft versus host disease (GVHD). The use of NK cells in non-transplant settings showed that infusion of NK cells from HLA-haploidentical donors in combination with IL-2 after lymphodepletion lead to remission in a number of patients with poor prognosis AML. Since then, various methods of activating and expanding NK cells for use in the clinical setting have been investigated. Preliminary studies show promise for the use of NK cells in a vast range of solid and liquid tumor settings including glioblastoma, colorectal cancer and ovarian cancer. Activation of peripheral blood derived NK cells with cytokines has been shown to induce a memory-like phenotype which results in expansion and persistence *in vivo* pre-clinical models as well as augmented response against tumor targets *in vitro*. These memory-like NK cells are currently being investigated in clinical trials for a range of cancer types and offer great promise for the future. Utilization of cord blood derived NK cells as well as iPSC-differentiated NK cells and immortalized NK cell lines are also being investigated with the hope to offer off-the shelf immunotherapies for malignant diseases. This chapter will discuss the biology of NK cells, their development from progenitor cells in the bone marrow and the balance of inhibitory and activating receptors that govern their interactions with both healthy and malignant cells. Methods for culture and expansion of NK cells both from peripheral blood cord blood and iPSC-differentiated NK cells will also be discussed as well as potential future directions for the use of CAR-NK cells.

G. C. Birch · R. Romee (✉)
Harvard School of Medicine, Dana-Farber Cancer Institute, Boston, MA, USA
e-mail: rizwan_romee@dfci.harvard.edu

T. F. Fehniger
Siteman Cancer Center, Washington University School of Medicine, St. Louis, MO, USA

© Springer Nature Switzerland AG 2022
A. Ghobadi, J. F. DiPersio (eds.), *Gene and Cellular Immunotherapy for Cancer*, Cancer Drug Discovery and Development,
https://doi.org/10.1007/978-3-030-87849-8_16

Keywords NK cells · Cytokine induced memory-like (CIML) NK cells · Graft versus leukemia (GvL) effect · Adoptive cellular therapy · Induced pluripotent stem cells (iPSC)

Introduction

Natural killer (NK) cells are large granular lymphocytes first identified in 1975 as a cytotoxic immune cell that could detect and destroy aberrant or infected cells without prior antigen stimulation or sensitization [1, 2]. Pre-clinical work using allograft rejection models, showed that NK cells could recognize and kill targets that lacked self-MHC class I expression [3, 4], this was termed the "missing self-hypothesis." In humans the ability to detect "missing self" is mediated by inhibitory killer Ig-like receptors (KIR) which recognize specific HLA- class I molecules [5], and the CD94/NKG2A heterodimer which is specific for the non-classical HLA-E molecule, often expressed on tumor cells [6]. NK cells also use germline DNA encoded receptors to recognizing stress-induced ligands, which in turn provide an activating signal. NK cells can therefore recognize cells virus-infected and malignant cells due to the reduced of MHC-I and stress-induced ligands. This provides the immune system a cell with the capacity to detect cells that escape T cell immunosurveillance.

The pivotal role that NK cells play in controlling viral infection is highlighted by human NK cell deficiencies. In the rare cases where humans are deficient in NK cells they present with recurrent herpes infections, particularly Epstein-Barr virus (EBV) and human cytomegalovirus (HCMV) [7, 8]. An alternative role that NK cells play is in the development of the placental vasculature [9].

NK cells constitute 5–15% of circulating lymphocytes in the peripheral blood and can be found in lymphoid and non-lymphoid organs including spleen, lung, and liver [10, 11]. In the peripheral blood, two distinct populations of NK cells exist that can be defined by the differential surface expression of CD56 and CD16, these are: CD56^{dim} (low expressing) CD16 positive and CD56^{bright} (high expressing), CD16 negative NK cells [10, 12, 13]. The dominant NK cell subset in the peripheral blood are CD56^{dim} NK cells, which account for 90% of circulating NK cells. CD56^{bright} NK cells can be found in higher numbers in the parafollicular regions of secondary lymphoid tissue including tonsils, lymph nodes and mucosal activated lymphoid tissue (MALT) where they sit alongside CD34$^+$CD45RA$^+$ pre-NK cells and antigen presenting cells (APC) [14]. Here CD56^{bright} NK cells respond to changes in the inflammatory milieu with the production of chemokines and cytokines including IFN-γ, TNF, GMSF, IL-10 and IL-13 [13–15]. The role of CD56^{bright} NK cells in activating APC and together with dendritic cells (DC), modulating the T cell response places them as a link between the rapidly activated innate immune system and the adaptive immune response [16, 17]. CD56^{bright} NK cells may also mature into CD56^{dim} NK cells following activation in SLT [13–15].

The predominant role of CD56^{dim} NK cells is to act as highly cytotoxic killer cells even in the resting state. These cells utilize perforin/granzyme or death receptor pathways to destroy target cells. CD56^{dim} NK cells can also respond to activating receptor ligands or cytokines (e.g. IL-12, IL- 15 and IL-18) to produce cytokines including IFN-γ, albeit at a lower level than CD56^{bright} NK cells [15]. The release of perforin/granzyme from activated CD56^{dim} NK cells relies on initiation of the cytotoxic immunological synapse between NK cells and target cells [18]. Initiation of the immunological synapse involves close cell-cell contact and adherence of the NK cells to its target. The actin cytoskeleton is rearranged and the microtubule organizing center of the NK cells is polarized towards the point of contact with the target cell [19–22]. Adhesion of the NK cells to the target cell involves integrins such as LFA-1. A signaling event in the cytoplasm from CD2, DNAM-1, NKG2D, 2B4 or Ly49 induces a conformational change within an integrin and primes it for activation [23–25]. LFA-1 then binds to ICAM-1 on the target cell activating signaling pathways within the cell [26]. A ring of peripheral actin forms around the synapse after activation. This is key to cytotoxic function; without reorganization of actin, NK cells are poorly cytotoxic [27]. Following activation, lytic granules rapidly converge to the MTOC, which polarizes to the immune synapse [28]. In this process the centrosome moves to and contacts the plasma membrane at the cSMAC [28]. An actin mesh is formed at the center of both inhibitory and activating synapses that periodically opens in specific regions, creating gaps for lytic granules to penetrate [29]. The movement of cytotoxic granules towards the secretion site depends upon kinesin-1, a microtubule dependent motor protein that transports cargo in a plus-end direction [30]. Kinesin forms a complex with Rab27a and slp3 to transport lyric granules towards the plus-ends of microtubules which are then inserted into the F-actin mesh [29, 30]. Myosin IIa is involved in transportation of cytotoxic granules through the actin mesh [31]. Secretory lysosomes dock at the plasma membrane and fuse with it, releasing their cytotoxic contents [21]. Perforin and granulisin facilitate the entry of granzymes from the secretory lysosomes into the cytoplasm of the target cell where they induce apoptosis [32].

The death receptor (DR) mediated apoptotic process is the second method of killing utilized by NK cells. This is a caspase enzymatic cascade induced apoptosis mediated by interactions between CD95/FasL and TNF-related apoptosis inducing ligand (TRAIL) expressed on NK cells which activate death receptors CD95/Fas and TRAIl-R1-R2 on the cell surface of target cells [33–36].

NK cells are also capable of antibody dependent cell-mediated cytotoxicity (ADCC), mediated by immunoglobulin G (IgG) in humans [37–39]. The Fab moiety of the IgG molecule binds to the tumor-associated antigens (TAAs) on tumor cells and the Fc moiety to CD16A (FcγRIIIA) on NK cells triggering their cytotoxic response.

NK cells develop from CD34$^+$ hematopoietic progenitor cells in the bone marrow and mature in secondary lymphoid tissue including the lymph nodes, tonsil and spleen [40]. NK cell differentiation has been divided into five stages distinguished by the expression of distinct cell surface markers, transcription factors and cytokines (Fig. 1) [41–43]. Unlike B or T cells, NK cells do not rearrange genes to acquire clonally arranged antigen-specific receptors. NK cell function is instead dictated by NK activating and inhibitory signals from various germline DNA-encoded activating and inhibitory receptors expressed on the cell surface [44, 45]. As technology advances it has become clear that a heterogeneous pool of NKCs exists in which over 1000 distinct specificities can be described [46].

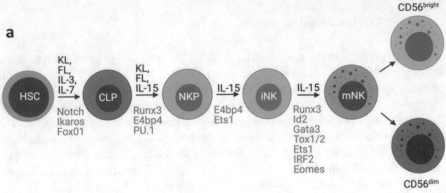

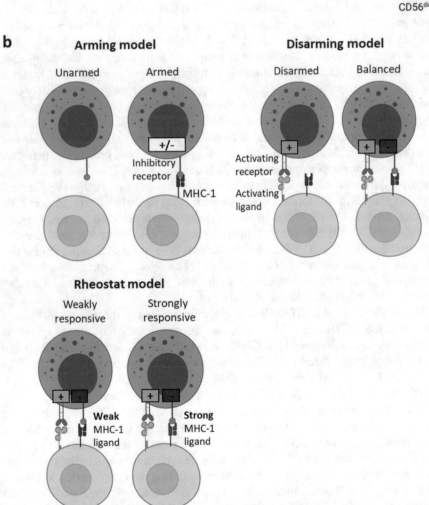

Fig. 1 Schematic representation of NK cell development and licensing/education. (**a**) NK cell development from hematopoietic stem cells (HSC) to common lymphoid progenitor (CLP), natural killer progenitor (NKP), immature NK (iNK) and mature NK (mNK) cells. (**b**) Models of NK cell licensing. The arming model in which cells become "armed" with the capability to respond to MHC-I on target cells. The disarming model in which cells become "disarmed" by lack of ligand-receptor interactions with target cells expressing MHC-I. The rheostat model in which NK cell reactivity is defined by the number of self-MHC-I inhibitory receptors expressed by each NK cell and the affinity of each of these receptors for the MHC-I ligands they bind

NK cells undergo an education process called licensing in order to gain functional competence. In this process, NK cells possessing inhibitory receptors specific to self-MHC-I functionally mature, and those that lack MHC-I specific receptors are rendered unlicensed and hypofunctional —they do not respond to MHC-I deficient or aberrant cells [47, 48]. There are three different models that have been proposed to describe this process of licensing (Fig. 1b). The first is NK cell "arming" in which NK cells gain functionality via ITIM dependent signaling following binding of specific MHC-I inhibitory receptors to cognate self MHC-I molecules and their ligands [47, 49]. An alternative mechanism proposes that rather than gaining a licensed function, NK cells lose the ability to respond through "disarming." In this model, all NKC are poised and activated, but cells that lack inhibitory receptors for MHC-I become hyporesponsive following continuous stimulatory signaling [50]. A third model for NK cell education/licensing is the "rheostat" model. This model suggests that NK cell reactivity can be defined by the number of self-MHC-I inhibitory receptors expressed by an NK cell and the affinity of each of these receptors for MHC-I [51]. NK cells expressing more than one inhibitory receptor for self-MHC-I are suggested to respond more robustly than NK cells with a single inhibitory receptor for self-MHC-I. The combined effect of an individual's KIR and HLA alleles therefore contributes to the overall NK cell activity in that individual [52]. This arming of NK cells is associated with structural organization within the endolysosomal compartment. NK cells possessing KIR that recognized self-MHC-I degranulated more readily towards K562 cells [53]. In accordance with this, educated, self-specific KIR expressing cells possessed large granzyme B rich secretory lysosomes close to the centrosome [53]. These cells also possessed higher chondroitin sulphate 4 (CS4) a glyosaminoglycan sidechain and perforin which suggests that the composition of secretory lysosomes is altered in educated cells [53]. The number of secretory lysosomes, however, is no different within educated and un-educated cells [53]. Inhibition of the lysosomal compartment in educated NK cells also affected production of cytokines in response to stimuli, suggesting that lysosomal derived signals expand beyond degranulation [53]. This study also offered a mechanism for disarming of NK cells through activation signals [53]. They showed that antagonizing the lysosomal calcium channel TRPML1 resulted in loss of granzyme B specific degranulation towards K562 target cells and loss of IFN-γ responses [53]. Silencing of TRPML1, however led to increased granzyme B production and enlargement of lysosomal structures, increased degranulation and IFN-γ production [53].

Inhibitory receptors that are specific to self MHC class include killer cell Ig-like receptors (KIR) and NKG2A. KIR receptors contain type 1 transmembrane glycoproteins with two or three C2 type IG-like domains (2D or 3D) and either a short (S) or long (L) cytoplasmic tails [54]. KIR with short cytoplasmic tails (no ITIMs) are activating and long tails (ITIM) inhibitory [55].

KIR interact with MHC-I ligands expressed on the cell-surface. These ligands have been divided into 3 categories according to the amino acid sequence that determines the KIR-binding epitope [56]. HLA-C alleles are denoted C1 (HLA-C group 1) or C2 (HLA-C group 2) depending on whether they possess an asparagine or lysine at position 80 of the alpha-1 domain of the alpha helix [57, 58]. HLA-B alleles can be distinguished by the presence of Bw4 and Bw6, where only Bw4 motif bearing HLA-B products can function as ligands for KIRs [56]. KIR are sensitive to the peptide bound by HLA-I, offering KIR⁺ NK cells the propensity to detect changes in the peptide and MHC-I repertoire which occurs during viral infection and tumorigenesis [59–61].

Other inhibitory NK cells receptors in humans include CD94/NGK2A heterodimers. These recognize non-classical HLA-I, HLA-E on the surface of target cells and prevent inappropriate activation of NK cells [6, 62]. A recent murine study has shown that NKG2A may also play a role in licensing of NK cells [63]. In this study it was shown that deletion of Ly49 receptors reduced the responsiveness of NKG2A negative cells but significantly increased the function of NKG2A⁺ cells, suggestive of a NKG2A dependent compensation for Ly49 deficiency. Using CRISPR/Cas9 gene editing it was shown that lack of NKG2A and Ly49 receptors C/G/I rendered NK cells functionally impaired an effect that was almost equivalent to that seen in $\beta 2m^{-/-}$ mice [63].

NKG2A signals via two ITIMS in its cytoplasmic tail [64]. HLA-E peptide complexes can bind to CD94 homodimers in the absence of NKG2A. This is thought to augment inhibitory signaling via CD94-NKG2A [62]. Peptides from viruses including EBV, HIV and CMV bind to HLA-E [65, 66]. Activating CD94/NKG2C molecules specific to HLA-E also exist, that associate with DAP-12, in a similar way as activating KIR bind to HLA-E. These complexes have a much lower affinity than the inhibitory CD94/NKG2A receptor but are involved in the response to CMV [67, 68]. In response to CMV an expansion of CD94/NKG2C expressing NK cells occurs. These cells are shown to possess an adaptive NK cell phenotype in which prolonged NKG2C+ NK cell expansion and augmented CD16A-mediated effector response occurs [69].

Leukocyte immunoglobulin-like receptors (LILRB1, ILT or CD85) are alternate type 1 transmembrane glycoprotein inhibitory receptors that bind to classical and non-classical HLA molecules as well as non-HLA ligands [70]. Ligand binding to LILRB inhibits NK cell activation by inhibiting polarization of lytic granules. HLA-G binding to LILRB1 on NK cells inhibits cytotoxicity towards trophoblasts in pregnancy, for example [71]. Inhibition of this receptor may be important in cancer therapy. Inhibition of LILRB1 as well as NKG2A can induce killing of AML and ALL cells by KIR-deficient NK cells. Blockade of LILRB1 alone has been shown to induce cytotoxicity of NK cells towards breast cancer cells [70, 72, 73].

Killer cell lectin-like receptor G1 (KLRG1) is another inhibitory receptor that is expressed by a large number of CD56 NK cells and terminally differentiated T cells [74]. Its ligands are ubiquitously expressed classical cadherins (E, N and R cadherins) which are present on healthy tissues [75]. This receptor has been shown to be increasingly expressed on NK cells in older individuals [74]. The inhibitory potential of this receptor is directly correlated to its cell surface expression. In individuals >70 years old that have a higher KLRG1 expression on both CD56^{dim} and CD56^{bright} cells an increased activation threshold of NK cells can be observed [76]. Cells with high KLRG1 were shown to spontaneously activate the metabolic sensor Amp-activated protein kinase (AMPK) which was shown to negatively regulate NK cell function. KLRG1 prevents the de-phosphorylation of AMPK by protein phosphatase PP2C, a phosphatase that normally de-phosphorylates AMPK *in vitro* and *in vivo*. KLRG1 was shown to internalize upon ligation and bind directly to AMPK to stimulate its function and inhibit PP2C-like phosphatase activity. It was shown however that KLRG1 requires pre-existing AMPK activity to stimulate the AMPK pathway, functioning as an "AMPK enhancer." This occurs in highly differentiated NK cells that exhibit senescence characteristics.

Key activating NK cells receptors include NKp30, NKp46 and CD16 which interact with transmembrane adaptor proteins with cytoplasmic ITAMS, CD3ζ and/or FcεRIγ or alternatively activating KIR, CD94/NKG2C and NKp44 which act via DAP12. CD3ζ and FcεRIγ are expressed either as homodimers or heterodimers, while DAP12 is always a homodimer [77]. Ligation of ITAM receptor complexes lead to recruitment and activation of tyrosine kinases SyK and ZAP70 initiating cytotoxicity and cytokine production [77].

NKG2D is an activating receptor which is important for recognizing virus-infected and transformed cells that express MICA, MICB and ULBP, signals via DAP10 in humans [77–79]. DAP10 contains amino acids that bind to the p85 subunit of PI3 kinase and Grb2 upon phosphorylation, stimulating phosphatidylinositol-3 kinase (PI3K) associated pathways [80]. NKG2D, only mediates cytotoxicity in the presence of a secondary inflammatory signal [81]. The function of this receptor is in regulating signaling of other receptors promoting CD16 signaling, ADCC as well as potentiating signaling via NKp46 and 2B4 [82–84].

CD160 is an Ig-like glycosyl phosphatidyl inositol (GPI)- anchored receptor that recognizes HLA-Ia and Ib molecules and recruits PI3-K to trigger cytotoxicity and cytokine secretion, including IFN-γ, TNF, IL-6, IL-8 and MIP1-β [85, 86]. It has been shown that this receptor is crucial for the production of IFN-γ by NK cells and subsequent tumor control in pre-clinical models of B16 melanoma and lymphoma [87]. Knockout of CD160 in these mice led to impaired tumor control that was resurrected with the introduction of CD160 positive NK cells. The authors concluded that CD160 is required by NK cells for efficient IFN-γ production [87].

Alongside the various activating and inhibitory receptors expressed by NK cells are co-stimulatory receptors which contribute to the activating or inhibitory signals. These include NKR-P1 receptors, DNAM-1 and PILR receptor [88, 89]. In humans, only one NKR-P receptor exists, NKR-P1A (KLRB1/CD161/CLEC5B [90]. This receptor functions via binding to Clr-related ligand, LLT1 (CLEC2D/OCIL/CLAX) [91]. DNAM-1 (CD226) is expressed on around 50% of NK cells and its ligands are CD155 and CD112 (Nectin-2), which are expressed at low levels on the cell surface of monocytes as well as on hematopoietic, epithelial and endothelial both humans and mice [88, 92, 93]. It has been implicated in anti-tumor responses and also in the recognition of both iDCs and mDCs [84]. DNAM-1 also plays a role in cell adhesion of NK and T effector cells to target cells [92]. Two paired Ig-like 2 receptors PILβ and PilRα are also expressed by NK cells which have a role in the recognition of carbohydrate chains on target cells, broadening the scope of targets that NK cells can recognize [94].

NK Cells in Cancer

As a result of their innate ability to detect and destroy tumor cells, NK cells stand out as an attractive candidate for cancer immunotherapies. At the same time as mounting cytotoxic responses against malignant target cells, NK cells secrete cytokines and chemokines that recruit other immune cells towards the tumor microenvironment. Secretion of chemokines including CCL 3, 4, 5 and 10 form a chemical gradient that directs immune effector cells to the tumor site. The secretion of IL-10 and IL-6 increase immune activity at the site of production. Secretion of CCL5, XCL1 and XCL2 from NK cells promotes the migration of DCs into the solid tumor microenvironment [95, 96]. NK cell activation in the lymph nodes aids in the recruitment of antigen-presenting cells towards the tumor microenvironment (TME), as well as in the activation of T cells in the lymph nodes via production of IFN-γ [37].

Following the advent of hematopoietic cell transplants (HCT) for cancer treatments, it was discovered that NK cells from HLA mismatched donors exerted a graft versus leukemia effect without initiating T cell mediated graft versus host disease (GVHD) [97, 98]. This may be due to the missing self-hypothesis, as alloreactive NK cells from an HLA haplotype-mismatched donor were shown to kill allogeneic leukemia [98]. Furthermore, transplants from KIR mismatched donors had higher engraftment rate. Miller et al. pioneered the use of NK cells in nontransplant settings [99]. Infusion of enriched NK cells from HLA-haploidentical donors in combination with subcutaneous IL-2 after lymphodepletion with high dose cyclophosphamide and fludarabine however, was successful leading to expansion of donor NK cells and complete remission in a quarter of patients with poor prognosis AML [99].

It is important to note that NK cell expansion and *in vivo* persistence was only observed in patients that received high-dose cyclophosphamide and fludarabine prior to NK cells infusion [99]. This nonmyeloablative conditioning chemotherapy is administered to deplete endogenous lymphocyte populations [99]. These endogenous populations would compete with infused NK cells for cytokines, and recipient T cells would otherwise immediately reject the allogeneic NK cells. Also, in patients with hematological malignancies, fludarabine/cyclophosphamide may also reduce the tumor burden, increasing the possibility for NK cells to be effective. Lymphodepleting agents are associated with toxicities which have negative impacts on the patients therefore, safer and more selective approaches are needed to improve clinical use of adoptive NK cells [100]. For example, one approach being exploited by CART therapeutics is to create CD52 knockout CART cells and utilize alemtuzumab, an anti-CD52 antibody as a lymphodepleting treatment that is less toxic than chemotherapy [101–103]. This method is being evaluated in trials investigating the use of UCART22 and UCART123, both of which have CD52 knocked out for the treatment of r/r ALL and r/r AML, respectively. This technique could also be utilized for NK cell immunotherapies as CD52 is expressed by NK cells.

The initial success in adoptive transfer in hematological cancers prompted efforts to evaluate its efficacy in the solid tumor setting. Solid tumors provide a number of further challenges to overcome including the tumor microenvironment (TME) which alters the phenotype, activation, persistence and function of NK cells [104, 105]. Another hurdle to overcome is getting NK cells to traffic towards and infiltrate the tumor. The TME is composed of Tregs, tumor associated macrophages (TAMs), regulatory γδT cells, myeloid-derived suppressor cells (MDSCs) soluble factors and the extracellular matrix, endothelial cells, stromal cells, and non-cellular components including collagen, fibronectin, hyaluronan and laminin [106–108]. Within that TME are secreted cytokines and immunosuppressive factors including prostaglandin E2 (PGE2) indoleamine, 2,3-dioxygenase (IDO), IL-10, TGF-β and vascular endothelial growth factor (VEGF) as well as chemokines such as CXCL8 or CCL2 which support the accumulation of Tregs, TAM and MDSCs in the tumor site [109]. These cells produce IL-10 and TGF-β which inhibit NK cell cytotoxicity [107]. Both Tregs and MDSCs also suppress NK cell activity via membrane bound TGF-β in a contact-dependent manner [110, 111]. MDSCs secrete soluble factors IDO, NO and adenosine, which limit the release of IFN-γ and TNF as well as inhibiting FASL and perforin and granzyme mediated cytotoxicity of NK cells [109, 112, 113]. Cancer associated fibroblasts also secrete IDO, PGE2 or TGF-β which leads to decreased NK cell expression of NKG2D, NKP30 and NKp44 as well as downregulating NK cell CD155 expression [114–116]. Despite this immunosuppressive TME, NK cell infiltration into solid tumor lesions has been associated with favorable prognosis [117]. A meta-analysis of 56 studies showed that high levels of NK cell associated markers CD56, CD57, NKP30 and NKp46 significantly correlated with better OS in solid cancer [117].

Finding ways to arm NK cells with the capability to overcome the suppressive TME and migrate towards the tumor site is therefore likely to be beneficial in the treatment of solid malignancies. One method of doing this is to add integrin or TGF-β inhibitors alongside NK cells in treatments or to arm them with TGF-β receptor gene editing, which inhibit the TGF-β axis and thereafter impeding the suppression from the TME [118]. This has shown promise in pre-clinical models of glioblastoma. Foltz et al. showed that TGF-β imprinting, induced by activation with TGF-β and IL-2 potently induces hypersecretion of IFN-y, TNF-α and GM-CSF in response to tumor targets and to cytokine stimulation [119]. This hypersecretion was shown to last for one month after imprinting, corresponding to changes in several IFN-y genes including JUN, Tbet and SMAD3. In a similar vein, engraftment of a dominant negative TGF-β receptor II (DNRII) on NK cells has shown promising results. In the context of glioblastoma, adoptively transferred cord blood NKCs that were retrovirally transduced to express the DNRII were shown to maintain perforin and NKG2D/DNMA1 expression in the presence of TGF-β. Henceforth, could kill glioblastoma tumor cells showing a functional advantage over control NK cells in the TGF-β secreting TME [120].

HLA-KIR mismatched NK cells have also been shown to be effective in a pre-clinical model of glioblastoma. In this study it was shown that HLA-KIR mismatched NK cells could target GBM cells both *in vitro* and *in vivo*. Further to this, it was shown that sorted KIR2DS2 positive NK cell populations showed increased cytotoxicity and persistence [121]. It is interesting to note that even in the absence of KIR-HLA ligand mismatch, treatment of GBM xenografts in NOD/SCID mice with NK cells from a KIR2DS2+ donor led to prolonged survival [121]. This was even longer than that observed for NK cells with multiple KIR-HLA ligand mismatches but lacking KIR2DS2 positivity [121]. This group concluded that KIR2DS2 can be used to identify potent alloreactive NK cells against GBM [121].

In colorectal cancer it was shown that umbilical cord blood (UCB) hematopoietic stem cell derived NK cells were more effective against colon cancer cells compared to peripheral blood NK cells, however it was noted that this could be due to the higher cytokine concentrations used to activate these cells [122]. In this study UCB-NK cells were tested against cetuximab-resistant human EGFR+Ras mutant colon cancer cells and shown to be effective *in vitro*. This finding was confirmed in an *in vivo* preclinical model where UCB-NK cells showed efficacy against tumor cells despite EGFR and RAS status, suggesting that UC-NK cells could be a promising treatment for cetuximab resistant colon cancer [122]. In an analysis of colorectal cancer patients undergoing surgery and chemotherapy, higher numbers of NK cell in the peripheral blood was associated with improved prognosis [123]. Xu et al. showed that NK cells expanded from UCB with membrane bound IL-21 (eUCB-NK cells) effectively lysed CRC cell lines *in vitro* and secreted higher levels of IFN-y, TNF and GM-CSF compared to IL-2 stimulated NK cells. Adoptive transfer of mbIL-21 activated NK cells significantly inhibited the growth of xenografts *in vivo* [124]. Interestingly this was only the case for HT29 xenografts, where LoVo tumors were not controlled by eUCB-NK cells. This is likely due to the lower numbers of infiltrating NK cells observed in LoVo tumors. Bevacizumab, however, was shown to increase NK cell extravasation into LoVo tumors, improving the therapeutic activity of eUCB-NK cells in this xenograft model. This study suggests that adoptive transfer of NK cells alone or in combination could offer promise in the clinic as a treatment for CRC [124]. Other studies utilizing iPSC derived NK cells have also shown promising results [125].

In a xenograft model of ovarian cancer, the efficacy of intraperitoneal (IP)-delivered NK cells was evaluated [126]. IP delivery of human NK cells in concert with cytokines led to high levels of circulating NK cells and clearance of ovarian cancer burden [126]. This original success in an *in vivo* model has been recapitulated in various other pre-clinical models including the use of iPSC-NK cells which were shown to be as effective as expanded PB-NK cells when administered three times intraperitoneally [127]. Umbilical cord derived HSPC NK cells were shown to efficiently target ovarian carcinoma spheroids and infiltrate intraperitoneal tumors *in vivo*, highlighting a potential role for these cells in ovarian cancer treatment [128]. In humans the frequency of NK cells within the lymphocyte fraction in ascites at diagnosis has been correlate with better overall survival in OC patients [129].

Isolation, Expansion and Stimulation of NK Cells

The promising safety profile and efficacy associated with NK cell-based immunotherapies have prompted a drive to develop "off-the-shelf" NK cell-based therapies. However, there are many logistic challenges to overcome. NK cells are notoriously difficult to expand *ex vivo*, and their persistence *in vivo* is variable. In recent years this has been a major focus of the field [100].

The source of NK cells for use in these therapies has also been subject to debate, with limitations associated with utilization of NK cells from each source. There are four major sources of NK cells—from the peripheral blood, the umbilical cord, IPSC-differentiated NK cells and immortalized NK cell lines.

The predominant source of NK cells in clinical trials currently is the peripheral blood collected via non mobilized apheresis. It is imperative that NK cells be purified prior to infusion to avoid GVHD caused by T cells [130], or passenger lymphocyte syndrome by B cells [131]. Purification methods vary. The most popular and efficient method is by magnetic bead selection to remove CD3$^+$ cells and enrich for CD56 positivity [132, 133]. An alternative method is to perform flow sorting CD56$^+$CD3$^-$ cells but this is time consuming and often reduces the yield of NK cells without prior enrichment [134]. An alternative method is to utilize a single step CD3/CD19 depletion to remove T and B cells [135]. If the NK cell source is only modestly enriched with many passenger cells, there may be a contribution of these additional immune cells to effects observed.

Cord blood is an alternative method for generating NK cells, however in cord blood there are a limited number of NK cells per cord blood unit [136]. These NK cells also express lower levels of KIRs and granzyme B as well as higher levels of the NKG2A receptor pertaining to a potentially more immature phenotype [136]. One advantage of cord blood NK cells is that they retain cytotoxicity following cryopreservation. This has been shown to be a problem with primary NK cells where cytotoxicity is reduced following freezing [137, 138].

It has been of recent interest in the field to develop iPSC-NK therapies to overcome the supply-chain bottlenecks associated with primary and cell line NK cell therapies. iPSCs can be generated from fibroblasts or peripheral blood and retain pluripotency during expansion [139]. Human embryonic stem cell derived NK cells (hESc-NK) or induced pluripotent stem cell (iPSC-NK) derived NK cells have advantages over peripheral blood derived or cord blood derived NK, coming from a stem cell population, they can be cultured to develop into a homogeneous population without having to worry about the presence of other immune cells. HESC/hiPSC-NK cells do however display a similar phenotype, transcriptome and function as primary NK cells, making them a very attractive target for therapeutic use [140, 141].

Methods used to generate iPSC-NK cells have improved significantly over the last 10 years [127, 140]. Initially, a two-stage stromal dependent culture system was utilized in which undifferentiated hESCs were cultured over a stromal cell line such as S17 or M2-10B4. Hematopoietic progenitor cells were then sorted and moved to culture over a second stromal cell line, AFT024 or ELO8-IDT cells, in media that was supplemented with SCF, FMs-like tyrosine kinase 3 ligand (FLT3L), IL-2, IL-15 and IL-7 to support their differentiation towards the NK cell lineage. This protocol was adapted to facilitate differentiation of NK cells in a serum-free, stromal-free environment to omit the need to use murine cells as stromal layers which could inhibit clinical translation [127, 141]. This method known as "spin embryoid body" uses recombinant protein-based, animal product-free medium and centrifugation to form embryoid bodies from hESC/iPSC [142]. The generation of spin EBs involved culture of hESC and iPSC that were lacking any signs of differentiation. Briefly, cells are passaged for a minimum of 10 times, in TrypLE select (Invitrogen) to a confluence of 60–70%, differentiated and filtered. To set up spin EB formation 3000 cells per well are added to a round bottom 96 well plate in bovine serum albumin polyvinyl alcohol essential lipids (BPEL) medium containing SCF, VEGF and BMP 4. Plates are spin aggregated at 1500 rpm for 5 minutes at room temperature and placed in an incubator for 3 days to ensure formation of EBs. After 11 days of differentiation, cells are transferred to a 24 well-plate where 6 wells of the 96 well plate constituted 1 well of the 24-well plate in differentiation media that contained SCF, FLT3L, IL-3, IL-15 and IL-7 for 4 weeks to generate CD45+ CD56+ NK cells [141]. These cells do not require sorting and are noted to form a homogeneous population of CD56+ NK cells. Recent updates to the method have been published to improve efficiency and reduce culture time [143].

NK cells derived from iPSCs have proven to be as effective as primary NK cells and NK-92 cells in ovarian tumor xenograft models [127]. Interestingly donor peripheral blood-iPSC-NK cells have shown greater cytotoxicity towards SKOV3, SW480, HCT-8, MCF7 and SCC-25 cancer cell lines compared to donor peripheral blood NK cells [144]. Zeng et al. have shown that PB-iPSC-NK cells are capable of ADCC, however it is not known if iPSC-NK cells utilize the same activation pathways to induce granule and cytokine secretion as PB-NK cells [144]. Further to this, Zhu et al. developed iPSC-NK cells with non-cleavable CD16a (hnCD16-iNK cells). These cells are highly resistant to activation-induced cleavage of CD16a and henceforth exhibit enhanced ADCC against multiple tumor targets [145]. These cells showed great promise when used in combination with mAB such as anti-CD20 for the treatment of B-cell lymphoma where hnCD16-iNK cells significantly improved regression. In an ovarian cancer xenograft model, in combination with anti-HER2 mAB hnCD16-iNK led to improved survival. This was in contrast to treatment with PB-NK cells and unmodified iNK cells which did not inhibit tumor growth. Interestingly treatment with hnCD16-iNK alone did not decrease tumor growth in this model. Fate therapeutics have a phase I clinical trial to investigate an "off-the-shelf" iPSC-NK product, FT500 that is derived from a clonal master iPSC line bank with the capacity to produce homogeneous, quality controlled iPSC-NK cells [146].

Expanding cells ex vivo using cytokines is a bone fide method of increasing NK cell product yield, however the optimal conditions for this are subject to much debate (Table 1). Utilizing IL-2/IL-15/IL-21 together can support the expansion of NK cells up to eight fold [147]. Most recent studies however, showed that ex vivo

Table 1 NK cell expansion protocols [162]

Stimulation	Stimulation	Fold expansion (time)	In clinical use	Considerations	Reference
	IL-15	~23 (21–23 days)	Yes	– Generate highly activated NK cells – Possibility of dependence on cytokine – Expansion is facilitated in the presence of autologous PBMC	[163]
	IL-21/IL-15	~2.3 fold (2 weeks)			[164]
	IL-21/IL-15	~4.3 (10–12 days)			[165]
	IL-2/IL-15/ IL-21	~8 (2 weeks)	No		[147]
	IL-15/IL-18/ IL-27	~17 (2 weeks)	No		[148]
	IL-2, IL-18	~500 (2 weeks)	No		[149]
Autologous feeder cells	OK432, RN-T cells	~600 (3 weeks)	Yes	RN-T cells were established by activation PBMC with OKT-3 and RetroNectin FN-CH296	[166]
Autologous feeder cell and activating antibodies	Anti-CD335 and anti CD2	~3800 (3 weeks)	No	CD2 and CD335 coated nanomatrices with commercially available cell stimulation beads (Miltenyi Biotec Kit)	Patent EP2824112b, 2007
	OKT-3 (Anti CD3), anti-CD52	~1537 (18 days)	Yes	PBMCs are typically irradiated 25 Gy or more GMP-grade antibody Anti CD3 is available	[167]
	OKT-3 (anti-CD3), IL-2	~1000 (2 weeks)	Yes		[168]
	Anti CD16	>500 (2 weeks)	No		[169]

(continued)

Table 1 (continued)

Stimulation	Stimulation	Fold expansion (time)	In clinical use	Considerations	Reference
Allogeneic feeder cells PBMC	+ PHA, Ionomycin, IL-2, IL-15	80–100	No	– Without selection final product may contain up to 40% T cells – PBMCs are typically irradiated 25 Gy or more	[170]
	+anti CD3, IL-2	~300	Yes		[171]
	Wilms tumor cell line (HFWT)	~113 (2 weeks)	Yes	– Feeder can be genetically modified to enhance activation – Feeder cells require irradiation and GMP-grade production – Final product needs to be feeder free assured	[172]
Allogeneic feeder cells (tumor)	Jurkat	~100 (2 weeks)	No	– Risk of bacterial and viral contamination derived from feeder cells	[173]
	EBV lymphoblastoid cell line (EBV-LCL)	~3000 (2 weeks)	Yes	– Feeder cells require irradiation – Safety considerations associated with feeder	[174]
Engineered feeder	K562 41-BB + IL-15	~1200 (2 weeks)	Yes	– Increased apoptosis of NK cells noted after extensive expansion	[151, 152, 175, 176]
	K562 41-BB + IL-21	~30,000 (3 weeks)	Yes	– Greatest rate of expansion reported so far – Lower dose of supportive IL-2 required	[152–155, 176]

(continued)

Table 1 (continued)

Stimulation	Stimulation	Fold expansion (time)	In clinical use	Considerations	Reference
Feeder particles	K562 4-1BB + IL21	~250 (2 weeks)		– Avoids the safety considerations associated with feeder cells – Laborious to produce	[177]
	Group A streptococcus and zoledronate	~1560 (3 weeks)	No	– >90% of NK cells – May not require magnetic cell sorting – Components IL2, streptococcus and zoledronate are FDA approved	[178]

stimulation of human NK cells with the combination of IL-15/IL-18/IL-27 can achieve 17-fold expansion [148], and the combination of IL-2 with IL-18 can achieve up to 500-fold expansion over in two weeks [149]. The presence of autologous feeder cells (typically CD3-depleted PBMCs) in culture also aids NK cell expansion [150]. Expanding NK cells ex vivo has been a subject of study for a long time, predominantly owing to the fact that in order to sustain NK cells in culture they must receive activation. Too much activation leads to exhaustion or changes in the phenotype of NK cells. Further, NK cells can become addicted to the mixture of growth factors used for expansion, thereby resulting in limited *in vivo* persistence following adoptive transfer.

Membrane-bound interleukins may offer a potential means for NK cell expansion that is more effective than soluble interleukins. Campana et al. showed that stimulation NK cells with K562 cells expressing 4-1BB and IL-15 could induce greater than 20-fold expansion over a 7-day period *in vitro* [151] Other studies have shown that up to 30,000-fold expansion can be achieved with K562 expressing membrane bound IL-21 (mbIL-21)and 4-1BB ligand [152–155]. These cells have been shown to be highly cytotoxic and cytokine producing, displaying a high expression of NCRs, CD16 and NKG2D [152, 156]. Further to this, the use of mbIL-21 promotes increased telomere length which is a suggested mechanism for the increased persistence *in vivo* observed when using NK cells expanded in this way. This protocol is currently being used in a phase I/II clinical trial (NCT01787474) utilizing haploid-identical NK cells for relapsed or refractory AML.

NK92 cells are an IL-2 dependent cell line established in 1992 from the peripheral blood of a 50-year-old male patient with non-Hodgkin's lymphoma. They are characterized by the expression of bright CD56 and CD2 and the lack of expression of CD3, CD8 and FCγRIII and CD16 [157]. They are however highly cytotoxic, displaying high cytotoxicity against tumor targets, notably higher than primary NK cells [158]. NK92 lack the expression of all KIR receptors apart from KIR2DL4. Owing to their lack of KIR and other receptors, these cells pose no risk for graft-versus-host disease in patients, therefore trials utilizing this potential "off-the-shelf" NK cell therapy have been conducted with NK92 cells expanded from a master cell bank, tested negative for blood pathogens and fungal and bacterial contaminants [158]. Early studies indicated a promising safety profile associated with the use of irradiated NK-92 in patients with advanced cancer [159, 160]. The caveat with use of these cells being that they must be irradiated before use, which limits their *in vivo* activity and persistence [160]. Arming NK-92 with CAR for better targeting of tumor subsets offers a promising off the shelf platform for cancer treatment [161] (Table 1).

Cytokine Induced Memory-Like (CIML) and Adaptive NK Cells

NK cells, unlike antigen specific T and B cells, have classically been considered to exert short-lived, non-specific responses with no capacity to retain memory like responses. However, in recent years studies have suggested that NK cells have the capacity to elicit memory-like behavior [133, 179–182]. This phenomenon has been shown to occur following hapten exposure, viral infection or cytokine activation with a combination of cytokines (IL- 12, IL-15 and IL-18) [183, 184].

The first evidence of a memory like NK cell response was shown in a murine model of hapten-mediated contact hypersensitivity [180]. In this model, an epithelial surface is exposed to organic or inorganic molecules that chemically modify proteins. These "haptenated" molecules are recognized by the immune system as foreign antigens, triggering a memory-like response. This memory response is known to be mediated by T and B cells, however in a Rag2 deficient mouse model, in which mice lack both B and T cells, a hapten-specific response was shown to be elicited by NK cells [180]. This NK cell response was long-lived and antigen specific with NK cells capable of acquiring memory of three distinct foreign molecular entities. Hepatic NK cells that were transferred to naïve mice retained memory-like features and antigen specificity [180]. Mechanisms responsible for hapten-related NK cell memory remain under investigation.

Evidence of a specific memory like NK cell subset came from studies of murine cytomegalovirus (MCMV) in which expansion of a Ly49H+ NK cell subset was observed in mice that were infected with this virus [185]. Further studies showed that the m157 glycoprotein that was expressed on MCMV-infected cells was recognized by this receptor and that expanded populations of Ly49H+ NK cells exerted a more prominent immune response upon subsequent infections [186–188].

In an analogous fashion, CMV infection in humans has been shown to induce expansion of a population of NK cells that express the receptor NKG2C [189]. These CD56^{dim}NKG2C$^+$ NK cells show enhanced proliferation and cytokine secretion in response to HCMV infected targets [189]. Similarly, in other viral infections such as Hepatitis C, HBV, EBV and HIV-1, an expansion of these NKG2C+ cells can be observed [190]. NK cell memory for CMV has been shown to be associated with chromatin modification and reduced DNA methylation as the IFN-γ gene locus, suggesting a differentiated adaptive state, with specialization for response via CD16a, NKG2C, and selected other activating receptors [191, 192].

Inflammatory cytokines which are known to play a role in the differentiation and function of NK cells also have the propensity to induce a memory-like adaptive response in the absence of antigen stimulation. Cooper et al. first showed that *in vitro* stimulation of NK cells with IL-2, IL-15 and IL-18 lead to an expansion of NK cells with enhanced IFN-γ secretion following adoptive transfer into syngeneic B6 or syngeneic Rag1$^{-/-}$ mice [182]. These cytokine induced memory-like NK cells display enhanced proliferation, prolonged persistence *in vivo* and increased IFN-γ production upon re-stimulation. Subsequently, human NK cells were shown to also exhibit cytokine-induced memory-like responses. Brief activation with IL-1, IL-15 and IL-18 endowed cells with the ability to exhibit enhanced IFN-γ production [133, 193], as well as an enhanced response upon stimulation with K562 cells *in vitro*. This was true of both CD56^{dim} and CD56^{bright} NK cells subsets. CD56^{dim} stimulated cells were described to increase expression of CD94 and NKG2A as well as NKp46 and CD69 and CD56^{bright} NK cells were shown to express NKp46 and CD69 [133]. One important feature of memory-like NK cell biology is that the enhanced function is passed on to daughter cells following cell division, suggesting an epigenetic mechanism for a distinct memory-like NK cell differentiation state.

The mechanisms underlying differentiation of CIML NK cells are not fully understood. One established mechanism is the demethylation of the IFN-γ locus. Stimulation with IL-12/15/18 increased the ability of these NK cells to maintain antitumor activity and IFN-γ production which coincided with demethylation of the conserved non-coding sequence (CNS) 1 in the IFN-γ locus [194]. This genetic imprinting lead to the persistence of an IFN-γ producing phenotype in a xenograft mouse model after adoptive transfer [194]. Additional epigenetic mechanisms are likely, and this remains an active area of investigation.

Leong et al. showed that human CIML activated NK cells CD25 the high affinity IL-2 receptor, elucidating a potential mechanism for their increased production of IFN-γ following further activation [195]. Adoptive transfer into immunodeficient NOD-SCID-γc$-/-$ mice showed that human CIML activated NK cells expand and respond to IL-2 with enhanced survival and functionality [195]. This complemented prior work by the Cerwenka laboratory, demonstrating that murine memory-like NK cells took advantage of T-cell derived IL-2 *in vivo*, to enhance function and persistence [193]. In addition, Wagner et al. demonstrated that memory-like differentiation rescued "unlicensed" hypofunctional cells, restoring their ability to respond to MHC-class I low target cells. In addition, CIML NK cells were shown to exhibit enhanced responses via CD16a, demonstrating their potential for antibody dependent responses [196].

CIML NK Cells in Cancer Treatment

CIML NK cells pose as an attractive target for cancer immunotherapies owing to their prolonged proliferation and persistence *in vivo* coupled with their augmented response against tumor targets *in vitro*.

In an *in vivo* mouse models of lymphoma and melanoma, adoptive transfer of IL-12, IL-15 and IL-18 activated NK cells in irradiated mice resulted in rapid NK cell proliferation and enhanced tumor control, compared to conventional NK cells [193]. In these mice activated NK cells proliferated rapidly, utilized T cell-derived IL-2, and resulted in reduced tumor growth and prolonged survival, compared to mice treated with conventional NK cells. This anti-tumor response persisted for months after adoptive transfer.

Studies with human NK cells showed similar results. In the first study purified human NK cells were stimulated with IL-12, IL-15 and IL-18 for 16 h *in vitro*. The cells were then rested *in vitro* with a low dose of IL-15 for 1–3 weeks. Following rest, these cells were shown to exhibit enhanced IFN-γ production following cytokine re-stimulation or, more importantly in response to tumor target cells blasts when compared to NK cells incubated with IL-12, IL-18 or IL-15 alone [133, 197]. This enhanced IFN-γ production was shown to be true for both CD56^{dim} and CD56^{bright} NK cell subsets. Cells displaying enhanced IFN-γ production had increased expression of CD94, NKG2A, NKG2C and CD69 as well as a lack of KIR and CD57. These cells were responsive to low concentrations of IL-2, where picomolar concentrations of IL-2 resulted in proliferation of these cells both *in vitro* and *in vivo* and enhanced IFN-γ production and cytotoxicity. Human CIML NK cells were shown to exhibit higher granzyme B protein expression and increased cytotoxicity against leukemia targets or AML blasts *in vitro* [197]. This was further investigated in a xenograft model where the injection CIML NK cells showed persistent expansion and trafficking to the bone marrow, spleen, liver and blood. In a model of leukemia CIML NK cells were shown to improve leukemia clearance supported by low dose IL-2 [197]. This effect was also shown *in vivo* in nonobese diabetic (NOD)/severe combined immunodeficient (SCID)/common gamma chain$^{-/-}$ ($\gamma c^{-/-}$) (NSG) mouse xenograft models of AML where CIML NK cells significantly reduced AML burden and improved overall survival [198].

In light of the pre-clinical evidence demonstrating improved anti-tumor responses by CIML NK cells, this approach was translated to the clinic as a cellular therapy. HLA-haploidentical adoptively transferred CIML NK cells were utilized in a phase I clinical trial [198, 199]. In this study, donor NK cells were purified by CD3 depletion and CD56 positive selection, pre-activated for 12–16 h with IL-12, IL-15 and IL-18, washed and infused into patients who had received fludarabine and cyclophosphamide for lymphodepletion. Low does (1 mIU/m^2 every other day x 7) IL-2 was administered following adoptive transfer. Memory-like NK cells were shown to peak in frequency between days 7 to 14 and decrease following recovery of the T cell compartment, persisting for at least 21 days [198]. In the bone marrow it was shown that at day 8 after infusion large percentages of donor NK cells were present.

It is important to note that there was heterogeneity here between donor and recipient pairs. Functional analysis revealed an increase in donor IFN-γ producing NK cells in the peripheral blood and in the bone marrow. The overall IWG response rate for this study was 67% with a CR/Cri rate of 47%, suggesting that allogeneic transfer of CIML activated NK cells may be a promising therapeutic intervention for r/r AML [198]. Further correlative studies used mass cytometry to define a unique multidimensional phenotype, that was confirmed using donor or recipient-specific HLA monoclonal antibodies. Utilizing this mass cytometry on *in vivo* differentiated CIML NK cells, it was observed that supraphysiologic NKG2A induction on donor CIML NK cells associated with treatment failure. *In vitro* studies confirmed NKG2A is a dominant transcriptionally-induced checkpoint that limits CIML NK cells response to leukemia, as CRISPR/Cas9 gene editing or antibody-blockade restored CIML NK cell function against HLA-E+ leukemia targets [199]. It was also shown that the presence of CD8α expression on CIML NK cells was associated with treatment failure, likely owing to reduced ability to proliferate in response to cytokine activation [199].

CIML NK cells have also shown promise in a pre-clinical models of solid cancers. For example, in an ovarian cancer model Uppendhal et al. showed that CIML NK cells displayed enhanced cytokine production and killing of ovarian cancer cells when compared to conventional NK cells [200]. This study showed that CIML NK cells exhibited enhanced effector function in the immunosuppressive TME [200]. Another recent study by Marin et al. demonstrated that CIML NK cells exhibit enhanced responses against human melanoma. Here, both allogeneic healthy donor and melanoma-patient memory-like NK cells exhibited enhanced IFN-γ and killing of melanoma targets, compared to conventional NK cells. This included enhanced autologous response of a melanoma patients' CIML NK cells against their own primary melanoma cells, and an *in vivo* model demonstrating CIML NK cells with improved melanoma control in NSG mice, compared to conventional NK cells [201].

Current clinical trials are investigating the potential for CIML NK cells in patients with myeloid malignancies to prevent relapse in the setting of allogenic HCT (NCT02782546), and for patients who have relapsed following haploidentical hematopoietic stem cell transplant (NCT03068819, NCT04024761). These studies are evaluating the use of CIML NK cells from the same stem cell donor to increase *in vivo* expansion and persistence of adoptively transferred CIML NK cells. The safety and efficacy of allogeneic CIML NK cells in patients with metastatic head and neck cancer is also under current investigation (NCT04290546). This study is evaluating the use of CTLA-4 inhibition with ipilumab prior to CIML NK cell infusion with an aim to deplete intratumoral Tregs [200]. Patients enrolled on this study are also receiving IL-15 super-agonist which has been shown to preferentially activate NK cells without affecting Tregs in an aim to maintain durable CIML activated NK cell responses [202].

CIML NK cells also represent an intriguing platform for cellular engineering. The initial report showing clinical safety and preliminary efficacy of cord-blood derived CD19-CAR expressing NK cells in B cell malignancies provided proof of concept that CAR-engineering NK cells was both possible and promising [203].

Gang et al., showed that memory-like NK cells engineered with a CD19-CAR (41bb/zeta) had superior *in vitro* functional responses, compared to conventional blood NK cells, against NK-resistant B cell lymphomas [204]. Healthy donor and lymphoma patient CIML NK cells exhibited enhanced CAR-directed responses, including against autologous lymphoma targets. *In vivo*, CD19CAR-ML NK cells expanded and persisted in NSG mice, and induced responses against a B cell lymphoma model *in vivo*.

Overcoming Tumor Evasion of the NK Cell Response

The interaction between NK cells and MHC-class I is important for the prevention of autoimmunity, however this mechanism is also hijacked by cancer cells to evade immune recognition and leads to energy of NK cells. One way that tumor cells evade NK cell control is to express inhibitory ligands HLA-E which acts via and NKG2A/CD94 to inhibit the activation of NK cells. Recently HLA-G has also been shown to bind to NKG2A/CD94 [205].

Monalizumab (previously IPH2201) is an anti-NKG2A checkpoint inhibitor that is currently under clinical investigation in head and neck cancer and ovarian cancer [206]. Blockade of NKG2A using monalizumab was shown to enhance NK cell activity against tumor targets [207]. In combination with PD-L1 blocking mAb durvalumab, monalizumab was shown to be effective in promoting both NKG2A+ NK cell and CD8+ T cell effector functions. Combination with anti-epidermal growth factor receptor (EGF-R) mAb also enhanced NK cell mediated ADCC adding weight to the benefit of its use in combination with other cancer mAb treatments [207].

Alternative methods of tumor cell evasion include expression of ligands that bind to NK cell and cytotoxic T cell inhibitory "checkpoint" receptors including PD-1, lymphocyte activation gene 3 (LAG3), T cell immunoglobulin and mucin-domain containing-3 (TIM3) and T cell immunoreceptor with Ig and ITIM domains (TIGIT) [208]. Tumor cells also shed NKG2D ligands MICA and MICB to evade NK cell control as well as producing TGF-β and kynurenine which act to downregulate the expression of NKG2D itself [209].

Cancer immune therapies aim to bypass this tumor evasion and enhance the anti-tumor effects of NK cells, the use of checkpoint inhibition is a promising means for this. Checkpoint inhibition utilizes blocking antibodies that bind to the checkpoint receptor and prevent ligand binding [208]. This prevents the inhibition associated with tumor binding to cytotoxic T and NK cells [208].

Inhibition of PD-1 has become the most promising approach to cancer immunotherapy in recent years [208]. *In vitro* treatment of patient-derived PD-1+ NK cells with an anti-PD-1 antibody (pidilizumab, CT-011) was shown to increased NK cell-mediated killing of autologous cancer cells [210, 211]. In an *in vitro* system, cytotoxicity of NK92 cells and primary NK cells towards PD-L1 positive cancer cell lines was enhanced in the presence of anti-PD-L1 mAB with ADCC [212].

TIM-3 is shown to increase in expression on NK cells with cancer progression. The ligand for TIM-3, GAL9 is expressed on the surface of tumor cells [213]. TIM-3+ NK cells display an exhausted phenotype correlated with poor prognosis [214]. *In vitro* studies have shown highlight the potential for TIM-3 blockade as an immunotherapy [206].

Activation of TIGIT an inhibitory receptor expressed on NK cells that binds CD115 and CD112 has been shown to prevent *in vitro* cell killing of target cells. Antibody-mediated blocking of TIGIT, however was shown to successfully increase NK cell cytotoxicity [207, 215]. Clinical trials are currently investigating the use of TIGIT blockade as a monotherapy or in concert with anti-PD1/PDL-1 mAbs in the treatment of solid malignancies [216].

The fact that tumor cells upregulate HLA-E and other inhibitory molecules for KIR has sparked interest in creating KIR-blocking monoclonal antibodies. A humanized (mAb), IPH2101, has been generated and is currently tested in clinical trials. Preclinical *in vitro* and *in vivo* studies showed IPH2101-mediated KIR blockade on human NK cells increased killing of tumor cells [217]. In clinical phase I and II studies no severe side effects were observed in patients with acute lymphoblastic leukemia or multiple myeloma [218–220]. Unfortunately, however, significant anti-tumor efficacy was not observed.

Efforts to reduce immune suppressive signaling from the tumor microenvironment such as neutralization of TGF-β signaling have also shown some success *in vitro* [221, 222]. Antibodies recognizing tumor-specific epitopes are an alternative strategy to direct the cytolytic activity of NK cells towards malignant cells. One approach is to harness *ADCC via CD16* (FcγRIIIA) with tumor specific IgG. There are currently, several ADCC therapies being tested in clinical trials in use in the clinic including, such as α-CD20, α-GD2, α-Her2, and α-EGFR mAbs. However, it is important to mention that CD16 is expressed not only on NK cells but also on activated myeloid subsets. This means that it is probable several hematopoietic lineages contribute to the observed therapeutic effects of ADCC [218–220]. Besides mAbs, bispecific or trispecific killer engagers (BiKEs and TriKEs) that are able to target one or two different antigens on the tumor cell as well as binding to an alternate epitope of the CD16 receptor are being developed. These have the promise of improved NK cell mediated ADCC effect [223]. When CD16 is activated it is shed by NK cells and recycled, thus reducing signaling for a period of time [224, 225]. This shedding is mediated by a metalloproteinase (MMP) ADAM17 also known as TNFα cleaving enzyme (TACE), a transmembrane protein that induces ectodomain protein shedding. Inhibition of this protein is associated with abrogated CD16 loss but has no effect on CD107a production by NK cells. Interestingly inhibition of ADAM17 actually leads to enhanced IFN-γ production following CD16 activation [225]. Utilizing ADAM17 inhibitors is therefore of interest in combination with NK cell therapies [226, 227]. Development of NK cells expressing clip resistant CD16 is also the subject of much interest in the field at present [145].

There has been overwhelming interest in the use of NK cells for cancer therapy in the past decade with extremely promising results associated with the use of NK cell associated haplo-identical stem cell transplants and efforts to generate "off-the-shelf" novel immunotherapies utilizing NK cells. With their innate tumor killing abilities and ability to functionally adapt in response to cytokine stimulation, these cells remain at the forefront of cancer immune cell therapy today.

References

1. Herberman RB, Nunn ME, Lavrin DH. Natural cytotoxic reactivity of mouse lymphoid cells against syngeneic acid allogeneic tumors. I. Distribution of reactivity and specificity. Int J Cancer. 1975;16(2):216–29.
2. Kiessling R, Klein E, Pross H, Wigzell H. "Natural" killer cells in the mouse. II. Cytotoxic cells with specificity for mouse moloney leukemia cells. characteristics of the killer cell. Eur J Immunol. 1975;5(2):117–21.
3. Karre K, Ljunggren HG, Piontek G, Kiessling R. Selective rejection of H-2-deficient lymphoma variants suggests alternative immune defence strategy. Nature. 1986;319(6055):675–8.
4. Ljunggren H-G, Kärre K. In search of the 'missing self': MHC molecules and NK cell recognition. Immunol Today. 1990;11:237–44. http://www.sciencedirect.com/science/article/pii/016756999090097S
5. Rajagopalan S, Long EO. Understanding how combinations of HLA and KIR genes influence disease. J Exp Med. 2005;201(7):1025–9. https://pubmed.ncbi.nlm.nih.gov/15809348
6. Braud VM, Allan DSJ, O'Callaghan CA, et al. HLA-E binds to natural killer cell receptors CD94/NKG2A, B and C. Nature. 1998;391(6669):795–9. https://doi.org/10.1038/35869.
7. Biron CA, Byron KS, Sullivan JL. Severe herpesvirus infections in an adolescent without natural killer cells. N Engl J Med. 1989;320(26):1731–5.
8. Orange JS. Natural killer cell deficiency. J Allergy Clin Immunol. 2013;132(3):515–25. https://pubmed.ncbi.nlm.nih.gov/23993353
9. Dosiou C, Giudice LC. Natural killer cells in pregnancy and recurrent pregnancy loss: endocrine and immunologic perspectives. Endocr Rev. 2005;26(1):44–62.
10. Freud AG, Mundy-Bosse BL, Yu J, Caligiuri MA. The broad spectrum of human natural killer cell diversity. Immunity. 2017;47(5):820–33. https://doi.org/10.1016/j.immuni.2017.10.008.
11. Björkström NK, Ljunggren H-G, Michaëlsson J. Emerging insights into natural killer cells in human peripheral tissues. Nat Rev Immunol. 2016;16(5):310–20.
12. Lanier LL, Testi R, Bindl J, Phillips JH. Identity of Leu-19 (CD56) leukocyte differentiation antigen and neural cell adhesion molecule. J Exp Med. 1989;169(6):2233–8. https://doi.org/10.1084/jem.169.6.2233.
13. Cooper MA, Fehniger TA, Caligiuri MA. The biology of human natural killer-cell subsets. Trends Immunol. 2001;22(11):633–40.
14. Freud AG, Becknell B, Roychowdhury S, et al. A human CD34(+) subset resides in lymph nodes and differentiates into CD56bright natural killer cells. Immunity. 2005;22(3):295–304.
15. Fehniger TA, Shah MH, Turner MJ, et al. Differential cytokine and chemokine gene expression by human NK cells following activation with IL-18 or IL-15 in combination with IL-12: implications for the innate immune response. J Immunol. 1999;162(8):4511 LP–4520. http://www.jimmunol.org/content/162/8/4511.abstract
16. Wallach D, Fellous M, Revel M. Preferential effect of gamma interferon on the synthesis of HLA antigens and their mRNAs in human cells. Nature. 1982;299(5886):833–6.
17. Vitale M, Chiesa MD, Carlomagno S, et al. The small subset of CD56brightCD16– natural killer cells is selectively responsible for both cell proliferation and interferon-γ production upon interaction with dendritic cells. Eur J Immunol. 2004;34(6):1715–22. https://doi.org/10.1002/eji.200425100.
18. Vyas YM, Mehta KM, Morgan M, et al. Spatial organization of signal transduction molecules in the NK cell immune synapses during MHC class I-regulated noncytolytic and cytolytic interactions. J Immunol. 2001;167(8):4358–67.

19. Katz P, Zaytoun AM, Lee JHJ. Mechanisms of human cell-mediated cytotoxicity. III. Dependence of natural killing on microtubule and microfilament integrity. J Immunol. 1982;129(6):2816–25.

20. Orange JS, Harris KE, Andzelm MM, Valter MM, Geha RS, Strominger JL. The mature activating natural killer cell immunologic synapse is formed in distinct stages. Proc Natl Acad Sci U S A. 2003;100(24):14151–6. https://www.ncbi.nlm.nih.gov/pubmed/14612578

21. Orange JS. The lytic NK cell immunological synapse and sequential steps in its formation. Adv Exp Med Biol. 2007;601:225–33.

22. Orange JS. Formation and function of the lytic NK-cell immunological synapse. Nat Rev Immunol. 2008;8(9):713–25. https://www.ncbi.nlm.nih.gov/pubmed/19172692

23. Osman MS, Burshtyn DN, Kane KP. Activating Ly-49 receptors regulate LFA-1-mediated adhesion by NK cells. J Immunol. 2007;178(3):1261–7.

24. Liu D, Bryceson YT, Meckel T, Vasiliver-Shamis G, Dustin ML, Long EO. Integrin-Dependent Organization and Bidirectional Vesicular Traffic at Cytotoxic Immune Synapses. Immunity. 2009;31(1):99–109. http://www.sciencedirect.com/science/article/pii/S1074761309002751

25. Hoffmann SC, Cohnen A, Ludwig T, Watzl C. 2B4 engagement mediates rapid LFA-1 and actin-dependent NK cell adhesion to tumor cells as measured by single cell force spectroscopy. J Immunol. 2011;186(5):2757–64.

26. Kim M, Carman CV, Springer TA. Bidirectional transmembrane signaling by cytoplasmic domain separation in integrins. Science. 2003;301(5640):1720–5.

27. Orange JS, Ramesh N, Remold-O'Donnell E, et al. Wiskott-Aldrich syndrome protein is required for NK cell cytotoxicity and colocalizes with actin to NK cell-activating immunologic synapses. Proc Natl Acad Sci U S A. 2002;99(17):11351–6.

28. Stinchcombe JC, Majorovits E, Bossi G, Fuller S, Griffiths GM. Centrosome polarization delivers secretory granules to the immunological synapse. Nature. 2006;443(7110):462–5.

29. Brown ACN, Oddos S, Dobbie IM, et al. Remodelling of cortical actin where lytic granules dock at natural killer cell immune synapses revealed by super-resolution microscopy. PLoS Biol. 2011;9(9):e1001152. https://doi.org/10.1371/journal.pbio.1001152.

30. Kurowska M, Goudin N, Nehme NT, et al. Terminal transport of lytic granules to the immune synapse is mediated by the kinesin-1/Slp3/Rab27a complex. Blood. 2012;119(17):3879–89. https://doi.org/10.1182/blood-2011-09-382556.

31. Krzewski K, Coligan JE. Human NK cell lytic granules and regulation of their exocytosis. Front Immunol. 2012;3:335. https://pubmed.ncbi.nlm.nih.gov/23162553

32. Lieberman J. The ABCs of granule-mediated cytotoxicity: new weapons in the arsenal. Nat Rev Immunol. 2003;3(5):361–70.

33. Screpanti V, Wallin RPA, Grandien A, Ljunggren H-G. Impact of FASL-induced apoptosis in the elimination of tumor cells by NK cells. Mol Immunol. 2005;42(4):495–9. https://www.sciencedirect.com/science/article/pii/S0161589004003086

34. Rouvier E, Luciani MF, Golstein P. Fas involvement in Ca(2+)-independent T cell-mediated cytotoxicity. J Exp Med. 1993;177(1):195–200.

35. Kagi D, Vignaux F, Ledermann B, et al. Fas and perforin pathways as major mechanisms of T cell-mediated cytotoxicity. Science (80-). 1994;265(5171):528 LP–530. http://science.sciencemag.org/content/265/5171/528.abstract

36. Strasser A, Jost PJ, Nagata S. The many roles of FAS receptor signaling in the immune system. Immunity. 2009;30(2):180–92.

37. Vivier E, Tomasello E, Baratin M, Walzer T, Ugolini S. Functions of natural killer cells. Nat Immunol. 2008;9(5):503–10. https://doi.org/10.1038/ni1582.

38. Malhotra A, Shanker A. NK cells: immune cross-talk and therapeutic implications. Immunotherapy. 2011;3(10):1143–66. https://pubmed.ncbi.nlm.nih.gov/21995569

39. Nigro CL, Macagno M, Sangiolo D, Bertolaccini L, Aglietta M, Merlano MC. NK-mediated antibody-dependent cell-mediated cytotoxicity in solid tumors: biological evidence and clinical perspectives. Ann Transl Med. 2019;7(5). http://atm.amegroups.com/article/view/23906

40. Eissens DN, Spanholtz J, van der Meer A, et al. Defining early human NK cell developmental stages in primary and secondary lymphoid tissues. PLoS One. 2012;7(2):e30930. https://doi.org/10.1371/journal.pone.0030930.

41. Wu Y, Tian Z, Wei H. Developmental and functional control of natural killer cells by cytokines. Front Immunol. 2017;8:930.
42. Wang D, Malarkannan S. Transcriptional regulation of natural killer cell development and functions. Cancers (Basel). 2020;12(6):1591.
43. Abel AM, Yang C, Thakar MS, Malarkannan S. Natural killer cells: development, maturation, and clinical utilization. Front Immunol. 2018;9:1869. https://www.frontiersin.org/article/10.3389/fimmu.2018.01869
44. Tassi I, Klesney-Tait J, Colonna M. Dissecting natural killer cell activation pathways through analysis of genetic mutations in human and mouse. Immunol Rev. 2006;214:92–105.
45. Bryceson YT, Chiang SCC, Darmanin S, et al. Molecular mechanisms of natural killer cell activation. J Innate Immun. 2011;3(3):216–26.
46. Horowitz A, Strauss-Albee DM, Leipold M, et al. Genetic and environmental determinants of human NK cell diversity revealed by mass cytometry. Sci Transl Med. 2013;5(208):208ra145.
47. Kim S, Poursine-Laurent J, Truscott SM, et al. Licensing of natural killer cells by host major histocompatibility complex class I molecules. Nature. 2005;436(7051):709–13.
48. Anfossi N, André P, Guia S, et al. Human NK Cell Education by Inhibitory Receptors for MHC Class I. Immunity 2006;25(2):331–42. Available from: https://doi.org/10.1016/j.immuni.2006.06.013.
49. Höglund P, Brodin P. Current perspectives of natural killer cell education by MHC class I molecules. Nat Rev Immunol. 2010;10(10):724–34. https://doi.org/10.1038/nri2835
50. Gasser S, Raulet DH. Activation and self-tolerance of natural killer cells. Immunol Rev. 2006;214:130–42.
51. Joncker NT, Fernandez NC, Treiner E, Vivier E, Raulet DH. NK cell responsiveness is tuned commensurate with the number of inhibitory receptors for self-MHC class I: the rheostat model. J Immunol. 2009;182(8):4572 LP–4580. http://www.jimmunol.org/content/182/8/4572.abstract
52. Kim S, Sunwoo JB, Yang L, et al. HLA alleles determine differences in human natural killer cell responsiveness and potency. Proc Natl Acad Sci U S A. 2008;105(8):3053 LP–058. http://www.pnas.org/content/105/8/3053.abstract
53. Goodridge JP, Jacobs B, Saetersmoen ML, et al. Remodeling of secretory lysosomes during education tunes functional potential in NK cells. Nat Commun. 2019;10(1):514. https://doi.org/10.1038/s41467-019-08384-x.
54. Colonna M, Samaridis J. Cloning of immunoglobulin-superfamily members associated with HLA-C and HLA-B recognition by human natural killer cells. Science. 1995;268(5209):405–8.
55. Campbell KS, Purdy AK. Structure/function of human killer cell immunoglobulin-like receptors: lessons from polymorphisms, evolution, crystal structures and mutations. Immunology. 2011;132(3):315–25.
56. Littera R, Piredda G, Argiolas D, et al. KIR and their HLA class I ligands: two more piecfile:///Users/gracebirch/Downloads/PMC3978238.rises towards completing the puzzle of chronic rejection and graft loss in kidney transplantation. PLoS One. 2017;12(7):e0180831. https://pubmed.ncbi.nlm.nih.gov/28686681
57. Uhrberg M, Valiante NM, Shum BP, et al. Human diversity in killer cell inhibitory receptor genes. Immunity. 1997;7(6):753–63.
58. Cerwenka A, Lanier LL. Ligands for natural killer cell receptors: redundancy or specificity. Immunol Rev. 2001;181:158–69.
59. Malnati MS, Peruzzi M, Parker KC, et al. Peptide specificity in the recognition of MHC class I by natural killer cell clones. Science. 1995;267(5200):1016–8.
60. Peruzzi M, Parker KC, Long EO, Malnati MS. Peptide sequence requirements for the recognition of HLA-B*2705 by specific natural killer cells. J Immunol. 1996;157(8):3350 LP–3356. http://www.jimmunol.org/content/157/8/3350.abstract
61. Cassidy SA, Cheent KS, Khakoo SI. Effects of peptide on NK cell-mediated MHC I recognition. Front Immunol. 2014;5:133. https://pubmed.ncbi.nlm.nih.gov/24744756

62. Cheent KS, Jamil KM, Cassidy S, et al. Synergistic inhibition of natural killer cells by the nonsignaling molecule CD94. Proc Natl Acad Sci U S A. 2013;110(42):16981 LP–16986. http://www.pnas.org/content/110/42/16981.abstract

63. Zhang X, Feng J, Chen S, Yang H, Dong Z. Synergized regulation of NK cell education by NKG2A and specific Ly49 family members. Nat Commun. 2019;10(1):5010. https://doi.org/10.1038/s41467-019-13032-5.

64. Carretero M, Cantoni C, Bellón T, et al. The CD94 and NKG2-A C-type lectins covalently assemble to form a natural killer cell inhibitory receptor for HLA class I molecules. Eur J Immunol. 1997;27(2):563–7.

65. Tomasec P, Braud VM, Rickards C, et al. Surface expression of HLA-E, an inhibitor of natural killer cells, enhanced by human cytomegalovirus gpUL40. Science (80-). 2000;287(5455):1031 LP–033. http://science.sciencemag.org/content/287/5455/1031.abstract

66. Nattermann J, Nischalke HD, Hofmeister V, et al. HIV-1 infection leads to increased HLA-E expression resulting in impaired function of natural killer cells. Antivir Ther. 2005;10(1):95–107.

67. Valés-Gómez M, Reyburn HT, Erskine RA, López-Botet M, Strominger JL. Kinetics and peptide dependency of the binding of the inhibitory NK receptor CD94/NKG2-A and the activating receptor CD94/NKG2-C to HLA-E. EMBO J. 1999;18(15):4250–60.

68. Pupuleku A, Costa-García M, Farré D, et al. Elusive role of the CD94/NKG2C NK cell receptor in the response to cytomegalovirus: novel experimental observations in a reporter cell system. Front Immunol. 2017;8:1317. https://www.frontiersin.org/article/10.3389/fimmu.2017.01317

69. Kovalenko EI, Streltsova MA, Kanevskiy LM, Erokhina SA, Telford WG. Identification of human memory-like NK cells. In: Current protocols in cytometry. John Wiley & Sons, Inc.; 2001. https://doi.org/10.1002/cpcy.13.

70. Kang X, Kim J, Deng M, et al. Inhibitory leukocyte immunoglobulin-like receptors: Immune checkpoint proteins and tumor sustaining factors. Cell Cycle. 2016;15(1):25–40. https://pubmed.ncbi.nlm.nih.gov/26636629

71. Ponte M, Cantoni C, Biassoni R, et al. Inhibitory receptors sensing HLA-G1 molecules in pregnancy: decidua-associated natural killer cells express LIR-1 and CD94/NKG2A and acquire p49, an HLA-G1-specific receptor. Proc Natl Acad Sci U S A. 1999;96(10):5674–9.

72. Godal R, Bachanova V, Gleason M, et al. Natural killer cell killing of acute myelogenous leukemia and acute lymphoblastic leukemia blasts by killer cell immunoglobulin-like receptor-negative natural killer cells after NKG2A and LIR-1 blockade. Biol Blood Marrow Transplant J Am Soc Blood Marrow Transplant. 2010;16(5):612–21.

73. Roberti MP, Juliá EP, Rocca YS, et al. Overexpression of CD85j in TNBC patients inhibits cetuximab-mediated NK-cell ADCC but can be restored with CD85j functional blockade. Eur J Immunol. 2015;45(5):1560–9. https://onlinelibrary.wiley.com/doi/abs/10.1002/eji.201445353

74. Müller-Durovic B, Lanna A, Covre LP, Mills RS, Henson SM, Akbar AN. Killer cell lectin-like receptor G1 inhibits NK cell function through activation of adenosine 5′-monophosphate-activated protein kinase. J Immunol. 2016;197(7):2891–9. https://pubmed.ncbi.nlm.nih.gov/27566818

75. Li Y, Hofmann M, Wang Q, et al. Structure of natural killer cell receptor KLRG1 bound to E-cadherin reveals basis for MHC-independent missing self recognition. Immunity. 2009;31(1):35–46.

76. Hotmann M, Schweier O, Pircher H. Different inhibitory capacities of human and mouse KLRG1 are linked to distinct disulfide-mediated oligomerizations. Eur J Immunol. 2012;42(9):2484–90.

77. Lanier LL. Natural killer cell receptor signaling. Curr Opin Immunol. 2003;15(3):308–14. http://www.sciencedirect.com/science/article/pii/S0952791503000396

78. Huntington ND, Vosshenrich CAJ, Di Santo JP. Developmental pathways that generate natural-killer-cell diversity in mice and humans. Nat Rev Immunol. 2007;7(9):703–14.

79. Spear P, Wu M-R, Sentman M-L, Sentman CL. NKG2D ligands as therapeutic targets. Cancer Immun. 2013;13:8. https://pubmed.ncbi.nlm.nih.gov/23833565

80. Upshaw JL, Arneson LN, Schoon RA, Dick CJ, Billadeau DD, Leibson PJ. NKG2D-mediated signaling requires a DAP10-bound Grb2-Vav1 intermediate and phosphatidylinositol-3-kinase in human natural killer cells. Nat Immunol. 2006;7(5):524–32.

81. Wensveen FM, Jelenčić V, Polić B. NKG2D: a master regulator of immune cell responsiveness. Front Immunol. 2018;9:441. https://www.frontiersin.org/article/10.3389/fimmu.2018.00441

82. Bryceson YT, March ME, Ljunggren H-G, Long EO. Synergy among receptors on resting NK cells for the activation of natural cytotoxicity and cytokine secretion. Blood. 2006;107(1):159–66.

83. Kim HS, Das A, Gross CC, Bryceson YT, Long EO. Synergistic signals for natural cytotoxicity are required to overcome inhibition by c-Cbl ubiquitin ligase. Immunity. 2010;32(2):175–86.

84. Parsons MS, Richard J, Lee WS, et al. NKG2D acts as a co-receptor for natural killer cell-mediated anti-HIV-1 antibody-dependent cellular cytotoxicity. AIDS Res Hum Retrovir. 2016;32(10–11):1089–96.

85. Touzani O, Boutin H, LeFeuvre R, et al. Interleukin-1 influences ischemic brain damage in the mouse independently of the interleukin-1 type I receptor. J Neurosci. 2002;22(1):38–43.

86. Le Bouteiller P, Tabiasco J, Polgar B, et al. CD160: a unique activating NK cell receptor. Immunol Lett. 2011;138(2):93–6.

87. Tu TC, Brown NK, Kim T-J, et al. CD160 is essential for NK-mediated IFN-γ production. J Exp Med. 2015;212(3):415–29.

88. Shibuya A, Campbell D, Hannum C, et al. DNAM-1, a novel adhesion molecule involved in the cytolytic function of T lymphocytes. Immunity. 1996;4(6):573–81. http://www.sciencedirect.com/science/article/pii/S1074761300700604

89. Lanier LL. Turning on natural killer cells. J Exp Med. 2000;191(8):1259–62. https://www.ncbi.nlm.nih.gov/pubmed/10770793

90. Kirkham CL, Carlyle JR. Complexity and diversity of the NKR-P1:Clr (Klrb1:Clec2) recognition systems. Front Immunol. 2014;5:214. https://pubmed.ncbi.nlm.nih.gov/24917862

91. Aldemir H, Prod'homme V, Dumaurier M-J, et al. Cutting edge: lectin-like transcript 1 is a ligand for the CD161 Receptor. J Immunol. 2005;175(12):7791 LP–7795. http://www.jimmunol.org/content/175/12/7791.abstract

92. Bottino C, Castriconi R, Pende D, et al. Identification of PVR (CD155) and nectin-2 (CD112) as cell surface ligands for the human DNAM-1 (CD226) activating molecule. J Exp Med. 2003;198(4):557 LP–567. http://jem.rupress.org/content/198/4/557.abstract

93. Pende D, Castriconi R, Romagnani P, et al. Expression of the DNAM-1 ligands, Nectin-2 (CD112) and poliovirus receptor (CD155), on dendritic cells: relevance for natural killer-dendritic cell interaction. Blood. 2006;107(5):2030–6.

94. Pegram HJ, Andrews DM, Smyth MJ, Darcy PK, Kershaw MH. Activating and inhibitory receptors of natural killer cells. Immunol Cell Biol. 2011;89(2):216–24.

95. Chiossone L, Dumas P-Y, Vienne M, Vivier E. Natural killer cells and other innate lymphoid cells in cancer. Nat Rev Immunol. 2018;18(11):671–88. https://doi.org/10.1038/s41577-018-0061-z.

96. Böttcher JP, Bonavita E, Chakravarty P, et al. NK cells stimulate recruitment of cDC1 into the tumor microenvironment promoting cancer immune control. Cell. 2018;172(5):1022–1037.e14. https://www.sciencedirect.com/science/article/pii/S0092867418300394

97. Ruggeri L, Capanni M, Casucci M, et al. Role of natural killer cell alloreactivity in HLA-mismatched hematopoietic stem cell transplantation. Blood. 1999;94(1):333–9.

98. Ruggeri L, Aversa F, Martelli MF, Velardi A. Allogeneic hematopoietic transplantation and natural killer cell recognition of missing self. Immunol Rev. 2006;214:202–18.

99. Miller JS, Soignier Y, Panoskaltsis-Mortari A, et al. Successful adoptive transfer and in vivo expansion of human haploidentical NK cells in patients with cancer. Blood. 2005;105(8):3051–7.

100. Myers JA, Miller JS. Exploring the NK cell platform for cancer immunotherapy. Nat Rev Clin Oncol. 2021;18(2):85–100. https://doi.org/10.1038/s41571-020-0426-7.
101. Zhao Y, Su H, Shen X, Du J, Zhang X, Zhao Y. The immunological function of CD52 and its targeting in organ transplantation. Inflamm Res. 2017;66(7):571–8.
102. Poirot L, Philip B, Schiffer-Mannioui C, et al. Multiplex Genome-edited T-cell manufacturing platform for "off-the-shelf" adoptive T-cell immunotherapies. Cancer Res. 2015;75(18):3853–64.
103. Benjamin R, Graham C, Yallop D, et al. Preliminary data on safety, cellular kinetics and anti-leukemic activity of UCART19, an allogeneic anti-CD19 CAR T-cell product, in a pool of adult and pediatric patients with high-risk CD19+ relapsed/refractory B-cell acute lymphoblastic leukemia. Blood. 2018;132(Suppl 1):–896.
104. Sun C, Sun H, Xiao W, Zhang C, Tian Z. Natural killer cell dysfunction in hepatocellular carcinoma and NK cell-based immunotherapy. Acta Pharmacol Sin. 2015;36(10):1191–9.
105. Melaiu O, Lucarini V, Cifaldi L, Fruci D. Influence of the tumor microenvironment on NK cell function in solid tumors. Front Immunol. 2020;10:3038. https://www.frontiersin.org/article/10.3389/fimmu.2019.03038
106. Chen H, He W. Human regulatory γδT cells and their functional plasticity in the tumor microenvironment. Cell Mol Immunol. 2018;15(4):411–3.
107. Trzonkowski P, Szmit E, Myśliwska J, Dobyszuk A, Myśliwski A. CD4+CD25+ T regulatory cells inhibit cytotoxic activity of T CD8+ and NK lymphocytes in the direct cell-to-cell interaction. Clin Immunol. 2004;112(3):258–67.
108. Baghban R, Roshangar L, Jahanban-Esfahlan R, et al. Tumor microenvironment complexity and therapeutic implications at a glance. Cell Commun Signal, 2020. 18(1):59. https://doi.org/10.1186/s12964-020-0530-4.
109. Zhang C, Hu Y, Shi C. Targeting natural killer cells for tumor immunotherapy. Front Immunol. 2020;11:60. https://pubmed.ncbi.nlm.nih.gov/32140153
110. Castriconi R, Cantoni C, Della Chiesa M, et al. Transforming growth factor beta 1 inhibits expression of NKp30 and NKG2D receptors: consequences for the NK-mediated killing of dendritic cells. Proc Natl Acad Sci U S A. 2003;100(7):4120–5.
111. Hoechst B, Voigtlaender T, Ormandy L, et al. Myeloid derived suppressor cells inhibit natural killer cells in patients with hepatocellular carcinoma via the NKp30 receptor. Hepatology. 2009;50(3):799–807.
112. Cekic C, Day Y-J, Sag D, Linden J. Myeloid expression of adenosine A2A receptor suppresses T and NK cell responses in the solid tumor microenvironment. Cancer Res. 2014;74(24):7250–9.
113. Chiu DK-C, Tse AP-W, Xu IM-J, et al. Hypoxia inducible factor HIF-1 promotes myeloid-derived suppressor cells accumulation through ENTPD2/CD39L1 in hepatocellular carcinoma. Nat Commun. 2017;8(1):517.
114. Li T, Yang Y, Hua X, et al. Hepatocellular carcinoma-associated fibroblasts trigger NK cell dysfunction via PGE2 and IDO. Cancer Lett. 2012;318(2):154–61.
115. Balsamo M, Scordamaglia F, Pietra G, et al. Melanoma-associated fibroblasts modulate NK cell phenotype and antitumor cytotoxicity. Proc Natl Acad Sci U S A. 2009;106(49):20847–52.
116. Inoue T, Adachi K, Kawana K, et al. Cancer-associated fibroblast suppresses killing activity of natural killer cells through downregulation of poliovirus receptor (PVR/CD155), a ligand of activating NK receptor. Int J Oncol. 2016;49(4):1297–304.
117. Zhang S, Liu W, Hu B, et al. Prognostic significance of tumor-infiltrating natural killer cells in solid tumors: a systematic review and meta-analysis. Front Immunol. 2020;11:1242. https://www.frontiersin.org/article/10.3389/fimmu.2020.01242
118. Shaim H, Sanabria MH, Basar R, et al. Inhibition of the αv integrin-TGF-β axis improves natural killer cell function against glioblastoma stem cells. bioRxiv. 2020. http://biorxiv.org/content/early/2020/03/31/2020.03.30.016667.abstract
119. Foltz JA, Moseman JE, Thakkar A, Chakravarti N, Lee DA. TGFβ imprinting during activation promotes natural killer cell cytokine hypersecretion. Cancers. 2018;10(11)

120. Yvon ES, Burga R, Powell A, et al. Cord blood natural killer cells expressing a dominant negative TGF-β receptor: implications for adoptive immunotherapy for glioblastoma. Cytotherapy. 2017;19(3):408–18.
121. Gras Navarro A, Kmiecik J, Leiss L, et al. NK cells with KIR2DS2 immunogenotype have a functional activation advantage to efficiently kill glioblastoma and prolong animal survival. J Immunol. 2014;193(12):6192–206.
122. Veluchamy JP, Lopez-Lastra S, Spanholtz J, et al. In vivo efficacy of umbilical cord blood stem cell-derived nk cells in the treatment of metastatic colorectal cancer. Front Immunol. 2017;8:87. https://doi.org/10.3389/fimmu.2017.00087.
123. Tang Y, Xie M, Li K, Li J, Cai Z, Hu B. Prognostic value of peripheral blood natural killer cells in colorectal cancerX. Oncogene. 2021;40(4):717–30. https://doi.org/10.1186/s12876-020-1177-8.
124. Xu C, Liu D, Chen Z, et al. Umbilical cord blood-derived natural killer cells combined with bevacizumab for colorectal cancer treatment. Hum Gene Ther. 2019;30(4):459–70.
125. Wang F, Lau JKC, Yu J. The role of natural killer cell in gastrointestinal cancer: killer or helper. Oncogene. 2021;40(4):717.–30. https://doi.org/10.1038/s41388-020-01561-z.
126. Geller MA, Knorr DA, Hermanson DA, et al. Intraperitoneal delivery of human natural killer cells for treatment of ovarian cancer in a mouse xenograft model. Cytotherapy. 2013;15(10):1297–306.
127. Hermanson DL, Bendzick L, Pribyl L, et al. Induced pluripotent stem cell-derived natural killer cells for treatment of ovarian cancer. Stem Cells. 2016;34(1):93–101.
128. Hoogstad-van Evert JS, Cany J, van den Brand D, et al. Umbilical cord blood CD34(+) progenitor-derived NK cells efficiently kill ovarian cancer spheroids and intraperitoneal tumors in NOD/SCID/IL2Rg(null) mice. Onco Targets Ther. 2017;6(8):e1320630.
129. Hoogstad-van Evert JS, Maas RJ, van der Meer J, et al. Peritoneal NK cells are responsive to IL-15 and percentages are correlated with outcome in advanced ovarian cancer patients. Oncotarget. 2018;9(78):34810–20.
130. Ferrara JLM, Levine JE, Reddy P, Holler E. Graft-versus-host disease. Lancet (London, England). 2009;373(9674):1550–61.
131. Berséus O, Boman K, Nessen SC, Westerberg LA. Risks of hemolysis due to anti-A and anti-B caused by the transfusion of blood or blood components containing ABO-incompatible plasma. Transfusion. 2013;53(Suppl 1):114S–23S.
132. Koehl U, Brehm C, Huenecke S, et al. Clinical grade purification and expansion of NK cell products for an optimized manufacturing protocol. Front Oncol. 2013;3:118.
133. Romee R, Schneider SE, Leong JW, et al. Cytokine activation induces human memory-like NK cells. Blood. 2012;120(24):4751–60.
134. Siegler U, Meyer-Monard S, Jörger S, et al. Good manufacturing practice-compliant cell sorting and large-scale expansion of single KIR-positive alloreactive human natural killer cells for multiple infusions to leukemia patients. Cytotherapy. 2010;12(6):750–63.
135. Cooley S, He F, Bachanova V, et al. First-in-human trial of rhIL-15 and haploidentical natural killer cell therapy for advanced acute myeloid leukemia. Blood Adv. 2019;3(13):1970–80.
136. Wang Y, Xu H, Zheng X, Wei H, Sun R, Tian Z. High expression of NKG2A/CD94 and low expression of granzyme B are associated with reduced cord blood NK cell activity. Cell Mol Immunol. 2007;4(5):377–82.
137. Mark C, Czerwinski T, Roessner S, et al. Cryopreservation impairs cytotoxicity and migration of NK cells in 3-D tissue: implications for cancer immunotherapy. bioRxiv. 2019;812172. http://biorxiv.org/content/early/2019/10/21/812172.abstract
138. Mehta RS, Shpall EJ, Rezvani K. Cord Blood as a Source of Natural Killer Cells. Front Med. 2015;2:93.
139. Valamehr B, Robinson M, Abujarour R, et al. Platform for induction and maintenance of transgene-free hiPSCs resembling ground state pluripotent stem cells. Stem cell reports. 2014;2(3):366–81.

140. Woll PS, Grzywacz B, Tian X, et al. Human embryonic stem cells differentiate into a homogeneous population of natural killer cells with potent in vivo antitumor activity. Blood. 2009;113(24):6094–101.
141. Knorr DA, Ni Z, Hermanson D, et al. Clinical-scale derivation of natural killer cells from human pluripotent stem cells for cancer therapy. Stem Cells Transl Med. 2013;2(4):274–83.
142. Ng ES, Davis R, Stanley EG, Elefanty AG. A protocol describing the use of a recombinant protein-based, animal product-free medium (APEL) for human embryonic stem cell differentiation as spin embryoid bodies. Nat Protoc. 2008;3(5):768–76. https://doi.org/10.1038/nprot.2008.42.
143. Zhu H, Kaufman DS. An improved method to produce clinical scale natural killer cells from human pluripotent stem cells. bioRxiv. 2019:614792. http://biorxiv.org/content/early/2019/04/21/614792.abstract
144. Zeng J, Tang SY, Toh LL, Wang S. Generation of "Off-the-Shelf" Natural Killer Cells from Peripheral Blood Cell-Derived Induced Pluripotent Stem Cells. Stem cell reports. 2017;9(6):1796–812.
145. Zhu H, Blum RH, Bjordahl R, et al. Pluripotent stem cell–derived NK cells with high-affinity noncleavable CD16a mediate improved antitumor activity. Blood. 2020;135(6):399–410. https://doi.org/10.1182/blood.2019000621.
146. Shankar K, Capitini CM, Saha K. Genome engineering of induced pluripotent stem cells to manufacture natural killer cell therapies. Stem Cell Res Ther. 2020;11(1):234. https://pubmed.ncbi.nlm.nih.gov/32546200
147. Oberschmidt O, Morgan M, Huppert V, et al. Development of automated separation, expansion, and quality control protocols for clinical-scale manufacturing of primary human NK cells and alpharetroviral chimeric antigen receptor engineering. Hum Gene Ther Methods. 2019;30(3):102–20.
148. Choi YH, Lim EJ, Kim SW, Moon YW, Park KS, An H-J. Correction to: IL-27 enhances IL-15/IL-18-mediated activation of human natural killer cells. J Immunother Cancer. 2019;7(1):211.
149. Tanaka Y, Nakazawa T, Nakamura M, et al. Ex vivo-expanded highly purified natural killer cells in combination with temozolomide induce antitumor effects in human glioblastoma cells in vitro. PLoS One. 2019;14(3):e0212455.
150. Torelli GF, Rozera C, Santodonato L, et al. A good manufacturing practice method to ex vivo expand natural killer cells for clinical use. Blood Transfus. 2015;13(3):464–71.
151. Fujisaki H, Kakuda H, Shimasaki N, et al. Expansion of highly cytotoxic human natural killer cells for cancer cell therapy. Cancer Res. 2009;69(9):4010–7.
152. Denman CJ, Senyukov VV, Somanchi SS, et al. Membrane-bound IL-21 promotes sustained ex vivo proliferation of human natural killer cells. PLoS One. 2012;7(1):e30264.
153. Ojo EO, Sharma AA, Liu R, et al. Membrane bound IL-21 based NK cell feeder cells drive robust expansion and metabolic activation of NK cells. Sci Rep. 9(2019, 1):14916. https://pubmed.ncbi.nlm.nih.gov/31624330
154. Shah N, Li L, McCarty J, et al. Phase I study of cord blood-derived natural killer cells combined with autologous stem cell transplantation in multiple myeloma. Br J Haematol. 2017;177(3):457–66.
155. Ciurea SO, Schafer JR, Bassett R, et al. Phase 1 clinical trial using mbIL21 ex vivo-expanded donor-derived NK cells after haploidentical transplantation. Blood. 2017;130(16):1857–68.
156. Koehl U, Kalberer C, Spanholtz J, et al. Advances in clinical NK cell studies: Donor selection, manufacturing and quality control. Onco Targets Ther. 2016;5(4):e1115178.
157. Maki G, Klingemann HG, Martinson JA, Tam YK. Factors regulating the cytotoxic activity of the human natural killer cell line, NK-92. J Hematother Stem Cell Res. 2001;10(3):369–83.
158. Tonn T, Becker S, Esser R, Schwabe D, Seifried F. Cellular immunotherapy of malignancies using the clonal natural killer cell line NK-92. J Hematother Stem Cell Res. 2001;10(4):535–44. https://doi.org/10.1089/15258160152509145.

159. Arai S, Meagher R, Swearingen M, et al. Infusion of the allogeneic cell line NK-92 in patients with advanced renal cell cancer or melanoma: a phase I trial. Cytotherapy. 2008;10(6):625–32. https://doi.org/10.1080/14653240802301872.

160. Tonn T, Schwabe D, Klingemann HG, et al. Treatment of patients with advanced cancer with the natural killer cell line NK-92. Cytotherapy. 2013;15(12):1563–70. https://doi.org/10.1016/j.jcyt.2013.06.017.

161. Mitwasi N, Feldmann A, Arndt C, et al. "UniCAR"-modified off-the-shelf NK-92 cells for targeting of GD2-expressing tumour cells. Sci Rep. 2020;10(1):2141. https://doi.org/10.1038/s41598-020-59082-4.

162. Liu S, Galat V, Galat Y, YKA L, Wainwright D, Wu J. NK cell-based cancer immunotherapy: from basic biology to clinical development. J Hematol Oncol. 2021;14(1):7. https://doi.org/10.1186/s13045-020-01014-w.

163. Iliopoulou EG, Kountourakis P, Karamouzis MV, et al. A phase I trial of adoptive transfer of allogeneic natural killer cells in patients with advanced non-small cell lung cancer. Cancer Immunol Immunother. 2010;59(12):1781–9.

164. Choi I, Yoon SR, Park S-Y, et al. Donor-derived natural killer cells infused after human leukocyte antigen–haploidentical hematopoietic cell transplantation: a dose-escalation study. Biol Blood Marrow Transplant. 2014;20(5):696–704. https://www.sciencedirect.com/science/article/pii/S1083879114000767

165. Heinze A, Grebe B, Bremm M, et al. The synergistic use of IL-15 and IL-21 for the generation of NK cells from CD3/CD19-depleted grafts improves their ex vivo expansion and cytotoxic potential against neuroblastoma: perspective for optimized immunotherapy post haploidentical stem cell tran. Front Immunol. 2019;10:2816.

166. Sakamoto N, Ishikawa T, Kokura S, et al. Phase I clinical trial of autologous NK cell therapy using novel expansion method in patients with advanced digestive cancer. J Transl Med. 2015;13:277.

167. Masuyama J, Murakami T, Iwamoto S, Fujita S. Ex vivo expansion of natural killer cells from human peripheral blood mononuclear cells co-stimulated with anti-CD3 and anti-CD52 monoclonal antibodies. Cytotherapy. 2016;18(1):80–90.

168. Parkhurst MR, Riley JP, Dudley ME, Rosenberg SA. Adoptive transfer of autologous natural killer cells leads to high levels of circulating natural killer cells but does not mediate tumor regression. Clin Cancer Res. 2011;17(19):6287 LP–6297. http://clincancerres.aacrjournals.org/content/17/19/6287.abstract

169. Lee H-R, Son C-H, Koh E-K, et al. Expansion of cytotoxic natural killer cells using irradiated autologous peripheral blood mononuclear cells and anti-CD16 antibody. Sci Rep. 2017;7(1):11075.

170. Luhm J, Brand J-M, Koritke P, Höppner M, Kirchner H, Frohn C. Large-scale generation of natural killer lymphocytes for clinical application. J Hematother Stem Cell Res. 2002;11(4):651–7. https://doi.org/10.1089/15258160260194794.

171. Kim E-K, Ahn Y-O, Kim S, Kim TM, Keam B, Heo DS. Ex vivo activation and expansion of natural killer cells from patients with advanced cancer with feeder cells from healthy volunteers. Cytotherapy. 2013;15(2):231–241.e1.

172. Ishikawa E, Tsuboi K, Saijo K, et al. Autologous natural killer cell therapy for human recurrent malignant glioma. Anticancer Res. 2004;24(3b):1861–71.

173. Lim SA, Kim T-J, Lee JE, et al. Ex vivo expansion of highly cytotoxic human NK cells by cocultivation with irradiated tumor cells for adoptive immunotherapy. Cancer Res. 2013;73(8):2598–607.

174. Granzin M, Stojanovic A, Miller M, Childs R, Huppert V, Cerwenka A. Highly efficient IL-21 and feeder cell-driven ex vivo expansion of human NK cells with therapeutic activity in a xenograft mouse model of melanoma. Onco Targets Ther. 2016;5(9):e1219007.

175. Imai C, Iwamoto S, Campana D. Genetic modification of primary natural killer cells overcomes inhibitory signals and induces specific killing of leukemic cells. Blood. 2005;106(1):376–83.

176. Szmania S, Lapteva N, Garg T, et al. Ex vivo-expanded natural killer cells demonstrate robust proliferation in vivo in high-risk relapsed multiple myeloma patients. J Immunother. 2015;38(1):24–36.

177. Oyer JL, Pandey V, Igarashi RY, et al. Natural killer cells stimulated with PM21 particles expand and biodistribute in vivo: clinical implications for cancer treatment. Cytotherapy. 2016;18(5):653–63.
178. Mu YX, Zhao YX, Li BY, et al. A simple method for in vitro preparation of natural killer cells from cord blood. BMC Biotechnol. 2019;19(1):80.
179. Cerwenka A, Lanier LL. Natural killer cell memory in infection, inflammation and cancer. Nat Rev Immunol. 2016;16(2):112–23. https://doi.org/10.1038/nri.2015.9.
180. O'Leary JG, Goodarzi M, Drayton DL, von Andrian UH. T cell- and B cell-independent adaptive immunity mediated by natural killer cells. Nat Immunol. 2006;7(5):507–16.
181. Sun JC, Beilke JN, Lanier LL. Adaptive immune features of natural killer cells. Nature. 2009;457:557. https://doi.org/10.1038/nature07665.
182. Cooper MA, Elliott JM, Keyel PA, Yang L, Carrero JA, Yokoyama WM. Cytokine-induced memory-like natural killer cells. Proc Natl Acad Sci U S A. 2009;106(6):1915 LP–1919. http://www.pnas.org/content/106/6/1915.abstract
183. Chu J, Deng Y, Benson DM, et al. CS1-specific chimeric antigen receptor (CAR)-engineered natural killer cells enhance in vitro and in vivo antitumor activity against human multiple myeloma. Leukemia. 2014;28(4):917–27.
184. Peng H, Tian Z. Natural killer cell memory: progress and implications. Front Immunol. 2017;8:1143.
185. Daniels KA, Devora G, Lai WC, O'Donnell CL, Bennett M, Welsh RM. Murine cytomegalovirus is regulated by a discrete subset of natural killer cells reactive with monoclonal antibody to Ly49H. J Exp Med. 2001;194(1):29–44.
186. Smith HRC, Heusel JW, Mehta IK, et al. Recognition of a virus-encoded ligand by a natural killer cell activation receptor. Proc Natl Acad Sci U S A. 2002;99(13):8826 LP–8831. http://www.pnas.org/content/99/13/8826.abstract
187. Voigt V, Forbes CA, Tonkin JN, et al. Murine cytomegalovirus m157 mutation and variation leads to immune evasion of natural killer cells. Proc Natl Acad Sci U S A. 2003;100(23):13483 LP–13488. http://www.pnas.org/content/100/23/13483.abstract
188. Forbes CA, Scalzo AA, Degli-Esposti MA, Coudert JD. Ly49C-dependent control of MCMV infection by NK cells is cis-regulated by MHC class I molecules. PLoS Pathog. 2014;10(5):e1004161. https://doi.org/10.1371/journal.ppat.1004161.
189. Lopez-Vergès S, Milush JM, Schwartz BS, et al. Expansion of a unique CD57+NKG2Chi natural killer cell subset during acute human cytomegalovirus infection. Proc Natl Acad Sci U S A. 2011;108(36):14725 LP–14732. http://www.pnas.org/content/108/36/14725.abstract
190. Malone DFG, Lunemann S, Hengst J, et al. Cytomegalovirus-driven adaptive-like natural killer cell expansions are unaffected by concurrent chronic hepatitis virus infections. Front Immunol. 2017;8:525. https://www.frontiersin.org/article/10.3389/fimmu.2017.00525
191. Tesi B, Schlums H, Cichocki F, Bryceson YT. Epigenetic regulation of adaptive NK cell diversification. Trends Immunol. 2016;37(7):451–61.
192. Lau CM, Adams NM, Geary CD, et al. Epigenetic control of innate and adaptive immune memory. Nat Immunol. 2018;19(9):963–72.
193. Ni J, Miller M, Stojanovic A, Garbi N, Cerwenka A. Sustained effector function of IL-12/15/18–preactivated NK cells against established tumors. J Exp Med. 2012;209(13):2351 LP–2365. http://jem.rupress.org/content/209/13/2351.abstract
194. Ni J, Hölsken O, Miller M, et al. Adoptively transferred natural killer cells maintain long-term antitumor activity by epigenetic imprinting and CD4+ T cell help. Onco Targets Ther. 2016;5(9):e1219009. https://doi.org/10.1080/2162402X.2016.1219009.
195. Leong JW, Chase JM, Romee R, et al. Preactivation with IL-12, IL-15, and IL-18 Induces CD25 and a functional high-affinity IL-2 receptor on human cytokine-induced memory-like natural killer cells. Biol Blood Marrow Transpl. 2014;20(4):463–73. https://doi.org/10.1016/j.bbmt.2014.01.006.
196. Wagner JA, Berrien-Elliott MM, Rosario M, et al. Cytokine-Induced memory-like differentiation enhances unlicensed natural killer cell antileukemia and fcγriiia-triggered responses. Biol blood marrow Transplant J Am Soc Blood Marrow Transplant. 2017;23(3):398–404.

197. Rosario M, Romee R, Schneider SE, Leong JW, Sullivan RP, Fehniger TA. Human cytokine-induced memory-like (CIML) NK cells are active against myeloid leukemia in vitro and in vivo. Blood. 2014;124(21):1117. https://doi.org/10.1182/blood.V124.21.1117.1117.
198. Romee R, Rosario M, Berrien-Elliott MM, et al. Cytokine-induced memory-like natural killer cells exhibit enhanced responses against myeloid leukemia. Sci Transl Med. 2016;8(357):357ra123.
199. Berrien-Elliott MM, Cashen AF, Cubitt CC, et al. Multidimensional analyses of donor memory-like NK cells reveal new associations with response after adoptive immunotherapy for leukemia. Cancer Discov. 2020;10(12):1854–71.
200. Uppendahl LD, Felices M, Bendzick L, et al. Cytokine-induced memory-like natural killer cells have enhanced function, proliferation, and in vivo expansion against ovarian cancer cells. Gynecol Oncol. 2019;153(1):149–57.
201. Marin ND, Krasnick BA, Becker-Hapak M, Conant L, Goedegebuure SP, Berrien-Elliott MM, Robbins KJ, Foltz JA, Foster M, Wong P, Cubitt CC, Tran J, Wetzel CB, Jacobs M, Zhou A, Russler-Germain D, Marsala L, Schappe T, Fields RCFT. Memory-like differentiation enhances NK cell responses to melanoma. Clin Cancer Res. 2021;27(17):4859–69.
202. Ha D, Tanaka A, Kibayashi T, et al. Differential control of human Treg and effector T cells in tumor immunity by Fc-engineered anti-CTLA-4 antibody. Proc Natl Acad Sci U S A. 2019;116(2):609–18.
203. Liu E, Marin D, Banerjee P, et al. Use of CAR-transduced natural killer cells in CD19-positive lymphoid tumors. N Engl J Med. 2020;382(6):545–53.
204. Gang M, Marin ND, Wong P, et al. CAR-modified memory-like NK cells exhibit potent responses to NK-resistant lymphomas. Blood. 2020;136(20):2308–18.
205. Hò G-GT, Celik AA, Huyton T, et al. NKG2A/CD94 is a new immune receptor for HLA-G and distinguishes amino acid differences in the HLA-G heavy chain. Int J Mol Sci. 2020;21(12):4362. https://pubmed.ncbi.nlm.nih.gov/32575403
206. Gleason MK, Lenvik TR, McCullar V, et al. Tim-3 is an inducible human natural killer cell receptor that enhances interferon gamma production in response to galectin-9. Blood. 2012;119(13):3064–72.
207. André P, Denis C, Soulas C, et al. Anti-NKG2A mAb is a checkpoint inhibitor that promotes anti-tumor immunity by unleashing both T and NK cells. Cell. 2018;175(7):1731–1743.e13.
208. Quatrini L, Mariotti FR, Munari E, Tumino N, Vacca P, Moretta L. The immune checkpoint PD-1 in natural killer cells: expression, function and targeting in tumour immunotherapy. Cancers (Basel). 2020;12(11):3285. https://pubmed.ncbi.nlm.nih.gov/33172030
209. Romee R, Cooley S, Berrien-Elliott MM, et al. First-in-human phase 1 clinical study of the IL-15 superagonist complex ALT-803 to treat relapse after transplantation. Blood. 2018;131(23):2515–27.
210. Benson DMJ, Bakan CE, Mishra A, et al. The PD-1/PD-L1 axis modulates the natural killer cell versus multiple myeloma effect: a therapeutic target for CT-011, a novel monoclonal anti-PD-1 antibody. Blood. 2010;116(13):2286–94.
211. Campbell KS, Hasegawa J. Natural killer cell biology: an update and future directions. J Allergy Clin Immunol. 2013;132(3):536–44. https://pubmed.ncbi.nlm.nih.gov/23906377
212. Park J-E, Kim S-E, Keam B, et al. Anti-tumor effects of NK cells and anti-PD-L1 antibody with antibody-dependent cellular cytotoxicity in PD-L1-positive cancer cell lines. J Immunother Cancer. 2020;8(2):e000873. http://jitc.bmj.com/content/8/2/e000873.abstract
213. da Silva IP, Gallois A, Jimenez-Baranda S, et al. Reversal of NK-cell exhaustion in advanced melanoma by Tim-3 blockade. Cancer Immunol Res. 2014;2(5):410–22.
214. Westin JR, Chu F, Zhang M, et al. Safety and activity of PD1 blockade by pidilizumab in combination with rituximab in patients with relapsed follicular lymphoma: a single group, open-label, phase 2 trial. Lancet Oncol. 2014;15(1):69–77.
215. van Hall T, André P, Horowitz A, et al. Monalizumab: inhibiting the novel immune checkpoint NKG2A. J Immunother Cancer. 2019;7(1):263. https://doi.org/10.1186/s40425-019-0761-3.

216. Stanietsky N, Simic H, Arapovic J, et al. The interaction of TIGIT with PVR and PVRL2 inhibits human NK cell cytotoxicity. Proc Natl Acad Sci U S A. 2009;106(42):17858–63.
217. Harjunpää H, Guillerey C. TIGIT as an emerging immune checkpoint. Clin Exp Immunol. 2020;200(2):108–19.
218. Benson DMJ, Hofmeister CC, Padmanabhan S, et al. A phase 1 trial of the anti-KIR antibody IPH2101 in patients with relapsed/refractory multiple myeloma. Blood. 2012;120(22):4324–33.
219. Benson DMJ, Cohen AD, Jagannath S, et al. A phase i trial of the anti-KIR antibody IPH2101 and lenalidomide in patients with relapsed/refractory multiple myeloma. Clin Cancer Res Off J Am Assoc Cancer Res. 2015;21(18):4055–61.
220. Vey N, Bourhis J-H, Boissel N, et al. A phase 1 trial of the anti-inhibitory KIR mAb IPH2101 for AML in complete remission. Blood. 2012;120(22):4317–23. https://doi.org/10.1182/blood-2012-06-437558.
221. Lazarova M, Steinle A. Impairment of NKG2D-mediated tumor immunity by TGF-β. Front Immunol. 2019;10:2689. https://pubmed.ncbi.nlm.nih.gov/31803194
222. Della Chiesa M, Carlomagno S, Frumento G, et al. The tryptophan catabolite L-kynurenine inhibits the surface expression of NKp46- and NKG2D-activating receptors and regulates NK-cell function. Blood. 2006;108(13):4118–25.
223. Wang W, Erbe AK, Hank JA, Morris ZS, Sondel PM. NK cell-mediated antibody-dependent cellular cytotoxicity in cancer immunotherapy. Front Immunol. 2015;6:368.
224. Lajoie L, Congy-Jolivet N, Bolzec A, et al. ADAM17-mediated shedding of FcγRIIIA on human NK cells: identification of the cleavage site and relationship with activation. J Immunol 2014;192(2):741 LP–741751. http://www.jimmunol.org/content/192/2/741.abstract.
225. Romee R, Lenvik T, Wang Y, Walcheck B, Verneris MR, Miller JS. ADAM17, a novel metalloproteinase, mediates CD16 and CD62L shedding in human NK cells and modulates IFNγ responses. Blood. 2011;118(21):2184. https://doi.org/10.1182/blood.V118.21.2184.2184.
226. Mishra HK, Pore N, Michelotti EF, Walcheck B. Anti-ADAM17 monoclonal antibody MEDI3622 increases IFNγ production by human NK cells in the presence of antibody-bound tumor cells. Cancer Immunol Immunother. 2018;67(9):1407–16. https://pubmed.ncbi.nlm.nih.gov/29978334
227. Pham D-H, Kim J-S, Kim S-K, et al. Effects of ADAM10 and ADAM17 inhibitors on natural killer cell expansion and antibody-dependent cellular cytotoxicity against breast cancer cells in vitro. Anticancer Res. 2017;37(10):5507–13.

Part VII
T/NK Cell Engagers

Biology and Clinical Evaluation of T/NK Cell Engagers

Rebecca Epperly, Stephen Gottschalk, and M. Paulina Velasquez

Abstract Bispecific engagers are cancer immunotherapeutics that incorporate at least two antigen recognition domains and engager both a tumor-associated antigen and an immune effector cell surface molecule to facilitate targeted antitumor activity. This strategy is most advanced for CD19+ B cell malignancies, where the CD19xCD3 bispecific T cell engager (BiTE) blinatumomab has achieved FDA approval. However, efforts are underway to expand the application of this technology to other malignancies. This chapter reviews design strategies to decrease immunogenicity, alter kinetics, enhance effector function, optimize antigen recognition, and direct specific assembly. Additionally, we explore alternative immune effector cell platforms and delivery methods. We describe the landscape of ongoing clinical studies of bispecific T cell and natural killer cell engagers for hematologic malignancies and solid tumors. As the clinical translation of bispecific immune cell engagers continues to advance, key additional considerations include the impact of the host immune environment, integration with other immune and conventional therapies, and mitigation of toxicities.

Keywords Bispecific antibody · Bispecific natural killer cell engager (BiKE) · Bispecific T cell engager (BiTE) · Cancer immunotherapy · Trispecific killer engagers (TriKE) · Dual affinity retargeting protein (DART) · Duobody · Diabody · Immune-mobilizing monoclonal T cell receptor against cancer (ImmTAC) · Monoclonal antibody

Introduction

The advent of immunotherapy has come to revolutionize the oncology field in the last decades. Strategies such as checkpoint inhibitors, chimeric antigen receptor (CAR) T cells, and bispecific engagers have been the object of preclinical and clinical evaluations [1, 2]. Bispecific engagers are bispecific antibodies that consist of at

R. Epperly · S. Gottschalk · M. P. Velasquez (✉)
St. Jude Children's Research Hospital, Memphis, TN, USA
e-mail: Paulina.Velasquez@STJUDE.ORG

© Springer Nature Switzerland AG 2022
A. Ghobadi, J. F. DiPersio (eds.), *Gene and Cellular Immunotherapy for Cancer*, Cancer Drug Discovery and Development,
https://doi.org/10.1007/978-3-030-87849-8_17

329

least two antigen recognition domains. One recognizes a tumor associated antigen (TAA) and the other an activating cell surface molecule on an immune effector cell (e.g., T cells, natural killer (NK) cells) [3]. Thus, bispecific engagers redirect immune cells to tumor cells, facilitating antitumor activity.

Bispecific engagers are off-the-shelf protein therapeutics, an advantage over adoptive cellular immunotherapies which rely on a resource-intensive process to generate autologous or off-the-shelf cellular products. Clinical application of bispecific engagers is most advanced for B cell malignancies, for which the CD19xCD3 bispecific T cell engager (BiTE) blinatumomab is FDA approved [4]. There has been much interest in building upon this success to develop bispecific engagers for other hematologic malignancies and solid tumors [3]. This chapter outlines bispecific antibody design, their biology considerations as well as ongoing clinical trials using T and NK cell engagers and combination strategies using innovative delivery systems [1, 2].

Bispecific Antibody Design

Naturally occurring antibodies consist of a constant fragment crystallizable (Fc) region, which binds common receptors and mediates effector function, and two antigen-binding fragment (Fab) regions, which confer specificity. Each Fab region is comprised of the variable domains of both a heavy (VH) and light (VL) chain [3]. Most antibodies found in nature can bind two or more identical binding epitopes (bivalent or multivalent molecules). Bispecific antibodies, on the other hand, are engineered to be able to recognize two different epitopes. For bispecific engagers, one binding site recognizes either an extracellular TAA or an intracellular TAA in the context of an MHC molecule, and the other an activating cell surface molecule on an immune effector cell. Bispecific antibodies can be generated by fusing antibody producing cell lines such as hybridomas, conjugating existing antibodies, or engineering recombinant proteins to allow for enhanced precision and control of structure [2]. Variations in bispecific engager design can modulate functional characteristics including immunogenicity, effector function, structure, and pharmacokinetics [2] (Figs. 1 and 2).

Immunogenicity

Non-human components of therapeutic antibodies include murine-derived sequences, or de novo engineered proteins, both of which can lead to immune responses. These responses can manifest as acute or delayed hypersensitivity reactions requiring close monitoring and management during infusion or formation of anti-drug antibodies which inhibit the therapeutic effect [5]. Early trials of bispecific antibodies were limited due to human anti-mouse antibody (HAMA) responses [4] and there has been interest in mitigating the effects of non-human components

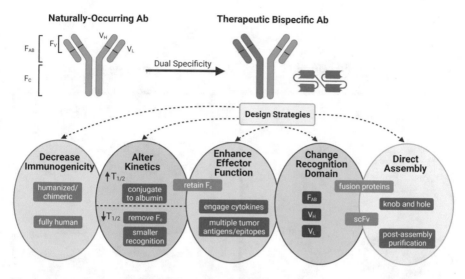

Fig. 1 Design strategies for bispecific T/NK cell engaging constructs. Components of naturally-occurring antibody (Ab) function are modified to render constructs bispecific. Strategies can decrease immunogenicity, alter kinetics by changing half-life ($T_{1/2}$), enhance effector function, change the antigen recognition domain, and direct correct assembly of heterogenous components. F_{AB} antigen binding fragment, F_v variable fragment, F_c constant fragment crystallizable region, *VH* variable heavy chain, *VL* variable light chain, *scFv* single chain variable fragment. *Figure generated using Biorender*

and decreasing immunogenicity of therapeutic antibodies. This has been achieved by replacing immunogenic components with human components, creating chimeric or humanized constructs [4]. Increasingly, fully human constructs are being generated using methods such as phage display to assess for anti-human reactivity and raising antibodies in mice transgenic for human IgG [2]. However, humanized constructs are still susceptible to anti-idiotype immune responses [6].

Structure

Bispecific engagers can be classified depending on structural elements such as the presence or absence of the Fc domain, their symmetry, and the number of binding sites. Bispecific antibodies incorporating the Fc domain are larger and can be designed to closely replicate a naturally occurring immunoglobulin or including additional binding sites [3]. Including the Fc domain can impact the kinetics and mechanism of action of the bispecific antibody, as detailed in the *Pharmacokinetics* section. Pairing heavy and light chains to generate a functional bispecific molecule is a challenge in bispecific antibody design [3]. Genetic modifications such as the "knob-in-hole" design can encourage heterodimerization of the heavy chains [7–11] and force association of coordinating heavy and light chains [12–14]. Additionally,

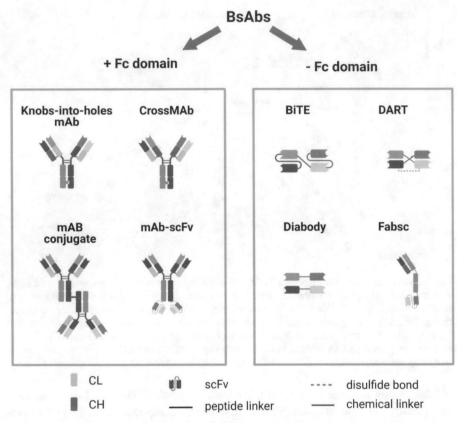

Fig. 2 Representative bispecific antibody (BsAbs) formats. BsAbs can be classified based on the presence or absence of a functional Fc domain. The addition of an Fc domain can impact $T_{1/2}$, BsAb flexibility and mechanisms of antitumor activity. *CL* constant light, *CH* constant heavy, *scFv* single chain variable fragment, *BiTE* bispecific T cell engager, *DART* dual-affinity retargeting. *Figure generated using Biorender*

modifications in the Fc portion can allow for post-assembly purification of heterodimers [15–17]. Modifications to the IgG structure creating symmetric forms include fusion of scFv to heavy or light chains [18] and fusion of additional domains are innovative configurations to confer dual specificity [3, 19].

Bispecific antibodies lacking the Fc domain are smaller molecules that use a single chain variable fragment (scFv) or a single domain (VH or VL) joined by a short linker, rather than a Fab region generated from 2 chains. This structure allows bypassing the challenges of directing cognate heavy and light chain pairing, BsAbs can be engineered without the Fc domain. Tandem scFv constructs joined by short linkers have been extensively studied [3, 20–22] and are the foundation of bispecific T cell engagers [23] and bispecific NK cell engagers (BiKEs) [24, 25]. Several other configurations have been explored, utilizing 1 to 3 binding sites per antigen [3]. Some examples include diabodies, which are bispecific antibodies comprised of 2 chains, each containing a VH and VL, with a short linker that doesn't allow for intrachain association [26–30]. Dual affinity retargeting (DART) proteins are a modification with covalent linkages between these chains [31]. Fusion proteins can link two antigen recognition regions in a fixed orientation without an Fc molecule [32–36]. Other methods fuse unique scFv regions or DARTs to Fc heterodimers [11, 37].The small size of these molecules also allows for variations with multiple specificities [3]. A summary of selected bispecific antibody formats is presented in Fig. 2.

Pharmacokinetics

The pharmacokinetics of antibodies are determined by molecular size. Smaller molecules have faster pharmacokinetics than larger molecules, with smaller molecules having predominantly renal clearance while larger molecules are predominantly cleared by the liver [2]. These molecules have a short half-life ($T_{1/2}$) of 1–2 h, and thus require administration via continuous infusion [38, 39]. One method of extending the half-life of bispecific engager molecules to allow for intermittent administration is conjugation to albumin [40–43].

Mechanism of Action

Monospecific antibodies act by activating Fc-mediated antibody effector functions such as complement-dependent cytotoxicity (CDC), antibody-dependent cellular cytotoxicity (ADCC), and antibody-dependent cellular phagocytosis (ADCP) [4]. Bispecific engaging antibodies activate the cytolytic capacity of immune cells and its mechanism of action depends on the presence or absence of the Fc region [3]. The mechanisms of bispecific antibodies that retain the Fc region involve Fc-mediated effector functions, similar to their monospecific counterparts, while bispecific antibodies engineered without an Fc domain act by establishing a cytolytic synapse between tumor cell and immune cell, leading to release of perforin and granzyme B [44, 45]. The presence or absence of the Fc region also impacts size and subsequently half-life. An additional strategy which has been employed to enhance effector function and specificity is targeting a third antigen such as an additional tumor marker or pro-inflammatory cytokine [46, 47].

Antigen Selection

As mentioned above, bispecific engagers bind to at least one TAA and one activating cell surface molecule on an effector immune cell. This brings the immune cell in proximity to the tumor, directing the cytolytic activity of the effector cell and inciting a local antitumor response. Optimal selection of TAA and activating cell surface molecule is key in establishing an effective engager therapy.

Tumor Antigens

The goal in selecting a TAA is to identify a marker which is differentially expressed on tumor cells with low to normal expression on healthy tissues to limit on-target off-tumor toxicity. Ideal TAAs have consistent homogenous expression throughout the tumor [48]. In contrast to naturally occurring T cell receptors (TCR) which recognize intracellular antigens in a major histocompatibility complex (MHC)-restricted manner, antibody-based therapies recognize cell surface antigens and are not restricted by MHC. Engagers couple this unrestricted antigen recognition with the cytolytic capacity of immune effector cells [49]. An alternative strategy is to engineer a soluble TCR to allow for recognition of an intracellular antigen, though these are MHC-restricted [50, 51]. ScFVs can also recognize peptides in the context of HLA that are derived from tumor-associated neoantigens [52, 53]. While any cell surface antigen can be sufficient for anchoring the engager complex, antigens which are essential to tumor growth, proliferation, and carcinogenesis may be less susceptible to immune escape as tumor cells are motivated to retain their expression.

Immune Cell Antigens

Currently the most common approach in immune effector cell engagers for cancer immunotherapy is engaging T cells via CD3ε, a component of the T cell receptor complex (CD3) universally expressed on T cells [2]. When a T cell engager binds both CD3 and a tumor associated antigen, a cytolytic synapse forms, prompting release of perforin and granzyme B and killing of the target cell [44, 45]. Most configurations are effective without including additional costimulatory molecules [54]. However, some models have shown enhanced activity with addition of costimulation [2, 55, 56] by methods such as engaging the T cell through the agonistic CD28 or 4-1BB receptors rather than CD3 [57, 58].

Additional approaches have involved engagement of NK cells. NK cell activity is regulated by a balance between activating and inhibitory receptors. A primary strategy for engaging NK cells through bispecific engagers is targeting the NK cell receptor CD16, also known as FcγRIII [24]. Incorporating additional stimulation through interleukin-15 (IL15) enhances proliferation and survival [59]. More recently, engagement of NK cells through NK cell receptor G2D (NKG2D) has also been described [60–62]. NKG2D is expressed not only on NK cells, but also on NK T cells, activated CD8$^+$ αβ T cells, γδ T cells, and activated macrophages [63]. Bispecific immunoligands which engage NK cells through the activating NKp30 receptor have also been evaluated in preclinical studies [64, 65]. Invariant natural killer T cells (iNKT), an immune effector subset with potent antitumor activity, have been harnessed through targeting CD1d [62, 66]. An alternative strategy to specifically direct innate immune responses to tumor cells using bispecific antibodies is by blocking inhibitory receptors on tumor cells. An example is a bispecific antibody targeting CD19 and CD47, a molecule upregulated on tumor cells which typically inhibits macrophage-mediated killing [67].

Clinical Translation of Bispecific Engagers

The clinical translation of bispecific engagers was initially dampened by limited antitumor activity and toxicities ranging from cytokine release syndrome [1] to severe immune-mediated hepatotoxicity [68, 69]. However, the success of blinatumomab, a CD19xCD3 BiTE in the treatment of B-cell malignancies, its FDA approval and rapid integration into clinical practice have propelled a robust pipeline developing T cell redirecting bispecific engagers [4], and selected clinical studies are highlighted in Table 1.

Table 1 Selected clinical trials using T cell Engagers

		Target	T cell engager type	Reference or Clinicaltrials.gov ID
Hematological malignancies	B-ALL/NHL	CD19	BiTE (blinatumomab)	[4, 71–74, 169, 170]
			Tandab (AFM11)	NCT02848911[a]
			DART (MGD011, duvortuxizumab)	NCT02454270[a]
		CD20	Triomab (FBTA05, lymphomun)	[83, 171–173]
			Duobody (epcoritamab)	NCT04628494 NCT04623541 NCT03625037
			BsAb (mosunetuzumab, glofitamab, odronextamab, plamotamab)	NCT02500407, [87] NCT03677154 NCT03075696, [85] NCT02290951, [84] NCT03888105 NCT02924402 [86]
	AML	CD123	DART (flotetuzumab)	[88–90]
			Duobody	NCT02715011
			XmAb (XmAb14045)	NCT02730312
		CD33	BiTE (AMG330)	[4, 91, 92]
			TandAb (AMV 564)	NCT03144245
		FLT3	BiTE	[93]
	MM	BCMA	BiTE	NCT02514239, NCT03287908
			Xmab (PF3135)	NCT03269136

(continued)

Table 1 (continued)

		Target	T cell engager type	Reference or Clinicaltrials.gov ID
Solid tumors	Colon carcinoma	CEA	CEAxCD3	[14, 105, 106]
	Neuroblastoma	GD2	Humanized 3F8 BsAb	NCT03860207
	Prostate cancer	PSMA	BiTE (Pasotuxizumab)	[112]
	Lung cancer	DLL3	BiTE (AMG 757)	[109]
	Breast, prostate	Her2	Ertumaxomab	[110, 111]
	Metastatic uveal or cutaneous melanoma	Gp100	Tebentafusp (gp100xCD3)	[113]

[a]Terminated due to strategic decision

T Cell Engagers

In addition to blinatumomab, clinical studies are advancing for other hematologic malignancies including non-Hodgkin lymphoma (NHL), acute myeloid leukemia (AML)/myelodysplastic syndrome (MDS), and multiple myeloma [1, 4]. While application to solid tumors has been challenged by identification of ideal antigens and the impact of an immune suppressive microenvironment, several strategies are in development to address these issues and are proceeding to clinical trials [1, 70].

Hematologic Malignancies

Blinatumomab, a CD19xCD3 BiTE, has become the bellwether for clinical application of bispecific T cell engagers. Blinatumomab can induce minimal residual disease-negative complete responses in patients with refractory B-ALL, though these responses are not sustained, and patients require additional consolidative therapy [38, 71]. Blinatumomab is administered via continuous infusion in 28-day cycles, reversible but serious immune-related adverse events including neurotoxicity and cytokine release syndrome have been described and counteracted by measures such as staged dose increase and dexamethasone prophylaxis [38]. A phase III study in adults with B-ALL demonstrated improved survival compared to conventional chemotherapy and blinatumomab was approved for adult patients in 2014. Safety and efficacy were established in pediatric patients [39], and approval was extended to pediatric patients in 2018 [72]. A subsequent randomized Phase III study in pediatric patients in first relapse through the Children's Oncology Group was stopped early due to superior efficacy in the blinatumomab arm, and ongoing studies are evaluating expanding indications for blinatumomab for higher-risk patients [4, 73, 74]. While initially evaluated in Ph[−] patients, subsequent investigation in Ph[+] patients demonstrated response [75]. Ongoing studies include evaluation of blinatumomab with tyrosine kinase inhibitors in this population [76–79]. While the safety of this combination strategy has been established, there is concern based on preclinical evidence that some tyrosine kinase inhibitors may limit efficacy of T cell-based therapies due to inhibition of TCR signaling [80]. Blinatumomab has also induced response in CD19+ non-Hodgkin lymphomas (NHL) including Diffuse Large B Cell Lymphoma (DLBCL), and phase II/III studies are underway [4, 81], in addition to combination therapies [82]. Other design variations of CD19xCD3 engagers are being clinically evaluated, including tetravalent diabodies, DARTs, tandem antibodies, bispecific antibodies, and trifunctional antibodies [4]. CD20xCD3 bispecifics have also been shown to induce moderate clinical response in B cell malignancies [83] and additional constructs are under evaluation with promising early results in Non-Hodgkin Lymphomas [84–87].

Translating targeted immune therapies to AML has been challenging because most common antigens in AML are also expressed on hematopoietic progenitors or mature neutrophils. Thus, the impact on hematopoietic recovery is an important consideration in clinical application of these therapies. Despite this challenge, CD123 and CD33 have emerged as attractive candidates in AML. Flotetuzumab is a humanized CD123xCD3 DART which is undergoing phase I/II evaluation. Early results have demonstrated clinical activity, with correlative analysis indicating that pre-treatment immune signatures and presence of TP53 mutations are associated with response [88–90]. Additional CD123xCD3 strategies include bispecific antibodies, duobody, and XmAb [4]. AMG330, a CD33xCD3 BiTE, has shown preclinical activity in AML and is undergoing phase I evaluation [4, 91, 92]. In addition, clinical evaluation is underway for CD33xCD3 TandAbs. Other AML antigens targeted with T cell engagers include early clinical studies for T cell engagers specific for FLT3 [93] and CLL1 (CLEC12A) [1], as well as preclinical development of CLL1xCD3 BiFabs [4].

B cell maturation antigen (BCMA) is an antigen almost exclusively specific to the malignant plasma cells of multiple myeloma, which makes it an attractive immunotherapeutic target. Several bispecific T cell-engaging BCMAxCD3 constructs being tested in early phase clinical trials, including BiTEs, bispecific Fab molecules, and XmAbs [4]. The bispecific antibody teclistamab had an acceptable toxicity profile in phase I evaluation and at therapeutic doses was able to generate durable remissions, prompting ongoing phase II evaluation and combination studies [94–96]. Additional bispecific antibodies PF06863135 and REGN5458 are being evaluated in phase I studies and have thus far been tolerated with some evidence of clinical activity [97, 98]. In a phase I study of AMG 420 a maximum tolerated dose was established, at which stringent complete responses were achieved, and is proceeding to further clinical studies [99]. TNB-383B incorporates 2 heavy-chain only BCMA recognition sequences coupled to 1 unique CD3 recognition sequence which aims to preferentially activate effector T cells [100]. A dose-dependent response has been observed in ongoing phase I evaluation [101]. Phase I studies are also underway evaluating FcRH5xCD3 and GPRC5DxCD3 in multiple myeloma [1].

Solid Tumors

Early clinical experience has shown feasibility and safety of T cell engagers in solid tumors, though with only modest efficacy [2]. Catumaxomab, an EpCamxCD3 tri-functional antibody administered via intraperitoneal injection, was evaluated in a phase II/III study and initially approved in the European Union for management of malignant ascites [102]. However, it was subsequently withdrawn from the US and European markets for commercial reasons. Escalation attempts of other EpCamxCD3 systemic therapies were hampered by dose limiting toxicities and did not demonstrate increased clinical efficacy [103, 104].

Due to the heterogeneity of solid tumors, tumor-associated antigens which are expressed on multiple tumor types are attractive targets. Examples of such antigens under investigation with T cell redirecting engagers include B7-H3, EGFR/EGFRvIII, GPC3, MUC1, P-cadherin, PRAME, PSCA, PD-L1, and 5T4 [1, 70]. Multiple carcinoembryonic antigen (CEA)xCD3 constructs are under clinical evaluation for CEA+ tumors including colorectal cancer, with early data supporting safety of combination therapy with the checkpoint inhibitor atezolizumab [14, 105, 106] and favoring continuous infusion for optimal therapeutic index [107, 108]. Additional antigens being targeted clinically with T cell engagers for gastrointestinal tumors include MUC17, GUCY2c, gpA33, and CLDN18.2 and for small cell lung carcinoma DLL3 [1, 109]. A SSTR2xCD3 engager is in early trials for neuroendocrine tumors, and a GD2xCD3 engager for neuroblastoma [1].

HER2 has been explored as a target for breast, prostate, and other solid tumors. Initial clinical experience with ertumaxomab, a HER2xCD3 antibody, provoked an immune response and had limited antitumor activity [110, 111]. Ongoing studies evaluate HER2xCD3 in combination with the checkpoint inhibitor pembrolizumab, in addition to HER2 targeting constructs engaging T cells via 4-1BB[70]. Pasotuxizumab, a PSMAxCD3 BiTE, was well tolerated and showed dose-dependent clinical response in a phase I study [112]. Ongoing studies are assessing the activity of PSMAxCD3 engagers in prostate as well as other solid tumors, both alone and in combination with pembrolizumab [70]. In addition to targeting PSMA, STEAP1xCD3 T cell engagers are undergoing early clinical evaluation in prostate cancer and MUC16 and MSLN in ovarian cancers.

A phase I/II study of tebentafusp, a gp100xCD3 bispecific agent utilizing a soluble TCR, in HLA-A2+ patients with metastatic uveal or cutaneous melanoma established the maximum tolerated dose with dose limiting toxicities related to cytokine release [113]. Efficacy was most notable in patients with uveal melanoma, and expanded clinical studies are underway in this population [113]. This platform fusing a tumor antigen-specific TCR and CD3 scFv, described as immune-mobilizing monoclonal T cell receptor against cancer (ImmTAC), has also been evaluated clinically targeting MAGE-A4 positive solid tumors [114].

Bispecific Innate Immune Cell Engagers

NK cells are a key component of cancer immunosurveillance which have been exploited for cancer immunotherapy. Their activity is modulated by a balance of activating and inhibitory receptors, with healthy cells expressing predominantly inhibitory receptors and some tumor cells increasing expression of activating receptors [24]. The goal of natural killer cell engager therapy is to add additional tumor-directed specificity to this response, along with stimulation of activating receptors. BiKEs have been generated against several tumor antigens, and have been given additional specificities including additional tumor-specific antigens or stimulatory cytokines to generate trispecific killer engagers (TriKE) trifunctional natural killer cell engagers (NKCE) or tetraspecific killer engagers (TetraKE) [24, 47, 59, 115–119]. Macrophage-mediated antitumor activity can be engaged using a bispecific CD19xCD47 antibody. CD47 is ubiquitously expressed and serves as an inhibitory signal for macrophages, and when co-engaged with a tumor antigen allows for antibody-dependent cellular phagocytosis [67].

Hematologic Malignancies

Like T cell engagers, the preclinical and clinical evaluation of NK engagers in hematological malignancies has focused on B-cell malignancies (CD19, CD22) and MDS/AML (CD33, CLEC12A). Preclinical evaluation of BiKEs and TriKEs specific for 1 (CD19xCD16) or 2 tumor-associated antigens (CD19xCD22xCD16) showed specific antitumor activity in B cell malignancies including ALL, B cell lymphoma, and chronic lymphocytic leukemia (CLL), with NK cell activation mediated through direct CD16 signaling [117, 120, 121]. CD19 has also been targeted with NK cells via NKG2D [61] and iNKT cells via CD1d[51]. A CD33xCD16 NK cell engager demonstrated antitumor activity in MDS/AML and was improved with the addition of IL15 [59, 122, 123]. GTB-3550, the CD33 x CD16 x IL15 TriKE, is being evaluated in an ongoing phase I/II clinical trial. CLEC12A is an additional antigen under evaluation as a TriKE for AML [124].

AFM13, a CD30xCD16 NK cell engager, was well tolerated in a phase I study for Hodgkin lymphoma, both as a single agent [30] and in combination with pembrolizumab [125] and is undergoing phase II evaluation. In multiple myeloma preclinical cytolytic activity has been demonstrated with CS1xNKG2D and BCMAxNKG2D bispecific antibodies, mediated through activation of NK cells along with other NKG2D+ effectors [60, 62].

Solid Tumors

The use of NK engagers against solid tumors has centered around breast cancer (HER2) and different carcinomas (EpCAM, CD133, CEA). Clinical evaluation of 2B1, a HER2xCD16 bispecific antibody in patients with refractory breast cancer induced an immune response but did not have notable antitumor activity [126, 127]. HER2xCD1d engagers have also been evaluated preclinically [62]. NK engagers targeting additional solid tumor antigens are under investigation, including BiKEs and TriKEs specific for B7-H3 which are applicable across a spectrum of solid tumor models [118, 128]. EpCAMxCD16 and CD133xCD16 engagers demonstrated activity in preclinical carcinoma models and have been augmented by addition of IL15 or used in combination (CD133xEpCAMxCD16xIL15) [25, 115, 116, 129]. Natural killer cells engaged through NKG2D have shown antitumor activity in various preclinical models [63] including targeting CEA in colon carcinoma [130] and CD24 in hepatocellular carcinoma [131].

Alternative Delivery Methods and Adoptive Cellular Therapies

Traditional delivery methods of bispecific immune effector cell engagers are limited by the reliance on an intact host immune system and requirement for frequent or continuous dosing. Coupling engagers with ex-vivo expanded adoptive cellular therapy products provides additional capacity to generate an antitumor immune response and is a platform on which costimulation or additional tumor antigen targeting for localization can be added. The endogenous generation of engagers through cellular products, nucleic acids, and oncolytic viruses allows for continuous exposure to molecules with a short half-life.

Bispecific Antibody Armed Activated T Cells

Armed activated T cells are generated by autologous pheresis, activation of T cells, incubation with a bispecific antibody, washing out any residual antibody, then infusing the activated T cells with bound bispecific antibody to the patient [132, 133]. This was first clinically described with local injection of T cells armed with a CD3 and anti-glioma antibody [132]. The technique was subsequently employed with intraperitoneal injection of Mov28xCD3 and folate receptor(FR)xCD3 armed T cells in patients with ovarian cancer [134]. In a pilot study, CD20xCD3 armed T cells were well tolerated after autologous hematopoietic cell transplant in patients with non-Hodgkin lymphoma [133, 135]. In a phase I studies HER2xCD3 armed T cells were tolerated in patients with breast and prostate cancer, in combination with granulocyte-macrophage colony stimulating factor (GM-CSF) and low dose IL2, with only modest antitumor activity [136, 137]. More recent clinical investigations have expanded to EGFRxCD3 armed T cells for pancreatic cancer [138]. CS1xCD3 armed T cells are under preclinical development for multiple myeloma [139]. To enhance the cytolytic capacity of armed T cells, preclinical work is evaluating CD19-CAR T cells armed with either HER2xCD3 or EGFRxCD3 antibodies to assess the ability to engage the intracellular signaling components of the CAR in CD19 negative targets [140].

T Cells Secreting Bispecific Engagers

T cells have been engineered to secrete bispecific engaging molecules to administer adoptive cellular therapy while engaging the local inflammatory response. An advantage of this method over systemic administration of bispecific engagers is that the engagers are secreted at the site of action, limiting systemic toxicities [141, 142]. In this method T cells are activated and expanded, engineered by transduction with a lentiviral or retroviral vector or electroporated with RNA encoding the bispecific engager, expanded, and then evaluated in functional assays or infused [141]. Because the engager molecule is then produced by the T cell, this allows for constant exposure to a small molecule with a short half-life without the requirement for continuous or frequent infusion. The secreted bispecific molecule can engage both the adoptively transferred T cells and bystander T cells, augmenting the antitumor effect [143]. In vitro and in vivo antitumor activity has been demonstrated across a range of tumors, including EphA2xCD3 and CEAxCD3 in solid tumors [143–145], CD19xCD3 in ALL [146, 147], and CD123xCD3 in AML[148]. One limitation to this strategy in comparison to other adoptive cellular therapies such as CAR-T cells is the lack of costimulation, which may dampen the magnitude of the antitumor response. This can be augmented by expressing additional ligands on the T cell which induce costimulation through CD28 or 4-1BB[56]. In AML models, activity of T cells secreting a CLEC12AxCD3 engager was enhanced by addition of a chimeric CD123.IL7Rα receptor, with a dual antigen-specific effect [149]. An additional strategy to utilize dual antigen specificity is secreting a bispecific engager from a CAR-T cell. This was demonstrated with CAR-T cells targeting tumor-specific epidermal growth factor receptor vIII (EGFRvIII) in glioblastoma secreting a wild type-specific EGFRxCD3 engager, with the goal that the engager would be secreted at the local tumor site to enhance antitumor activity while minimizing systemic on-target off-tumor toxicity [150].

Alternative Delivery Methods

In addition to T cells, other cell types have been engineered as delivery mechanisms for T cell engagers allowing for sustained exposure after a one-time infusion. Macrophages secreting an EGFRvIII specific T cell engager had *in vivo* activity in glioblastoma models, which was enhanced when macrophages also secreted IL12, with a hypothesis that macrophages will preferentially localize to tumor sites optimizing local delivery [151]. Alternative strategies have utilized mesenchymal stem cells (MSC) as a vehicle for expression of engager molecules. Confined to an extracellular matrix scaffold, engineered MSCs secreted a CEAxCD3 diabody which generated systemic in vivo antitumor activity [152]. In a hepatocellular carcinoma model, MSCs engineered to secrete GPC3xCD3 engagers had *in vitro* and *in vivo* antitumor activity which was enhanced by added costimulation through CD28 or 4-1BB [153].

Non-cellular based delivery methods have been explored to improve sustained delivery of engager molecules. Synthetic nucleic acids including mRNA and DNA vectors have generated endogenous production of engager molecules which demonstrate antitumor activity comparable to corresponding purified bispecific antibodies [154–156]. Oncolytic viruses are an attractive delivery method as a single agent therapeutic which enhances the local antitumor immune response through multiple mechanisms. Oncolytic viruses which have been engineered to secrete T cell engagers demonstrated antitumor activity in preclinical solid tumor models and are undergoing further development [157–160].

Challenges and Future Directions for Engager Therapy

Despite successes such as the expanding use of blinatumomab in B-ALL, there are challenges to be addressed to improve bispecific immune effector cell therapies and effectively apply them in other malignancies. Engager therapies rely on the host immune system and hence, quantitative or qualitative deficiencies in host immune cells resulting from the underlying malignancy or prior treatment can limit efficacy. In addition, resident T cell exhaustion and expression of inhibitory ligands can blunt the effectiveness of T cell-based immunotherapies, either preventing or limiting antitumor activity [1, 14].

Combining bispecific engager with adoptive cellular therapies or small molecules, as well as modifications to the timing of engager therapy within a treatment regimen may support the host immune system and increase the chance of success. Strategies to mitigate exhaustion include combining engagers with checkpoint inhibitors and targeting specific subsets of immune effector cells [70, 100, 105, 106, 161, 162]. In addition to intrinsic qualities of immune effector cells, the immunosuppressive microenvironment limits efficacy of engager therapies, particularly in solid tumors. This includes cellular components, cytokines and other soluble factors, and structural considerations [1]. Targeting stromal components, immune suppressive cells, and exploring combination therapies are all strategies to mitigate the inhibitory impact of the microenvironment [1].

One strategy to improve specificity is designing engager prodrugs that are specifically activated in the tumor microenvironment or assembled in the presence of tumor antigens [163–166]. When considering bispecific engager therapies beyond CD19-targeted BsAbs, antigen selection is crucial for guaranteeing the effectiveness bispecific engager therapy. Low levels of tumor antigen expression contribute to suboptimal potency, and immune escape is a key mechanism of resistance to or relapse after immune effector engager therapies. Shared expression between tumor antigens and healthy tissues can lead to on-target off-tumor toxicity. Targeting more than one antigen is a strategy which is being employed to increase specificity, apply additional selective pressure to prevent immune escape, and improve safety profile [1, 117, 148]. While immune-mediated side effects including cytokine release syndrome continue to be a common concern with immune effector cell-redirecting therapies, the understanding of optimal management strategies continues to advance [167, 168]. As this robust pipeline of enhancement strategies translates to the clinic, it is likely that the indications for bispecific immune effector cell engaging therapies will continue to expand.

References

1. Singh A, Dees S, Grewal IS. Overcoming the challenges associated with CD3+ T-cell redirection in cancer. Br J Cancer. 2021;
2. Suurs FV, Lub-de Hooge MN, de Vries EGE, de Groot DJA. A review of bispecific antibodies and antibody constructs in oncology and clinical challenges. Pharmacol Ther. 2019;201:103–19.
3. Brinkmann U, Kontermann RE. The making of bispecific antibodies. MAbs. 2017;9:182–212.
4. Thakur A, Huang M, Lum LG. Bispecific antibody based therapeutics: strengths and challenges. Blood Rev. 2018;32:339–47.
5. Ulitzka M, Carrara S, Grzeschik J, Kornmann H, Hock B, Kolmar H. Engineering therapeutic antibodies for patient safety: tackling the immunogenicity problem. Protein Eng Des Sel. 2020;33
6. Grosserichter-Wagener C, Kos D, van Leeuwen A, et al. Biased anti-idiotype response in rabbits leads to high-affinity monoclonal antibodies to biologics. MAbs. 2020;12:1814661.
7. Ridgway JB, Presta LG, Carter P. 'Knobs-into-holes' engineering of antibody CH3 domains for heavy chain heterodimerization. Protein Eng. 1996;9:617–21.
8. Merchant AM, Zhu Z, Yuan JQ, et al. An efficient route to human bispecific IgG. Nat Biotechnol. 1998;16:677–81.
9. Junttila TT, Li J, Johnston J, et al. Antitumor efficacy of a bispecific antibody that targets HER2 and activates T cells. Cancer Res. 2014;74:5561–71.
10. Shahied LS, Tang Y, Alpaugh RK, Somer R, Greenspon D, Weiner LM. Bispecific minibodies targeting HER2/ncu and CD16 exhibit improved tumor lysis when placed in a divalent tumor antigen binding format. J Biol Chem. 2004;279:53907–14.
11. Xie Z, Guo N, Yu M, Hu M, Shen B. A new format of bispecific antibody: highly efficient heterodimerization, expression and tumor cell lysis. J Immunol Methods. 2005;296:95–101.
12. Koerber JT, Hornsby MJ, Wells JA. An improved single-chain fab platform for efficient display and recombinant expression. J Mol Biol. 2015;427:576–86.
13. Klein C, Sustmann C, Thomas M, et al. Progress in overcoming the chain association issue in bispecific heterodimeric IgG antibodies. MAbs. 2012;4:653–63.
14 Bacac M, Fauti T, Sam J, et al. A novel carcinoembryonic antigen T-cell bispecific antibody (CEA TCB) for the treatment of solid tumors. Clin Cancer Res. 2016;22:3286–97.
15. Smith EJ, Olson K, Haber LJ, et al. A novel, native-format bispecific antibody triggering T-cell killing of B-cells is robustly active in mouse tumor models and cynomolgus monkeys. Sci Rep. 2015;5:17943.
16. Tustian AD, Endicott C, Adams B, Mattila J, Bak H. Development of purification processes for fully human bispecific antibodies based upon modification of protein a binding avidity. MAbs. 2016;8:828–38.

17. Fischer N, Elson G, Magistrelli G, et al. Exploiting light chains for the scalable generation and platform purification of native human bispecific IgG. Nat Commun. 2015;6:6113.
18. Asano R, Watanabe Y, Kawaguchi H, et al. Highly effective recombinant format of a humanized IgG-like bispecific antibody for cancer immunotherapy with retargeting of lymphocytes to tumor cells. J Biol Chem. 2007;282:27659–65.
19. Lu CY, Chen GJ, Tai PH, et al. Tetravalent anti-CD20/CD3 bispecific antibody for the treatment of B cell lymphoma. Biochem Biophys Res Commun. 2016;473:808–13.
20. Hayden MS, Linsley PS, Gayle MA, et al. Single-chain mono- and bispecific antibody derivatives with novel biological properties and antitumour activity from a COS cell transient expression system. Ther Immunol. 1994;1:3–15.
21. Mallender WD, Voss EW Jr. Construction, expression, and activity of a bivalent bispecific single-chain antibody. J Biol Chem. 1994;269:199–206.
22. Gruber M, Schodin BA, Wilson ER, Kranz DM. Efficient tumor cell lysis mediated by a bispecific single chain antibody expressed in Escherichia coli. J Immunol. 1994;152:5368–74.
23. Huehls AM, Coupet TA, Sentman CL. Bispecific T-cell engagers for cancer immunotherapy. Immunol Cell Biol. 2015;93:290–6.
24. Hodgins JJ, Khan ST, Park MM, Auer RC, Ardolino M. Killers 2.0: NK cell therapies at the forefront of cancer control. J Clin Invest. 2019;129:3499–510.
25. Schmohl JU, Gleason MK, Dougherty PR, Miller JS, Vallera DA. Heterodimeric bispecific single chain variable fragments (scFv) killer engagers (BiKEs) enhance NK-cell activity against CD133+ colorectal cancer cells. Target Oncol. 2016;11:353–61.
26. Cochlovius B, Kipriyanov SM, Stassar MJ, et al. Cure of Burkitt's lymphoma in severe combined immunodeficiency mice by T cells, tetravalent CD3 x CD19 tandem diabody, and CD28 costimulation. Cancer Res. 2000;60:4336–41.
27. Holliger P, Brissinck J, Williams RL, Thielemans K, Winter G. Specific killing of lymphoma cells by cytotoxic T-cells mediated by a bispecific diabody. Protein Eng. 1996;9:299–305.
28. Reusch U, Burkhardt C, Fucek I, et al. A novel tetravalent bispecific TandAb (CD30/CD16A) efficiently recruits NK cells for the lysis of CD30+ tumor cells. MAbs. 2014;6:728–39.
29. Reusch U, Harrington KH, Gudgeon CJ, et al. Characterization of CD33/CD3 tetravalent bispecific tandem Diabodies (TandAbs) for the treatment of acute myeloid leukemia. Clin Cancer Res. 2016;22:5829–38.
30. Rothe A, Sasse S, Topp MS, et al. A phase 1 study of the bispecific anti-CD30/CD16A antibody construct AFM13 in patients with relapsed or refractory Hodgkin lymphoma. Blood. 2015;125:4024–31.
31. Johnson S, Burke S, Huang L, et al. Effector cell recruitment with novel Fv-based dual-affinity re-targeting protein leads to potent tumor cytolysis and in vivo B-cell depletion. J Mol Biol. 2010;399:436–49.
32. Schoonjans R, Willems A, Schoonooghe S, Leoen J, Grooten J, Mertens N. A new model for intermediate molecular weight recombinant bispecific and trispecific antibodies by efficient heterodimerization of single chain variable domains through fusion to a Fab-chain. Biomol Eng. 2001;17:193–202.
33. Qu Z, Goldenberg DM, Cardillo TM, Shi V, Hansen HJ, Chang CH. Bispecific anti-CD20/22 antibodies inhibit B-cell lymphoma proliferation by a unique mechanism of action. Blood. 2008;111:2211–9.
34. Kellner C, Bruenke J, Horner H, et al. Heterodimeric bispecific antibody-derivatives against CD19 and CD16 induce effective antibody-dependent cellular cytotoxicity against B-lymphoid tumor cells. Cancer Lett. 2011;303:128–39.
35. Rozan C, Cornillon A, Petiard C, et al. Single-domain antibody-based and linker-free bispecific antibodies targeting FcgammaRIII induce potent antitumor activity without recruiting regulatory T cells. Mol Cancer Ther. 2013;12:1481–91.
36. Rossi DL, Rossi EA, Cardillo TM, Goldenberg DM, Chang CH. A new class of bispecific antibodies to redirect T cells for cancer immunotherapy. MAbs. 2014;6:381–91.
37. Xu Y, Lee J, Tran C, et al. Production of bispecific antibodies in "knobs-into-holes" using a cell-free expression system. MAbs. 2015;7:231–42.

38. Topp MS, Gokbuget N, Stein AS, et al. Safety and activity of blinatumomab for adult patients with relapsed or refractory B-precursor acute lymphoblastic leukaemia: a multicentre, single-arm, phase 2 study. Lancet Oncol. 2015;16:57–66.
39. von Stackelberg A, Locatelli F, Zugmaier G, et al. Phase I/phase II study of Blinatumomab in pediatric patients with relapsed/refractory acute lymphoblastic leukemia. J Clin Oncol. 2016;34:4381–9.
40. Dave E, Adams R, Zaccheo O, et al. Fab-dsFv: a bispecific antibody format with extended serum half-life through albumin binding. MAbs. 2016;8:1319–35.
41. Sleep D, Cameron J, Evans LR. Albumin as a versatile platform for drug half-life extension. Biochim Biophys Acta. 1830;2013:5526–34.
42. Muller D, Karle A, Meissburger B, Hofig I, Stork R, Kontermann RE. Improved pharmaco-kinetics of recombinant bispecific antibody molecules by fusion to human serum albumin. J Biol Chem. 2007;282:12650–60.
43. Fang M, Zhao R, Yang Z, et al. Characterization of an anti-human ovarian carcinomaxanti-human CD3 bispecific single-chain antibody with an albumin-original interlinker. Gynecol Oncol. 2004;92:135–46.
44. Offner S, Hofmeister R, Romaniuk A, Kufer P, Baeuerle PA. Induction of regular cytolytic T cell synapses by bispecific single-chain antibody constructs on MHC class I-negative tumor cells. Mol Immunol. 2006;43:763–71.
45. Haas C, Krinner E, Brischwein K, et al. Mode of cytotoxic action of T cell-engaging BiTE antibody MT110. Immunobiology. 2009;214:441–53.
46. Austin RJ, Lemon BD, Aaron WH, et al. TriTACs, a novel class of T-cell-engaging protein constructs designed for the treatment of solid tumors. Mol Cancer Ther. 2021;20:109–20.
47. Sarhan D, Brandt L, Felices M, et al. 161533 TriKE stimulates NK-cell function to overcome myeloid-derived suppressor cells in MDS. Blood Adv. 2018;2:1459–69.
48. Middelburg J, Kemper K, Engelberts P, Labrijn AF, Schuurman J, van Hall T. Overcoming challenges for CD3-bispecific antibody therapy in solid tumors. Cancers (Basel). 2021;13
49. Epperly R, Gottschalk S, Velasquez MP. Harnessing T cells to target pediatric acute myeloid leukemia: CARs, BiTEs, and beyond. Children (Basel). 2020;7
50. Liddy N, Bossi G, Adams KJ, et al. Monoclonal TCR-redirected tumor cell killing. Nat Med. 2012;18:980–7.
51. Dao T, Pankov D, Scott A, et al. Therapeutic bispecific T-cell engager antibody targeting the intracellular oncoprotein WT1. Nat Biotechnol. 2015;33:1079–86.
52. Hsiue EH, Wright KM, Douglass J, et al. Targeting a neoantigen derived from a common TP53 mutation. Science. 2021;371
53. Herrmann AC, Im JS, Pareek S, et al. A novel T-cell engaging bi-specific antibody targeting the leukemia antigen PR1/HLA-A2. Front Immunol. 2018;9:3153.
54. Dreier T, Lorenczewski G, Brandl C, et al. Extremely potent, rapid and costimulation-independent cytotoxic T-cell response against lymphoma cells catalyzed by a single-chain bispecific antibody. Int J Cancer. 2002;100:690–7.
55. Liu R, Jiang W, Yang M, et al. Efficient inhibition of human B-cell lymphoma in SCID mice by synergistic antitumor effect of human 4-1BB ligand/anti-CD20 fusion proteins and anti-CD3/anti-CD20 diabodies. J Immunother. 2010;33:500–9.
56. Velasquez MP, Szoor A, Vaidya A, et al. CD28 and 41BB Costimulation enhances the effector function of CD19-specific engager T cells. Cancer Immunol Res. 2017;5:860–70.
57. Otz T, Grosse-Hovest L, Hofmann M, Rammensee HG, Jung G. A bispecific single-chain antibody that mediates target cell-restricted, supra-agonistic CD28 stimulation and killing of lymphoma cells. Leukemia 2009;23:71 7.
58. Grosse-Hovest L, Hartlapp I, Marwan W, Brem G, Rammensee HG, Jung G. A recombi-nant bispecific single-chain antibody induces targeted, supra-agonistic CD28-stimulation and tumor cell killing. Eur J Immunol. 2003;33:1334–40.
59. Vallera DA, Felices M, McElmurry R, et al. IL15 Trispecific killer engagers (TriKE) make natural killer cells specific to CD33+ targets while also inducing persistence, in vivo expan-sion, and enhanced function. Clin Cancer Res. 2016;22:3440–50.

60. Wang Y, Li H, Xu W, et al. BCMA-targeting bispecific antibody that simultaneously stimu-lates NKG2D-enhanced efficacy against multiple myeloma. J Immunother. 2020;43:175–88.
61. Zhao Q, Pang J, Yan F, et al. Production of a novel bispecific protein ULBP1xCD19-scFv targeting the NKG2D receptor and CD19 to promote the activation of NK cells. Protein Expr Purif. 2021;178:105783.
62. Chan WK, Kang S, Youssef Y, et al. A CS1-NKG2D bispecific antibody collectively activates cytolytic immune cells against multiple myeloma. Cancer Immunol Res. 2018;6:776–87.
63. Godbersen C, Coupet TA, Huehls AM, et al. NKG2D ligand-targeted bispecific T-cell engagers Lead to robust antitumor activity against diverse human tumors. Mol Cancer Ther. 2017;16:1335–46.
64. Pekar L, Klausz K, Busch M, et al. Affinity maturation of B7-H6 translates into enhanced NK cell-mediated tumor cell lysis and improved proinflammatory cytokine release of bispecific immunoligands via NKp30 engagement. J Immunol. 2021;206:225–36.
65. Kellner C, Gunther A, Humpe A, et al. Enhancing natural killer cell-mediated lysis of lym-phoma cells by combining therapeutic antibodies with CD20-specific immunoligands engag-ing NKG2D or NKp30. Onco Targets Ther. 2016;5:e1058459.
66. Das R, Guan P, Wiener SJ, et al. Enhancing the antitumor functions of invariant natural killer T cells using a soluble CD1d-CD19 fusion protein. Blood Adv. 2019;3:813–24.
67. Buatois V, Johnson Z, Salgado-Pires S, et al. Preclinical development of a bispecific antibody that safely and effectively targets CD19 and CD47 for the treatment of B-cell lymphoma and leukemia. Mol Cancer Ther. 2018;17:1739–51.
68. Mau-Sorensen M, Dittrich C, Dienstmann R, et al. A phase I trial of intravenous catumax-omab: a bispecific monoclonal antibody targeting EpCAM and the T cell coreceptor CD3. Cancer Chemother Pharmacol. 2015;75:1065–73.
69. Borlak J, Langer F, Spanel R, Schondorfer G, Dittrich C. Immune-mediated liver injury of the cancer therapeutic antibody catumaxomab targeting EpCAM, CD3 and Fcgamma receptors. Oncotarget. 2016;7:28059–74.
70. Fuca G, Spagnoletti A, Ambrosini M, de Braud F, Di Nicola M. Immune cell engagers in solid tumors: promises and challenges of the next generation immunotherapy. ESMO Open. 2021;6:100046.
71. Topp MS, Kufer P, Gokbuget N, et al. Targeted therapy with the T-cell-engaging antibody blinatumomab of chemotherapy-refractory minimal residual disease in B-lineage acute lym-phoblastic leukemia patients results in high response rate and prolonged leukemia-free sur-vival. J Clin Oncol. 2011;29:2493–8.
72. Kantarjian H, Stein A, Gokbuget N, et al. Blinatumomab versus chemotherapy for advanced acute lymphoblastic leukemia. N Engl J Med. 2017;376:836–47.
73. Brown P, Ji L, Xu X, et al. A Randomized phase 3 trial of blinatumomab Vs. chemotherapy as post-reinduction therapy in high and intermediate risk (HR/IR) first relapse of B-acute lym-phoblastic leukemia (B-ALL) in children and adolescents/young adults (AYAs) demonstrates superior efficacy and tolerability of blinatumomab: a report from children's oncology group study AALL1331. Blood 2019;134.
74. Queudeville M, Schlegel P, Heinz AT, et al. Blinatumomab in pediatric patients with relapsed/refractory B-cell precursor acute lymphoblastic leukemia. Eur J Haematol. 2020;
75. Martinelli G, Boissel N, Chevallier P, et al. Complete hematologic and molecular response in adult patients with relapsed/refractory Philadelphia chromosome-positive B-precursor acute lymphoblastic leukemia following treatment with blinatumomab: results from a phase II, single-arm, multicenter study. J Clin Oncol. 2017;35:1795–802.
76. Assi R, Kantarjian H, Short NJ, et al. Safety and efficacy of blinatumomab in combina-tion with a tyrosine kinase inhibitor for the treatment of relapsed Philadelphia chromosome-positive leukemia. Clin Lymphoma Myeloma Leuk. 2017;17:897–901.
77. Foa R, Bassan R, Vitale A, et al. Dasatinib-blinatumomab for Ph-positive acute lymphoblas-tic leukemia in adults. N Engl J Med. 2020;383:1613–23.
78. Sharma R, Takemoto C, Waller B, Holland A, Pui CH, Inaba H. Reduced intensity chemother-apy with tyrosine kinase inhibitor and blinatumomab in a pediatric patient with Philadelphia chromosome-positive ALL and mechanical heart valves. Pediatr Blood Cancer. 2021:e28924.

79. King AC, Pappacena JJ, Tallman MS, Park JH, Geyer MB. Blinatumomab administered concurrently with oral tyrosine kinase inhibitor therapy is a well-tolerated consolidation strategy and eradicates measurable residual disease in adults with Philadelphia chromosome positive acute lymphoblastic leukemia. Leuk Res. 2019;79:27–33.

80. Leonard J, Kosaka Y, Malla P, et al. Concomitant use of a dual ABL/Src kinase inhibitor eliminates the in vitroefficacy of blinatumomab against Ph+ ALL. Blood 2021;137(7):939-944.

81. Viardot A, Goebeler ME, Hess G, et al. Phase 2 study of the bispecific T-cell engager (BiTE) antibody blinatumomab in relapsed/refractory diffuse large B-cell lymphoma. Blood. 2016;127:1410–6.

82. Lussana F, Gritti G, Rambaldi A. Immunotherapy of acute lymphoblastic leukemia and lymphoma with T cell-redirected bispecific antibodies. J Clin Oncol. 2021;39:444–55.

83. Schuster FR, Stanglmaier M, Woessmann W, et al. Immunotherapy with the trifunctional anti-CD20 x anti-CD3 antibody FBTA05 (Lymphomun) in paediatric high-risk patients with recurrent CD20-positive B cell malignancies. Br J Haematol. 2015;169:90–102.

84. Bannerji R, Allan J, Arnason J, et al. Clinical activity of REGN1979, a bispecific human, anti-CD20 x anti-CD3 antibody, in patients with relapsed/refractory (R/R) B-cell non-Hodgkin lymphoma (B-NHL). Blood. 2019;134

85. Hutchings M, Iacoboni G, Morschhauseer F, et al. CD20-Tcb (RG6026), a novel "2:1" format T-cell-engaging bispecific antibody, induces complete remissions in relapsed/refractory B-cell non-Hodgkin's lymphoma: preliminary results from a phase I first in human trial. Blood. 2018;132

86. Patel K, Michot J, Chanan A, et al. Preliminary safety and anti-tumor activity of XmAb13676, an anti-CD20 x anti-CD3 bispecific antibody, in patients with relapsed/refractory non-Hodgkin's lymphoma and chronic lymphocytic leukemia. Blood. 2019;134

87. Schuster S, Bartlett N, Assouline S, et al. Mosunetuzumab induces complete remissions in poor prognosis non-Hodgkin lymphoma patients, including those who are resistant to or relapsing after chimeric antigen receptor T-cell (CAR-T) therapies, and is active in treatment through multiple lines. Blood. 2019;134

88. Vadakekolathu J, Lai C, Reeder S, et al. TP53 abnormalities correlate with immune infiltration and associate with response to flotetuzumab immunotherapy in AML. Blood Adv. 2020;4:5011–24.

89. Uy G, Aldoss I, Foster M, et al. Flotetuzumab, an investigational CD123 x CD3 bispecific Dart® protein, in salvage therapy for primary refractory and early relapsed acute myeloid leukemia (AML) patients. Blood. 2019;134

90. Uy G, Rettig MP, Vey N, et al. Phase 1 cohort expansion of Flotetuzumab, a CD123×CD3 bispecific Dart® protein in patients with relapsed/refractory acute myeloid leukemia (AML). Blood. 2018;132

91. Friedrich M, Henn A, Raum T, et al. Preclinical characterization of AMG 330, a CD3/CD33-bispecific T-cell-engaging antibody with potential for treatment of acute myelogenous leukemia. Mol Cancer Ther. 2014;13:1549–57.

92. Laszlo GS, Gudgeon CJ, Harrington KH, et al. Cellular determinants for preclinical activity of a novel CD33/CD3 bispecific T-cell engager (BiTE) antibody, AMG 330, against human AML. Blood. 2014;123:554–61.

93. Brauchle B, Goldstein RL, Karbowski CM, et al. Characterization of a novel FLT3 BiTE molecule for the treatment of acute myeloid leukemia. Mol Cancer Ther. 2020;19:1875–88.

94. Garfall A, Usmani S, Mateos M-V, et al. Updated phase 1 results of Teclistamab, a B-cell maturation antigen (BCMA) x CD3 bispecific antibody, in relapsed and/or refractory multiple myeloma (RRMM) Blood. 2020;136

95. Usmani S, Mateos M, Nahi H, et al. Phase I study of teclistamab, a humanized B-cell maturation antigen (BCMA) x CD3 bispecific antibody, in relapsed/refractory multiple myeloma (R/R MM). J Clin Oncol. 2020;38

96. Pillarisetti K, Powers G, Luistro L, et al. Teclistamab is an active T cell-redirecting bispecific antibody against B-cell maturation antigen for multiple myeloma. Blood Adv. 2020;4:4538–49.

97. Raje N, Jakubowiak A, Gasparetto C, et al. Safety, clinical activity, pharmacokinetics, and pharmacodynamics from a phase I study of PF-06863135, a B-cell maturation antigen (BCMA)-CD3 bispecific antibody, in patients with relapsed/refractory multiple myeloma (RRMM). Blood. 2019;134

98. Cooper D, Madduri D, Lentzsch S, et al. Safety and preliminary clinical activity of REGN5458, an anti-Bcma x anti-CD3 bispecific antibody, in patients with relapsed/refractory multiple myeloma. Blood. 2019;134

99. Topp M, Duell J, Zugmaier G, et al. Evaluation of AMG 420, an anti-BCMA bispecific T-cell engager (BiTE) immunotherapy, in R/R multiple myeloma (MM) patients: updated results of a first-in-human (FIH) phase I dose escalation study. J Clin Oncol. 2019;37

100. Buelow B, Choudry P, Clarke S, et al. Pre-clinical development of TNB-383B, a fully human T-cell engaging bispecific antibody targeting BCMA for the treatment of multiple myeloma. J Clin Oncol. 2018;36

101. Rodriguez C, D'Souza A, Shah N, et al. Initial results of a phase I study of TNB-383B, a BCMA × CD3 bispecific T-cell redirecting antibody, in relapsed/refractory multiple myeloma. Blood. 2020;136

102. Heiss MM, Murawa P, Koralewski P, et al. The trifunctional antibody catumaxomab for the treatment of malignant ascites due to epithelial cancer: results of a prospective randomized phase II/III trial. Int J Cancer. 2010;127:2209–21.

103. Kebenko M, Goebeler ME, Wolf M, et al. A multicenter phase 1 study of solitomab (MT110, AMG 110), a bispecific EpCAM/CD3 T-cell engager (BiTE(R)) antibody construct, in patients with refractory solid tumors. Onco Targets Ther. 2018;7:e1450710.

104. Kroesen BJ, Nieken J, Sleijfer DT, et al. Approaches to lung cancer treatment using the CD3 x EGP-2-directed bispecific monoclonal antibody BIS-1. Cancer Immunol Immunother. 1997;45:203–6.

105. Segal N, Saro J, Melero I, et al. Phase I studies of the novel carcinoembryonic antigen T-cell bispecific (CEA-CD3 TCB) antibody as a single agent and in combination with atezolizumab: preliminary efficacy and safety in patients (pts) with metastatic colorectal cancer (mCRC). Ann Oncol. 2017;28:v134.

106. Tabernero J, Melero I, Ros W, et al. Phase Ia and Ib studies of the novel carcinoembryonic antigen (CEA) T-cell bispecific (CEA CD3 TCB) antibody as a single agent and in combination with atezolizumab: preliminary efficacy and safety in patients with metastatic colorectal cancer (mCRC). J Clin Oncol. 2017;35:3002.

107. Moek K, Fiedler W, von Einem J, et al. Phase I study of AMG 211/MEDI-565 administered as continuous intravenous infusion (cIV) for relapsed/refractory gastrointestinal (GI) adenocarcinoma. Ann Oncol. 2018;29:viii139–40.

108. Pishvaian M, Morse MA, McDevitt J, et al. Phase 1 dose escalation study of MEDI-565, a bispecific T-cell engager that targets human carcinoembryonic antigen, in patients with advanced gastrointestinal adenocarcinomas. Clin Colorectal Cancer. 2016;15:345–51.

109. Giffin MJ, Cooke K, Lobenhofer EK, et al. AMG 757, a half-life extended, DLL3-targeted bispecific T-cell engager, shows high potency and sensitivity in preclinical models of small-cell lung cancer. Clin Cancer Res. 2021;27:1526–37.

110. Haense N, Atmaca A, Pauligk C, et al. A phase I trial of the trifunctional anti Her2 x anti CD3 antibody ertumaxomab in patients with advanced solid tumors. BMC Cancer. 2016;16:420.

111. Kiewe P, Hasmuller S, Kahlert S, et al. Phase I trial of the trifunctional anti-HER2 x anti-CD3 antibody ertumaxomab in metastatic breast cancer. Clin Cancer Res. 2006;12:3085–91.

112. Hummel H, Kufer P, Grullich C, et al. Phase 1 study of pasotuxizumab (BAY 2010112), a PSMA-targeting bispecific T cell engager (BiTE) immunotherapy for metastatic castration-resistant prostate cancer (mCRPC). J Clin Oncol. 2019;37

113. Middleton MR, McAlpine C, Woodcock VK, et al. Tebentafusp, a TCR/anti-CD3 bispecific fusion protein targeting gp100, potently activated antitumor immune responses in patients with metastatic melanoma. Clin Cancer Res. 2020;26:5869–78.

114. Blumenschein G, Davar D, Gutierrez R, et al. A phase I/II first-in-human study of a novel anti-MAGE-A4 TCR/anti-CD3 bispecific (IMC-C103C) as monotherapy and in combination with atezolizumab in HLA-A*02:01-positive patients with MAGE-A4-positive advanced solid tumors (IMC-C103C-101). J Clin Oncol. 2020;38

115. Schmohl JU, Felices M, Oh F, et al. Engineering of anti-CD133 Trispecific molecule capable of inducing NK expansion and driving antibody-dependent cell-mediated cytotoxicity. Cancer Res Treat. 2017;49:1140–52.

116. Schmohl JU, Felices M, Todhunter D, Taras E, Miller JS, Vallera DA. Tetraspecific scFv construct provides NK cell mediated ADCC and self-sustaining stimuli via insertion of IL-15 as a cross-linker. Oncotarget. 2016;7:73830–44.

117. Gleason MK, Verneris MR, Todhunter DA, et al. Bispecific and trispecific killer cell engagers directly activate human NK cells through CD16 signaling and induce cytotoxicity and cytokine production. Mol Cancer Ther. 2012;11:2674–84.

118. Vallera DA, Ferrone S, Kodal B, et al. NK-cell-mediated targeting of various solid tumors using a B7-H3 tri-specific killer engager in vitro and in vivo. Cancers (Basel). 2020;12

119. Gauthier L, Morel A, Anceriz N, et al. Multifunctional natural killer cell engagers targeting NKp46 trigger protective tumor immunity. Cell. 2019;177:1701–13. e16

120. Felices M, Kodal B, Hinderlie P, et al. Novel CD19-targeted TriKE restores NK cell function and proliferative capacity in CLL. Blood Adv. 2019;3:897–907.

121. Cheng Y, Zheng X, Wang X, et al. Trispecific killer engager 161519 enhances natural killer cell function and provides anti-tumor activity against CD19-positive cancers. Cancer Biol Med. 2020;17:1026–38.

122. Gleason MK, Ross JA, Warlick ED, et al. CD16xCD33 bispecific killer cell engager (BiKE) activates NK cells against primary MDS and MDSC CD33+ targets. Blood. 2014;123:3016–26.

123. Wiernik A, Foley B, Zhang B, et al. Targeting natural killer cells to acute myeloid leukemia in vitro with a CD16 x 33 bispecific killer cell engager and ADAM17 inhibition. Clin Cancer Res. 2013;19:3844–55.

124. Arvindam US, van Hauten PMM, Schirm D, et al. A trispecific killer engager molecule against CLEC12A effectively induces NK-cell mediated killing of AML cells. Leukemia. 2020;

125. Bartlett NL, Herrera AF, Domingo-Domenech E, et al. A phase 1b study of AFM13 in combination with pembrolizumab in patients with relapsed or refractory Hodgkin lymphoma. Blood. 2020;136:2401–9.

126. Borghaei H, Alpaugh RK, Bernardo P, et al. Induction of adaptive anti-HER2/neu immune responses in a phase 1B/2 trial of 2B1 bispecific murine monoclonal antibody in metastatic breast cancer (E3194): a trial coordinated by the eastern cooperative oncology group. J Immunother. 2007;30:455–67.

127. Weiner LM, Clark JI, Davey M, et al. Phase I trial of 2B1, a bispecific monoclonal antibody targeting c-erbB-2 and Fc gamma RIII. Cancer Res. 1995;55:4586–93.

128. Liu J, Yang S, Cao B, et al. Targeting B7-H3 via chimeric antigen receptor T cells and bispecific killer cell engagers augments antitumor response of cytotoxic lymphocytes. J Hematol Oncol. 2021;14:21.

129. Vallera DA, Zhang B, Gleason MK, et al. Heterodimeric bispecific single-chain variable-fragment antibodies against EpCAM and CD16 induce effective antibody-dependent cellular cytotoxicity against human carcinoma cells. Cancer Biother Radiopharm. 2013;28:274–82.

130. Rothe A, Jachimowicz RD, Borchmann S, et al. The bispecific immunoligand ULBP2-aCEA redirects natural killer cells to tumor cells and reveals potent anti-tumor activity against colon carcinoma. Int J Cancer. 2014;134:2829–40.

131. Han Y, Sun F, Zhang X, et al. CD24 targeting bi-specific antibody that simultaneously stimulates NKG2D enhances the efficacy of cancer immunotherapy. J Cancer Res Clin Oncol. 2019;145:1179–90.

132. Nitta T, Sato K, Yagita H, Okumura K, Ishii S. Preliminary trial of specific targeting therapy against malignant glioma. Lancet. 1990;335:368–71.

133. Lum LG, Thakur A, Pray C, et al. Multiple infusions of CD20-targeted T cells and low-dose IL-2 after SCT for high-risk non-Hodgkin's lymphoma: a pilot study. Bone Marrow Transplant. 2014;49:73–9.

134. Lamers CH, Bolhuis RL, Warnaar SO, Stoter G, Gratama JW. Local but no systemic immunomodulation by intraperitoneal treatment of advanced ovarian cancer with autologous T lymphocytes re-targeted by a bi-specific monoclonal antibody. Int J Cancer. 1997;73:211–9.

135. Lum LG, Thakur A, Liu Q, et al. CD20-targeted T cells after stem cell transplantation for high risk and refractory non-Hodgkin's lymphoma. Biol Blood Marrow Transplant. 2013;19:925–33.

136. Lum LG, Thakur A, Al-Kadhimi Z, et al. Targeted T-cell therapy in stage IV breast cancer: a phase I clinical trial. Clin Cancer Res. 2015;21:2305–14.

137. Vaishampayan U, Thakur A, Rathore R, Kouttab N, Lum LG. Phase I study of anti-CD3 x anti-Her2 bispecific antibody in metastatic castrate resistant prostate cancer patients. Prostate Cancer. 2015;2015:285193.

138. Lum LG, Thakur A, Choi M, et al. Clinical and immune responses to anti-CD3 x anti-EGFR bispecific antibody armed activated T cells (EGFR BATs) in pancreatic cancer patients. Onco Targets Ther. 2020;9:1773201.

139. Lum LG, Thakur A, Elhakiem A, Alameer L, Dinning E, Huang M. Anti-CS1 x anti-CD3 bispecific antibody (BiAb)-armed anti-CD3 activated T cells (CS1-BATs) kill CS1(+) myeloma cells and release Type-1 cytokines. Front Oncol. 2020;10:544.

140. Thakur A, Scholler J, Schalk DL, June CH, Lum LG. Enhanced cytotoxicity against solid tumors by bispecific antibody-armed CD19 CAR T cells: a proof-of-concept study. J Cancer Res Clin Oncol. 2020;146:2007–16.

141. Blanco B, Ramirez-Fernandez A, Alvarez-Vallina L. Engineering immune cells for in vivo secretion of tumor-specific T cell-redirecting bispecific antibodies. Front Immunol. 2020;11:1792.

142. Velasquez MP, Bonifant CL, Gottschalk S. Redirecting T cells to hematological malignancies with bispecific antibodies. Blood. 2018;131:30–8.

143. Iwahori K, Kakarla S, Velasquez MP, et al. Engager T cells: a new class of antigen-specific T cells that redirect bystander T cells. Mol Ther. 2015;23:171–8.

144. Blanco B, Holliger P, Vile RG, Alvarez-Vallina L. Induction of human T lymphocyte cytotoxicity and inhibition of tumor growth by tumor-specific diabody-based molecules secreted from gene-modified bystander cells. J Immunol. 2003;171:1070–7.

145. Compte M, Blanco B, Serrano F, et al. Inhibition of tumor growth in vivo by in situ secretion of bispecific anti-CEA x anti-CD3 diabodies from lentivirally transduced human lymphocytes. Cancer Gene Ther. 2007;14:380–8.

146. Velasquez MP, Torres D, Iwahori K, et al. T cells expressing CD19-specific engager molecules for the immunotherapy of CD19-positive malignancies. Sci Rep. 2016;6:27130.

147. Liu X, Barrett DM, Jiang S, et al. Improved anti-leukemia activities of adoptively transferred T cells expressing bispecific T-cell engager in mice. Blood Cancer J. 2016;6:e430.

148. Bonifant CL, Szoor A, Torres D, et al. CD123-engager T cells as a novel immunotherapeutic for acute myeloid leukemia. Mol Ther. 2016;24:1615–26.

149. Krawczyk E, Zolov SN, Huang K, Bonifant CL. T-cell activity against AML improved by dual-targeted T cells stimulated through T-cell and IL7 receptors. Cancer Immunol Res. 2019;7:683–92.

150. Choi BD, Yu X, Castano AP, et al. CAR-T cells secreting BiTEs circumvent antigen escape without detectable toxicity. Nat Biotechnol. 2019;37:1049–58.

151. Gardell JL, Matsumoto LR, Chinn H, et al. Human macrophages engineered to secrete a bispecific T cell engager support antigen-dependent T cell responses to glioblastoma. J Immunother Cancer. 2020;8

152. Compte M, Cuesta AM, Sanchez-Martin D, et al. Tumor immunotherapy using gene-modified human mesenchymal stem cells loaded into synthetic extracellular matrix scaffolds. Stem Cells. 2009;27:753–60.

153. Szoor A, Vaidya A, Velasquez MP, et al. T cell-activating mesenchymal stem cells as a bio-therapeutic for HCC. Mol Ther Oncolytics. 2017;6:69–79.

154. Stadler CR, Bahr-Mahmud H, Celik L, et al. Elimination of large tumors in mice by mRNA-encoded bispecific antibodies. Nat Med. 2017;23:815–7.

155. Pang X, Ma F, Zhang P, et al. Treatment of human B-cell lymphomas using Minicircle DNA vector expressing anti-CD3/CD20 in a mouse model. Hum Gene Ther. 2017;28:216–25.

156. Perales-Puchalt A, Duperret EK, Yang X, et al. DNA-encoded bispecific T cell engagers and antibodies present long-term antitumor activity. JCI Insight. 2019;4

157. de Sostoa J, Fajardo CA, Moreno R, Ramos MD, Farrera-Sal M, Alemany R. Targeting the tumor stroma with an oncolytic adenovirus secreting a fibroblast activation protein-targeted bispecific T-cell engager. J Immunother Cancer. 2019;7:19.

158. Fajardo CA, Guedan S, Rojas LA, et al. Oncolytic adenoviral delivery of an EGFR-targeting T-cell engager improves antitumor efficacy. Cancer Res. 2017;77:2052–63.

159. Freedman JD, Duffy MR, Lei-Rossmann J, et al. An oncolytic virus expressing a T-cell engager simultaneously targets cancer and immunosuppressive stromal cells. Cancer Res. 2018;78:6852–65.

160. Speck T, Heidbuechel JPW, Veinalde R, et al. Targeted BiTE expression by an oncolytic vector augments therapeutic efficacy against solid tumors. Clin Cancer Res. 2018;24:2128–37.

161. Zebley CC, Gottschalk S, Youngblood B. Rewriting history: epigenetic reprogramming of CD8(+) T cell differentiation to enhance immunotherapy. Trends Immunol. 2020;41:665–75.

162. Osada T, Patel SP, Hammond SA, Osada K, Morse MA, Lyerly HK. CEA/CD3-bispecific T cell-engaging (BiTE) antibody-mediated T lymphocyte cytotoxicity maximized by inhibition of both PD1 and PD-L1. Cancer Immunol Immunother. 2015;64:677–88.

163. Geiger M, Stubenrauch KG, Sam J, et al. Protease-activation using anti-idiotypic masks enables tumor specificity of a folate receptor 1-T cell bispecific antibody. Nat Commun. 2020;11:3196.

164. Trang VH, Zhang X, Yumul RC, et al. A coiled-coil masking domain for selective activation of therapeutic antibodies. Nat Biotechnol. 2019;37:761–5.

165. Desnoyers LR, Vasiljeva O, Richardson JH, et al. Tumor-specific activation of an EGFR-targeting probody enhances therapeutic index. Sci Transl Med. 2013;5:207ra144.

166. Banaszek A, Bumm TGP, Nowotny B, et al. On-target restoration of a split T cell-engaging antibody for precision immunotherapy. Nat Commun. 2019;10:5387.

167. Kauer J, Horner S, Osburg L, et al. Tocilizumab, but not dexamethasone, prevents CRS without affecting antitumor activity of bispecific antibodies. J Immunother Cancer. 2020;8

168. Khadka RH, Sakemura R, Kenderian SS, Johnson AJ. Management of cytokine release syndrome: an update on emerging antigen-specific T cell engaging immunotherapies. Immunotherapy. 2019;11:851–7.

169. Topp MS, Gokbuget N, Zugmaier G, et al. Long-term follow-up of hematologic relapse-free survival in a phase 2 study of blinatumomab in patients with MRD in B-lineage ALL. Blood. 2012;120:5185–7.

170. Goebeler ME, Knop S, Viardot A, et al. Bispecific T-cell engager (BiTE) antibody construct Blinatumomab for the treatment of patients with relapsed/refractory non-Hodgkin lymphoma: final results from a phase I study. J Clin Oncol. 2016;34:1104–11.

171. Stanglmaier M, Faltin M, Ruf P, Bodenhausen A, Schroder P, Lindhofer H. Bi20 (fBTA05), a novel trifunctional bispecific antibody (anti-CD20 x anti-CD3), mediates efficient killing of B-cell lymphoma cells even with very low CD20 expression levels. Int J Cancer. 2008;123:1181–9.

172. Buhmann R, Michael S, Juergen H, Horst L, Peschel C, Kolb HJ. Immunotherapy with FBTA05 (Bi20), a trifunctional bispecific anti-CD3 x anti-CD20 antibody and donor lymphocyte infusion (DLI) in relapsed or refractory B-cell lymphoma after allogeneic stem cell transplantation: study protocol of an investigator-driven, open-label, non-randomized, uncontrolled, dose-escalating phase I/II-trial. J Transl Med. 2013;11:160.

173. Buhmann R, Simoes B, Stanglmaier M, et al. Immunotherapy of recurrent B-cell malignancies after allo-SCT with Bi20 (FBTA05), a trifunctional anti-CD3 × anti-CD20 antibody and donor lymphocyte infusion. Bone Marrow Transplant. 2009;43:383–97.

Part VIII
Logistics

Roadmap for Starting an Outpatient Cellular Therapy Program

Mariana Lucena, Katie S. Gatwood, Bipin N. Savani, and Olalekan O. Oluwole

Abstract Cellular therapy has made a landmark change within the treatment paradigm of several solid and hematologic malignancies. Novel cellular therapy products, such as chimeric antigen receptor (CAR) T-cell, have demonstrated impressive efficacy and produced durable responses. However, cellular therapies have been associated with significant toxicities as well as financial burden. Most of these therapies have been administered in the inpatient setting due to their toxicity profile particularly with cytokine release syndrome and neurological complications. Improved toxicity management strategies and better understanding of cellular therapy processes have been recently established. Therefore, efforts to transition cellular therapies to the outpatient setting are warranted with the potential to translate into enhanced patient quality of life as well as cost-savings. A successful launch of outpatient cellular therapies requires several components including a multidisciplinary cellular therapy team, and an outpatient center with appropriate clinical space and personnel. Additionally, a plan for patient workflow, criteria for admission upon clinical decompensation, toxicity management guidelines, and incorporation of telemedicine should be implemented. Effective education about cellular therapy and toxicity management is imperative especially for the Emergency Department and Intensive Care Unit teams. This information will be discussed to support patients as cellular therapy programs transition to outpatient treatments.

Keywords Cellular therapy · Outpatient · Chimeric antigen receptor (CAR) T-cell · Cost-savings · Education · Quality of life · Toxicity management · Cytokine release syndrome (CRS) · Immune effector cell-associated neurotoxicity syndrome (ICANS) · Supportive care · Telemedicine

M. Lucena
Department of Pharmacy, Medexus Pharmaceuticals, Inc., Chicago, IL, USA

K. S. Gatwood
Department of Pharmacy, Vanderbilt University Medical Center, Nashville, TN, USA

B. N. Savani · O. O. Oluwole (✉)
Vanderbilt University Medical Center, Nashville, TN, USA
e-mail: olalekan.oluwole@vumc.org

© Springer Nature Switzerland AG 2022
A. Ghobadi, J. F. DiPersio (eds.), *Gene and Cellular Immunotherapy for Cancer*, Cancer Drug Discovery and Development,
https://doi.org/10.1007/978-3-030-87849-8_18

Introduction

Cellular therapy products hold the promise of providing an unmet therapeutic need for several resistant solid and hematologic malignancies. The use of cellular therapy, particularly with chimeric antigen receptor (CAR) T-cell therapy, has greatly impacted the treatment paradigm of large cell lymphoma, acute lymphoblastic leukemia, mantle cell lymphoma, and multiple myeloma [1–3]. Tumor infiltrating lymphocytes (TIL) is another form of cellular therapy which though still being developed in solid tumors, has shown great promise in the treatment of melanoma [4] Although these cellular therapy products are producing robust responses with promising efficacy, treatment is associated with various mild to serious adverse events. CAR T-cell therapy has peculiar toxicities that occur within the first few days to weeks of treatment namely cytokine release syndrome (CRS) and immune effector cell-associated neurotoxicity syndrome (ICANS) have necessitated treatment in the inpatient setting during each of the pivotal trials [5]. Now that there are data-driven management guidelines for patient care, and several products are approved for commercial use, it seems reasonable to explore mechanisms to transition that care to the outpatient setting [5].

The term outpatient therapy connotes a situation in which the evaluations and interventions in patient care are provided in a designated space that is not considered to be an inpatient setting because it is unable to provide medical care for 24 h. The type and degree of interventions, equipment(s) used in that setting, length of time that the area is staffed and the number of days that it is open can be quite variable. Although cellular immunotherapy in lymphoma is new, cellular therapy in general is not. Allogeneic hematopoietic cell transplant (HCT) is a form of cellular therapy that started many decades ago exclusively in the inpatient setting. It has now moved largely to the outpatient setting, at least in part, in many centers especially for matched related transplants. Other forms of transplants such as haploidentical HCT are also being transitioned to the outpatient setting with planned admissions for toxicity management. Other forms of cellular therapies include but not limited to T cell receptor gene modified T cells (TCR-T cells), viral CTLs (cytotoxic T lymphocytes), unmodified or genetically modified natural killer (NK) cells, and tumor infiltrating lymphocytes (TILs). In the case of the approved cellular therapy products for lymphoma, namely axicabtagene ciloleucel (Yescarta®), tisagenlecleucel (Kymriah®), and lisocabtagene maraleucel (Breyanzi®), the early trials were done in the inpatient setting [6–8]. However, the management protocols have improved to the extent that some form of outpatient therapy or at least an exploration of such is warranted (Fig. 1).

Rationale

The ultimate goal of developing an outpatient cellular therapy center is to deliver optimal patient care and at the same time utilize health care resources judiciously.

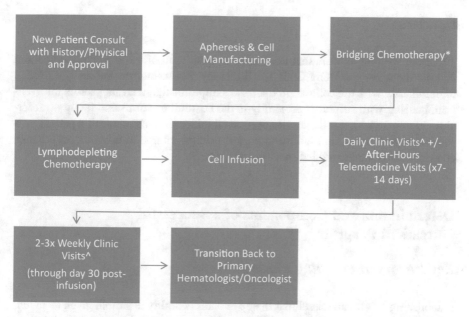

Fig. 1 Outpatient cellular therapy workflow for CAR-T. *If needed based on disease burden. ^Each visit should include key laboratory monitoring including but not limited to CBC, CMP, LDH, CRP, ferritin, PT, PTT, INR, and fibrinogen

There are many reasons why outpatient therapy is preferred if it can be done as safely as in the inpatient setting [9, 10]. Many hospitals operate under conditions in which they have to be judicious with the use of resources. This lack of redundancy makes it problematic to accommodate unplanned admissions which are likely to occur in patients receiving cellular therapy in the outpatient setting. On a positive note, the ability to treat patients in the outpatient setting will free up hospital beds that can then be used to care for other patients with acute complications.

There are also economic factors that need to be considered. For example, Medicare reimbursement for CAR T-cell therapy done in the inpatient setting often leaves the healthcare facility at a cost deficit. Contrarily, outpatient care does not attract nearly as much of a deficit. Reimbursement contracts are less favorable if patients end up being admitted within 3 days of receiving a drug (including CAR T-cell therapy) because the institution is reimbursed at a lower rate. Additionally, each center may have different workflows in terms of acquiring tocilizumab insurance approval. Some centers are able to bundle the authorization as part of the entire CAR T-cell therapy case agreement or case rate. Other centers may need to submit a claim for tocilizumab coverage separately and ensure it is approved in anticipation of needing to use it emergently in the outpatient setting.

Finally, there are patient comfort considerations that argue in favor of outpatient therapy. The treatment paradigm for CAR T-cell therapy is similar to autologous HCT and there is evidence that quality of life and patient satisfaction is better with outpatient compared to inpatient transplant [11–13].

Barriers

There are specific barriers that need to be overcome in order to provide outpatient cellular therapies including CAR T-cell therapy. These include but are not limited to, familiarity with the cellular product and symptoms that warrant prompt intervention, housing with sufficient proximity to the hospital or admission facility (preferably 30 min to 1 h), a reliable caregiver, availability of beds to admit a patient on a semi emergent basis, and ability to ensure prompt intervention with tocilizumab, corticosteroids, and extended spectrum antibiotics.

Determinants and Components of a Successful Outpatient Program

Key Factors in Planning Phase

Establishing an outpatient cellular therapy center is highly desirable given its potential for improving patient quality of life as well as beneficial financial implications for health care systems. Cellular therapy programs preparing for establishing outpatient cellular therapy centers should perform careful evaluations to ensure adequate resources including clinical space and health care workforce are provided and properly allocated. Additionally, a comprehensive Standard Operating Procedure (SOP) Manual needs to be prepared and updated regularly as one of the main requirements of FACT (Foundation for the Accreditation of Cellular Therapy) accreditation for cellular therapy centers. The dedicated outpatient cellular therapy center should ensure it is capable of fully supporting the needs of these patients across each phase of outpatient therapy. Any remaining gaps should be addressed and resolved before initiating the launch of outpatient cellular therapy program.

Clinical Space and Logistics of Patient Care

The implementation of a successful outpatient cellular therapy program requires a significant logistical planning and execution. In regards to physical location, an outpatient cellular therapy center should be the dedicated place for the primary components of cellular therapy including lymphodepletion therapy/conditioning chemotherapy infusion of cellular products, patient and provider visits, and toxicity monitoring and management. Ideally, the center should have open hours 7 days a week for at least daily patient's visit for the first 2 weeks post infusion to ensure specialized providers can evaluate and manage potential toxicities for example CRS and ICANS in patients receiving CAR T-cell [5, 14]. If the dedicated infusion center does not support weekend open hours, an alternative option is for the team to offer telemedicine visits provided by on-call physicians, hematology/oncology fellows, or advanced practice providers (APPs).

Workforce

A cohesive cellular therapy multidisciplinary healthcare team is by far the most important component of an outpatient cellular therapy program. This core group should consist of multiple entities including cellular therapy physicians plus a medical director, cellular therapy coordinators, APPs, nurses, financial coordinators, apheresis and cellular therapy lab personnel, clinical pharmacy specialists, social workers, case managers, and procurement personnel. Alliances to this central group include pharmacy informatics, emergency department (ED) staff and intensive care unit (ICU) staff, and hospitalists [15].

The members of the core cellular therapy team will assume certain roles and responsibilities, but the cellular therapy program should ensure each responsibility has a designated member to be carried out appropriately. The cellular therapy physicians and APPs should confirm that patients meet criteria to proceed with outpatient treatment. The providers will also be heavily involved in monitoring and managing cellular therapy related toxicities. Once the need for cellular therapy is identified, the financial and procurement coordinators should be in charge of developing case rates/agreements, placing orders for the products, and verifying the submission and reimbursement of claims. The case managers and social workers are primarily focused on arranging plans for dedicated caregivers and local housing if patients need temporary housing near the outpatient cellular therapy center. The cellular therapy coordinators are heavily involved in scheduling patient visits, educating patients and caregivers on appropriate on-call contacts, and logistics regarding the treatment. The apheresis and cellular therapy lab personnel will work together to collect, process, ship, store, and transfer the cellular products to the outpatient cellular therapy center. They are also fundamental in coordinating the time of cell infusion given most products have short expiration times. The clinical pharmacy specialists are involved in creating and verifying the lymphodepleting chemotherapy orders. They also serve as key educators to the patients, caregivers, and cellular therapy team on adverse event management and supportive care strategies. The pharmacists are also involved in securing enough tocilizumab supply for patients and communicating with procurement personnel to maintain appropriate inventory. In some centers, the pharmacists may also be tasked with ensuring the cellular therapy program meets Risk Evaluation and Mitigation Strategy (REMS) program criteria [6–8, 16, 17]. Depending on state regulations, pharmacists may also be required to label the cellular product including CAR T-cell product before it is infused to the patient. Nurses are tasked with the administration of cellular product and supportive care medication and coordination of the time of infusion with the cellular therapy lab personnel (see Fig. 2). The cellular therapy program should also have a contingency plan implemented for treating patients who remain ineligible for outpatient cellular therapy for any reason.

Each member of the cellular therapy team is indeed an invaluable guide to support outpatient treatment. However, alliances should be forged with other health care groups who may come across these patients requiring an immediate intervention for toxicities such as CRS and/or ICANS. If patients or caregivers recognize

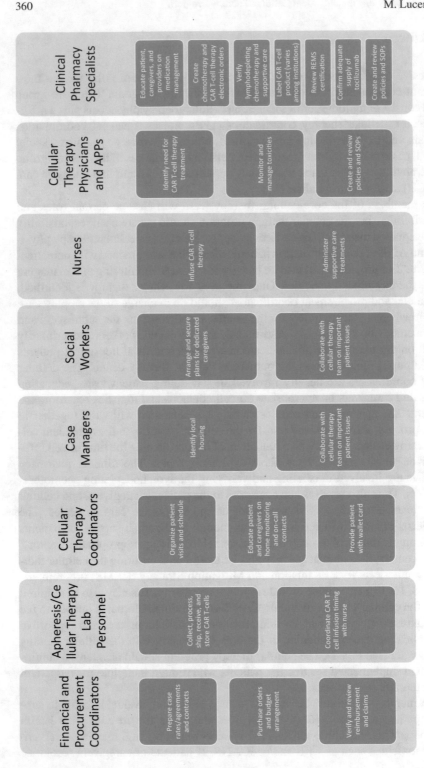

Fig. 2 Outpatient cellular therapy team roles and responsibilities. *APPs* advanced practice providers, *SOPs* standard operating procedures, *REMS* risk evaluation and mitigation strategy

worsening symptoms of CRS and/or ICANS, they could present to the ED, prompt a direct admission to the ICU, or be admitted to the cellular therapy floor. Healthcare professionals staffing ED and ICU should be aware of the severity of CAR T-cell therapy associated toxicities as they can often times present similar to sepsis or encephalopathy; they need to recognize the need for tocilizumab or corticosteroids and have quick access to cellular therapy specialists on call [5, 18]. Therefore, the cellular therapy team should engage with key leaders of the ED, ICU, and hospitalists to provide education specific to cellular therapies including CAR T-cell and anticipated toxicities. Effective communication amongst these teams is crucial for appropriate medical management. The ED, ICU, and hospitalist teams should be provided with a point of contact designated to discuss the need for tocilizumab or corticosteroids. This may vary from center to center, but one example is to create a virtual pager that is forwarded to the on-call cell therapy provider when he/she is covering the inpatient service. This can ensure one pager number is distributed to the ED, ICU, and hospitalist teams instead of multiple pagers or staff numbers which can lead to confusion. Furthermore, depending on the institution's electronic medical record (EMR) certain features could be attached to the patient's profile serving as alerts to any provider. For example, the patient's header on the EMR chart may be flagged with a different color or an additional text box stating "CAR T-cell therapy patient." Another feature may be to create a complex condition letter with information on the type of CAR T-cell therapy, date of infusion, anticipated toxicities and management, and cell therapy on-call provider pager. This complex condition letter can then be added to a best practice alert (BPA) which can inform providers, remind them of prior education, and provide appropriate CAR T-cell therapy resources. Similarly, an alert to prevent the administration of corticosteroids for reasons other than ICANS could be added to the patient's chart by including corticosteroids as a conditional allergy for a specified timeframe. If tocilizumab or corticosteroids are warranted, they must also be promptly ordered and dispensed for administration. Corticosteroids are commonly found in most hospital departments, but the clinical pharmacy specialist and nursing teams can ensure that the most readily used agents (e.g., intravenous dexamethasone and methylprednisolone) are available in the Pyxis or Omnicell stations. Ordering of corticosteroids are typically not restricted, but the correct doses and frequencies for CRS and ICANS should be reinforced through educational materials. The acquisition of tocilizumab faces more challenges but can be appropriately ordered with education and informatics support. Each institution may have distinct oncology based EMR systems (e.g., EPIC Beacon) allowing for different functionalities for chemotherapy ordering. Per REMS program requirements, tocilizumab should be administered immediately (within 2 h of observed toxicity) [5, 14]. Pharmacy informatics specialists could help build tocilizumab orders to be available for quicker dispensing and administration. For example, individual tocilizumab orders with correct dose, indication, and frequency could be placed within EPIC Beacon treatment plan orders to appear daily for hematology/oncology providers to access. For non-EPIC Beacon providers, an order panel with the correctly prepared tocilizumab order could be created for easier searching and access. The coordination of the dispensing, compounding, and administration of tocilizumab between providers, pharmacists, and nurses is crucial for prompt delivery and infusion. Education on REMS, tocilizumab ordering, and workflow is paramount for appropriate CAR T-cell patient management.

Telemedicine visits are highly encouraged for patients undergoing outpatient cellular therapy to help monitor toxicities after hours. Depending on the institution's bandwidth and staffing, telemedicine visits can be coordinated twice a day (e.g., 4 pm and 10 pm) as well as on weekends if the center is not open 7 days per week. Telemedicine should include both audio and video components to do a review of systems and focused physical exam. A basic neurological functional assessment can be done including viewing a signature. These telemedicine visits can help to identify signs and symptoms of toxicities including CRS/ICANS and guide the patient to appropriate management strategies (e.g., continue to monitor, or direct to hospital for administration of tocilizumab and/or corticosteroids).

Additionally, some centers may be able to offer patients wearable devices. Because of the relatively noninvasive nature of wearable devices, they can be worn for prolonged periods of time (for up to 30 days), and they can give valuable real time data that are actionable. It is recommended to use devices that measure heart rate, body surface temperature, and blood pressure if possible. Furthermore, some CAR T-cell therapy pharmaceutical companies provide support for outpatient treatments with digital platforms to provide pertinent information on personalized product and patient support (e.g., Cell Therapy 360) [19].

As with a variety of other clinical applications, SOPs and policies should be created to document and follow appropriate practices. It is highly recommended that the cell therapy program builds the SOPs outlining the studies and evidence for cellular therapy, patient selection, criteria and eligibility for outpatient administration, assigned staffing roles and responsibilities, patient follow up requirements, toxicity management, and supportive care strategies. These policies will help the cell therapy program ensure the internal guidelines are followed for each patient undergoing outpatient cellular therapy. Some institutions have adopted the use of quick reference guides (QRG) to have available for certain diseases, indications, therapeutic management and one can be created for outpatient cellular therapy workflow. Nevertheless, cellular therapy is changing rapidly and new findings from clinical experience may lead to changes for improved patient management. Thus, the SOPs and policies are dynamic and should be subject to annual revisions to fine tune any outdated areas.

Resource Utilization and Tracking

Transitioning a cellular product from the clinical trial setting to a commercial process is complex and can be a big strain on health care systems. Cellular products including CAR T-cell processes require multiple resources which in most institutions are shared resources. Traditionally, clinical trial teams function independently and do not often talk to those who govern commercially approved products. This paradigm is unlikely to work with cellular products including CAR T-cell. Apheresis labs and cellular therapy labs are shared resources used by both outpatient and inpatient cellular therapy programs; therefore, their management team needs to be engaged in the planning and implantation of establishing an outpatient cellular therapy program ensuring adequate communication and staffing. Periodic strategy meetings should be held with all stakeholders and upcoming infusions discussed so that appropriate resources are made available. Periodic quality metric reviews and regulatory processes should be implemented for immune effector cell (IEC) accreditation. Additionally, the cellular therapy program should ensure resources are appropriately shared and available to support commercial, clinical trial, outpatient, and inpatient services.

It is important to have quality metrics with any outpatient program. Since there are numerous CAR T-cell products, the choice of metrics should not be dependent on the properties of a specific product. Examples of metrics include time from screening to apheresis, rate of catheter infections, non-relapse mortality, time to admission if necessary, and time to tocilizumab administration [20, 21]. Additionally, the cellular therapy program should also specify and track outcomes of interest such as rates of grade 3 or higher CRS/ICANS in CAR T-cell patients and incidence of major infections.

Setting up an Outpatient Cellular Therapy Center

Patient selection is an important component to the successful running of an outpatient program. Each program should establish its criteria of minimum requirements for a patient to qualify for outpatient therapy. Regular team meetings are essential to review patients as they go through cellular therapy to ensure that they remain eligible for outpatient therapy. Those who become ineligible (e.g. due to rapidly progressive disease that warrants cytotoxic therapy before CAR T-cell is ready) should have an alternative way to receive salvage chemotherapy, lymphodepleting chemotherapy/preparative chemotherapy and cellular product in the hospitalized setting.

The cellular therapy program should be able to support clinic visits to the outpatient unit daily in the morning with the purpose to do a complete physical exam including detailed neurological exam, review of systems, and laboratory tests. If patients are asymptomatic, they can safely be sent back to their local housing. Institutions will have their own series of parameters that guide admission to the hospital [22]. Patients should be considered for admission if they have a fever (evidenced by a temperature greater than or equal to 38 °C or 100.4 °F. At a minimum, a fever should prompt immediate workup for sepsis (e.g., blood cultures, urine cultures, chest X-ray) and initiation of broad or extended spectrum antibiotics. However, patients who have been evaluated may also be managed outpatient with close monitoring if all other vital signs are stable. Potential strategies include starting Tocilizumab combined with a short course of dexamethasone 10 mg/day for

3 days for grade 1 CRS or dexamethasone 10 mg/day for 3 days for grade 1 ICANS in the appropriate instance per institution practice [18].

The process for admission will also vary by institution. One recommendation is to implement a 'scatter' hospital bed that can be made available for the patient to be admitted. Additionally, this bed should be in a designated unit where specific interventions like tocilizumab and high dose corticosteroids are available. Admission through the ED is an option so long as the ED is set up as able to rapidly evaluate the patient and administer specific interventions. The ED physicians will also need to be REMS trained and keep up with other regulatory requirements.

Cellular Therapy Educational Considerations

The unique toxicities of CAR T-cell and other cellular therapies and the associated monitoring warrants provision of extensive education to patients and caregivers by various members of the multidisciplinary team [23, 24]. Ideally, this education should begin several weeks prior to cell infusion to prepare them for the various phases of the treatment journey and some of its life-altering aspects. There are several phases to cellular therapy treatment, including initial consultation, apheresis, potential bridging chemotherapy, lymphodepleting chemotherapy, cell infusion, and close outpatient follow-up and each of these has unique educational considerations [25–27].

During consultation and initial evaluation, the patient should be informed of the need to identify a 24/7 caregiver as well as making plans for alternative caregivers in the event of primary caregiver emergency [23]. The caregiver should be someone who knows the patient well and is able to provide direct assistance and care to the patient. Caregivers will need to transport patients to appointments following cell infusion given restrictions on patient driving following infusion of some cellular products and patients deconditioning, as well as assist with medication management and administration, meal preparation, cleaning, and telemedicine visits (Beaupierre 2019 #106) [23]. Caregivers are also essential in aiding the medical team in identifying potential adverse effects of therapy, such as fever (indicator of CRS) and subtle neurologic changes that may indicate ICANS in CAR T-cell recipients [24]. The patient will also need to be educated on the need to stay within 2 h (preferably 30 min) of the hospital or clinic where the patient will receive the cellular therapy product for at least 4 weeks following infusion as this may require the patient to identify and secure local housing [6–8, 16, 17]. Patients should also receive preliminary education on the cellular therapy treatment journey and the most serious adverse effects of cellular therapy products, such as CRS and ICANS [23, 24]. Patient coordinators, APPs, and the cellular therapy physician are the most likely and most well suited providers to carry out education at this stage in the cellular therapy process (Beaupierre, 2019 #106) [23].

Once the patient has cleared evaluation and ready to undergo apheresis, they should receive education on the apheresis process and its potential risks, such as the potential need for central line placement, hypocalcemia, and hypotension [28]. They also should be informed of the possibility of a second apheresis in the event of a cell manufacturing failure. Following successful manufacturing, the patient will begin lymphodepleting chemotherapy/conditioning chemotherapy. This is a crucial time point for educating both patients and caregivers. Nurses, APPs, physicians, and pharmacists should all be involved in providing information related to the logistics of administration and most common side effects of chemotherapy including pancytopenia, infection risk, fatigue, nausea/vomiting, and alopecia as well as how to manage them [24, 27, 29]. They should also be educated of when and how to report serious side effects of chemotherapy to the medical team, ideally through the provision of a 24/7 number that is staffed by an APP or hematology/oncology fellow. Best practice should include pharmacist education on the supportive medications the patient will be required to take including but not limited to infection prophylaxis, seizure prophylaxis, and tumor lysis syndrome prevention [24, 27, 29]. The patient and caregiver should be provided with a medication list or chart to aid in correct administration of medications as this responsibility falls uniquely on the patient when administering cellular therapy in the outpatient setting.

On the day of cell infusion, patients and caregivers should be informed of the infusion process and all providers should assist in education regarding the logistics of continued close outpatient follow-up, including the need for any routine at-home monitoring of vital signs and neurologic status [23, 24]. They should also be extensively re-educated on the adverse effects of cellular therapy, particularly CRS and ICANS in CAR T-cell recipients, and how and when to report these symptoms to the medical team. All CAR T-cells products currently approved by the FDA have associated REMS programs in place due to the risk for CRS and neurologic toxicities [6–8, 16, 17]. A component of all of these REMS programs is the requirement of providing the patient with a Patient Wallet Card to inform them of signs and symptoms of CRS and ICANS and the requirement to stay within 2 h of the hospital or clinic where the patient received the CAR T-cell product for at least 4 weeks following infusion [6–8, 16, 17]. The patient and caregiver should be given this card on the day of or several days prior to the cell infusion (e.g., at the start of lymphodepleting chemotherapy) and keep it with them at all times for appropriate notification and identification in the event of an emergency.

At the point of care transition from the cellular therapy team back to the primary oncologist, APPs and patient coordinators should educate patients and caregivers on the need to refrain from driving or operating heavy machinery for at least 8 weeks after cell infusion due to the risk for late neurologic side effects [6–8, 16, 17]. They should also be informed of the risk of infection due to cytopenias and/or B-cell aplasia. This should include education on appropriate infection prevention practices, monitoring for signs/symptoms of infection, and any required infection prophylaxis [29].

Materials and techniques that can be useful to consider for providing patient and caregiver education include a class or pre-recorded webinar covering all of the above topics and/or a folder or binder that includes educational information, patient treatment calendars, monitoring information and logs, and medication lists [23].

Summary

Outpatient therapy represents the future for cellular therapy. It requires careful thought for a successful roll out so that patient safety and satisfaction is preserved, and resources are not wasted. It will start with stringent patient selection and multiple evaluations during the day and night. As data is accumulated, exclusion criteria or requirements will be relaxed, patient selection process will be more streamlined, and the degree of monitoring will be risk adapted to make it less intense for those with a lower risk profile. Hospital resource utilization will also be reduced, and the financial implications of cellular therapy delivery will show a more favorable profile. It is anticipated that the distance to the hospital will be extended, and more patients will be able to access this life saving intervention from the comfort of their homes.

The implementation of outpatient cellular therapy requires an outpatient infusion center able to support the needs of the patients during each phase of treatment. Most importantly, the cellular therapy program should have a core workgroup of members with dedicated roles and responsibilities to provide optimal care for these patients from start to finish. The members encompassing this workgroup consist of cellular therapy physicians, cellular therapy coordinators, APPs, nurses, financial coordinators, apheresis and cellular therapy lab personnel, clinical pharmacy specialists, social workers, case managers, and procurement personnel. Pharmacy informatics, emergency department staff and ICU staff, and hospitalists are also healthcare professionals who may care for these patients and will require education on how to manage toxicities of cellular therapies including CAR T-cells. Additional steps may be necessary to logistically prepare and administer tocilizumab and other supportive care agents for non-oncology providers. Institutions should also incorporate telemedicine visits to be able to provide guidance to outpatient CAR T-cell patients if signs/symptoms of CRS or ICANS arise. Wearable technology and other pharmaceutical company specific platforms could be useful to track vital signs on these patients. The cellular therapy program should also document the workflow for outpatient cellular therapy via policies and SOPs and perform routine updates with dynamic changes based on experience. Additionally, successful implementation of an outpatient cellular therapy program requires extensive patient and caregiver education as the share of responsibility in providing care shifts substantially onto the patient and caregiver. All members of the healthcare team should be involved in providing this education at multiple crucial time points along the cellular therapy journey.

References

1. Neelapu SS, Locke FL, Bartlett NL, et al. Axicabtagene Ciloleucel CAR T-cell therapy in refractory large B-cell lymphoma. N Engl J Med. 2017;377:2531–44.

2. Schuster SJ, Bishop MR, Tam CS, et al. Tisagenlecleucel in adult relapsed or refractory diffuse large B-cell lymphoma. N Engl J Med. 2019;380:45–56.
3. Wang M, Munoz J, Goy A, et al. KTE-X19 CAR T-cell therapy in relapsed or refractory mantle-cell lymphoma. N Engl J Med. 2020;382:1331–42.
4. Sarnaik AA, Hamid O, Khushalani NI, et al. Lifileucel, a tumor-infiltrating lymphocyte therapy, in metastatic melanoma. J Clin Oncol. 2021;39(24):2656–66.
5. Lee DW, Santomasso BD, Locke FL, et al. ASTCT consensus grading for cytokine release syndrome and neurologic toxicity associated with immune effector cells. Biol Blood Marrow Transpl. 2019;25:625–38.
6. Corp. NP. Tisagenlecleucel (Kymriah) [prescribing information]. East Hanover, NJ2020.
7. Juno Therapeutics I, a Bristol Myers Squibb Company. Lisocabtagene maraleucel (Breyanzi) [prescribing information]. Bothell, WA2021.
8. Kite Pharma I. Axicabtagene autoleucel (Yescarta) [prescribing information]. Santa Monica. CA2021.
9. Owattanapanich W, Suphadirekkul K, Kunacheewa C, Ungprasert P, Prayongratana K. Risk of febrile neutropenia among patients with multiple myeloma or lymphoma who undergo inpatient versus outpatient autologous stem cell transplantation: a systematic review and meta-analysis. BMC Cancer. 2018;18:1126.
10. Tan XN, Yew CY, Ragg SJ, Harrup RA, Johnston AM. Outpatient autologous stem cell transplantation in Royal Hobart Hospital, Tasmania: a single-centre, retrospective review in the Australian setting. Intern Med J. 2021;
11. Dhir V, Zibdawi L, Paul HK, et al. Quality of life and caregiver burden in patients and their caregivers undergoing outpatient autologous stem cell transplantation compared to inpatient transplantation. Blood. 2019;134:62.
12. Schulmeister L, Quiett K, Mayer K. Quality of life, quality of care, and patient satisfaction: perceptions of patients undergoing outpatient autologous stem cell transplantation. Oncol Nurs Forum. 2005;32:57–67.
13. Summers N, Dawe U, Stewart DA. A comparison of inpatient and outpatient ASCT. Bone Marrow Transplant. 2000;26:389–95.
14. Brudno JN, Kochenderfer JN. Toxicities of chimeric antigen receptor T cells: recognition and management. Blood. 2016;127:3321–30.
15. Alexander M, Culos K, Roddy J, et al. Chimeric antigen receptor T cell therapy: a comprehensive review of clinical efficacy, toxicity, and best practices for outpatient administration. Transpl Cell Therpy. 2021;
16. Company BMS. Idecabtagene vicleucel (Abecma) [prescribing information]. Summit, NJ2021.
17. Kite Pharma I. Brexucabtagene autoleucel (Tecartus) [prescribing information]. Santa Monica, CA2021.
18. Maus MV, Alexander S, Bishop MR, et al. Society for Immunotherapy of cancer (SITC) clinical practice guideline on immune effector cell-related adverse events. J Immunother Cancer. 2020;8
19. Cell Therapy 360. 2021. https://www.breyanzi.com/support/cell-therapy-360/. Accessed 25 May 25 2021
20. Dulan SO, Viers KL, Wagner JR, et al. Developing and monitoring a standard-of-care chimeric antigen receptor (CAR) T cell clinical quality and regulatory program. Biol Blood Marrow Transpl. 2020;26:1386–93.
21. Maus MV, Nikiforow S. The why, what, and how of the new FACT standards for immune effector cells. J Immunother Cancer. 2017;5:36.
22. Myers GD, Verneris MR, Goy A, Maziarz RT. Perspectives on outpatient administration of CAR-T cell therapy in aggressive B-cell lymphoma and acute lymphoblastic leukemia. J Immunother Cancer. 2021;9
23. Beaupierre A, Kahle N, Lundberg R, Patterson A. Educating multidisciplinary care teams, patients, and caregivers on CAR T-cell therapy. J Adv Pract Oncol. 2019;10:29–40.

24. Neelapu SS, Tummala S, Kebriaei P, et al. Chimeric antigen receptor T-cell therapy - assessment and management of toxicities. Nat Rev Clin Oncol. 2018;15:47–62.
25. Perica K, Curran KJ, Brentjens RJ, Giralt SA. Building a CAR garage: preparing for the delivery of commercial CAR T cell products at memorial Sloan Kettering cancer center. Biol Blood Marrow Transpl. 2018;24:1135–41.
26. Salter AI, Pont MJ, Riddell SR. Chimeric antigen receptor-modified T cells: CD19 and the road beyond. Blood. 2018;131:2621–9.
27. Shank BR, Do B, Sevin A, Chen SE, Neelapu SS, Horowitz SB. Chimeric antigen receptor T cells in hematologic malignancies. Pharmacotherapy. 2017;37:334–45.
28. Philip J, Sarkar RS, Pathak A. Adverse events associated with apheresis procedures: incidence and relative frequency. Asian J Transfus Sci. 2013;7:37–41.
29. Hill JA, Seo SK. How I prevent infections in patients receiving CD19-targeted chimeric antigen receptor T cells for B-cell malignancies. Blood. 2020;136:925–35.

Index

Printed in the United States
by Baker & Taylor Publisher Services